EMPA

AND

PSYCHIC ABILITIES

Meditations for Highly Sensitive People.

6 BOOKS IN 1

A Beginner's Guide to Third Eye Development, Mind Power, Aura Reading, Mindfulness, Telepathy, and Clairvoyance

Kundalini Spiritual Awakening Study – Chakra & Reiki Healing Academy

BOOK 1

Introduction

Empath and psychic abilities are not the same thing.

The ability to feel and understand other people is called empathy. You can be empathic without being psychic. Empathy lets you know what someone else is feeling without that person having to say a word or show any physical signs. It's an intuitive form of emotional intelligence that helps you identify with other people and genuinely care about them in a way that doesn't require much effort yet can have profound effects on their well-being and your own self-worth.

You don't have to be empathic to have psychic powers, but empaths usually have at least some forms of psychic ability. That's because they are natural feelers, and many people who are naturally good at feeling things also seem to be able to feel into the future.

Whether you're an empath or a psychic, you are very sensitive to other people's energy and surroundings. You tend to absorb everything in your surroundings even if you don't consciously realize it. If someone is feeling sad or angry, you'll probably start feeling the same thing once you register that person's energy on some level.

Empaths can be extremely sensitive to negative energy and emotions, in fact it's commonly believed that empaths are more intuitively sensitive than non-empaths, but this is probably a matter of degree and doesn't necessarily mean that empaths have better psychic or empathic abilities, though they definitely do. If you are a strong empath, though, negative emotions more easily affect you than most people are able to consciously notice.

Empaths often feel things they don't quite understand. They have an overactive sensitivity to other people's moods and body language, so they are often prone to experience the negative emotions they pick up on in others, even if the other person isn't aware of what he or she is feeling.

Empaths don't just feel what you feel - they also feel what you are going to say and do before it happens. These feelings can make life difficult for someone with overly active empathy abilities, but it's possible to learn how to control your powers if you know how. Learning how to manage your intuitive sensitivity is important if your natural empathy is overwhelming for you or others around you.

If you're an empath or a psychic, you might find that your feelings and intuitions get stronger around certain people. You might feel more intuitive around friends or family members who treat you well. This may be a subconscious response to the need to protect yourself, though this is not to be confused with not trusting people who aren't close to you. It is not a sign of distrust to feel a little more intuitive around strangers as a way to protect yourself until you learn more about them.

Empaths tend to be more intuitive around people who treat them badly, and this usually has an internal root. This can make it difficult for empaths to deal with abusive personalities because their desire to help can make them feel responsible for the abuser's actions and emotions or cause them to take on too much of the abuser's energy and feelings. Empaths may feel like they are being abused even when it doesn't appear that way on the surface. In situations like this, it can be difficult for empaths to find a balance between helping people and not hurting themselves in the process.

The sooner you learn to be aware of your intuition, the easier it will be for you to control and understand the powerful sensations you experience on a daily basis. Your level of empathy or psychic ability depends largely on your level of emotional intelligence. Empaths have high emotional intelligence because they naturally care about other people and feel a strong desire to help those in need. They are often very compassionate, giving people who truly understand what it means to love unconditionally - even if they don't know that's what they're doing.

Some empaths come into this world with a strong sense of light and a desire to help others, while others develop their powers later in life. Most empaths are sensitive to emotional energy, and they are able to feel the feelings of others, but some may also experience premonitions or see spirits in dreams or visions.

If you enjoy helping other people and you want your sensitivity to come from a place of love instead of stress, learn how to manage it so that you can use your empathic abilities when needed without giving too much or absorbing negativity when it's not necessary. Take care of yourself first, and you'll be able to give back more and feel better about yourself at the same time.

The best way to develop your empathic abilities is by learning more about them and understanding how you are naturally wired. To use your empathy effectively, focus on the good feelings in others, not the negative ones. Try practicing a little emotional management every day so that you can avoid absorbing bad energy or falling prey to negative emotions in others.

Empathic Abilities vs. Psychic Abilities

If you're an empath, you are able to pick up on the emotions of others even when they aren't aware of it. Sometimes this can be overwhelming for empaths who feel like they are feeling everything that everyone else is feeling. If you have psychic abilities, you may see and hear things before other people do. You have the ability to see spirits, read minds and communicate with people in your dreams or visions. These abilities are similar to intuitiveness but differ in that they are more passive and come from a place of thought rather than emotion. Psychic abilities are more similar to intuition than empath abilities.

In either case, learning how to use your natural ability to help you through tough times is the best thing you can do to take control of your life and be happy. Being an empath will help you become a more compassionate and empathic person, which in turn will allow you to feel for others and become a kinder, more successful person by default. When you are able to listen with your heart instead of with your mind, it also gives you the gift of understanding rather than judgment or assumptions. Empaths make good counselors because they are able to understand others' perspectives easily without relying on intellectual knowledge.

Once you learn how to control your empathic abilities, you will be able to care for others and love yourself at the same time. By using these six steps, you'll be less overwhelmed by the emotions of others and more in control of your own happiness.

Chapter 1. How Do You Discover Your Intuitive Type?

The first step towards discovering your intuitive type is to know how to invest time in understanding your intuitive abilities. This will help you develop a particular intuitive skill set, hence become more accurate. It is good to mention that everybody has an intuitive type that is more dominant in their life. The moment you understand what your dominant type of intuitive you are; it will become easy to concentrate on developing that strength.

Intuition is part of the mind that supports one's predictions; it is more of an internal source, rather than a logical one. Some people are intuitive, others are not. Intuitive people use their inner knowing to make decisions. They will easily discover what needs to be done and will do it effortlessly. They have a strong gut feeling about their decisions, and therefore make it easier for them and everyone around them.

Understanding your intuitive type will help you to be a step ahead when it comes to making business decisions, relationships, friendships and even in intimate matters. Intuitive people use their natural intuition as a source of motivation for making decisions and plan their life accordingly.

Intuition is a very useful skill that should not be ignored; however, one should also acknowledge his or her weak spots when it comes to making decisions based on instinct. Making irrational choices based on instinct can often lead to problems as well as result in unsatisfactory results.

You will also discover that the way you read something intuitively is not the same way your friends and colleagues do it. This is because everyone has a different innate intuitive ability and uses it differently, which is okay. When you understand your awakening intuition, you can use it to out your dominant intuition type. With regular practice, you will develop it, and find it easy to believe what you feel or sense intuitively, and become more present, less reactive, and much calmer.

- **Listen to your inner voice**
The number one thing that you must learn to do to discover your type of intuition is to listen to the guidance of your hunches and gut feelings. Everybody is connected to their intuition, but most people dismiss or ignore their inner voice, hence paying no attention to their intuition. Your intuition serves to bridge the gap between your instinct and your rational thinking.

- **Take time for solitude**
In the same way that solitude helps to enhance your creativity, it will help you to connect with your most profound wisdom. Taking time to engage in deep reflection and connect with yourself can help you discover your intuitive type.

- **Practice mindfulness**
Such practices help you to tune into your intuition, weigh your options objectively, and filter out mental clatter. They promote self-knowledge that allows you to connect to your intuition.

- **Observe everything**
Observe and notice everything. This will enable you to see when odd things happen. You will be keen to notice when there are surprising connections, coincidences, or immediate intuition in your life. You will start to tap into your intuition.

- **Pay attention to your dreams**

By paying attention to your dreams, you get in touch with your subconscious thinking process. Since both dreams and intuition spring from the unconscious, you will be receiving information from that intuitive or unconscious part of your brain. Attuning to your dreams can, therefore, connect you to your intuition.

- **Mindfully get rid of negative emotions**

Strong negative emotions can cloud your intuition. With such negative feelings, you feel out of sorts, and like you are not yourself because they disconnect you with your intuition. When you are stressed and depressed, your intuition, you will find your intuition failing. Letting go of emotions clears you to connect with your intuition more intimately.

Chapter 2. How to develop your Psychic Abilities?

Developing your psychic abilities can be a hard nut to crack if you have got no plans of how to do it. There are myriads of techniques that are of great importance in your journey of developing strong psychic abilities. With these techniques at hand, you might still find it very hard. The secret to this is that you have to practice only one technique per day. You do not necessarily have to practice these exercises in a given order as they all have one aim, that is, the development of your psychic abilities.

The following are the various ways in which you can develop your psychic abilities:

Take a walk in a park

Taking a walk in a park or any other place surrounded by nature is one of the best ways of meditating. This is where you get a chance to concentrate on your steps while walking. As you walk, keep focusing on each step you take while uttering the word 'step' after each step. This will help you a great deal in clearing the mind of confusion and jumbles.

Practice Staring at Auras

You can easily learn to always stare at an aura, and this is one of the best ways of developing your psychic abilities. The best way of coming up with an aura is having a friend standing in front of a wall with only one-colored paint. You are then required to step back approximately eight feet. Now you have to stare on his or her forehead while imagining that you are looking through her behind the wall. At this point, you will notice that there is an aura layer formed around their heads. This, therefore, will have greatly developed your psychic ability.

Pray Often

Praying is one of the greatest tools for developing your psychic abilities. Prayer is a tool that many employs in relieving themselves of burdens as they talk to a Supreme being; they believe in. This also makes you feel supported and loved. Therefore, having some time designated for prayers daily will be of help to a great deal.

Make A Symbol

There is a variety of ways in which you can obtain psychic information. They are usually not literal and thus have to look at symbolically. Everyone has got Spirit guides, and thus yours will guide you through the interpretation of information. You will, therefore, develop your psychic abilities in the process.

Make Your Tarot

In case you are using tarot to develop your psychic abilities, then you can get a tarot deck and make your tarot. Use your imaginations to make your meanings of the cards rather than looking at the meanings that come with them. You can also spend time with one card a day and meditate upon it the note down all you think about the card. This, therefore, will help you in developing your psychic abilities using a tarot.

Keep Your Vibration High

When developing your psychic abilities, it is imperative to have your vibrations high. This is because like is always attracted to like, and thus you will also be able to attract other souls that are spiritually aware. Apart from that, the frequency at which the spirits vibrate is very high.

Activities That Help in Psychic Progress

The more knowledge you have of people, the abler you are to pick up on messages from others. For example, if you are empathetic, you are able to place yourself into their situation and see things in a much clearer way. If you are inexperienced with different kinds of people, you are less likely to be able to read them or to give them accurate readings. Thus, there are some activities that you can do to help you to develop your psychic abilities:

Observation Exercises – Understanding Body Language

Observation is a wonderful tool. You are able to observe people and to see the different ways in which they react to certain situations. This gives you many clues when it comes to being able to assure them while giving them a reading or consultation. Body language is one way in which you can learn if people are being honest with you. It shows on their faces and the movement of muscles when someone is deliberately lying to you and as a psychic it's important that you know who you are dealing with. Try to learn from the body language of people and the best way to do this is to look out for the following things:

Crossed arms – This shows a defensive stance. The person may not be open to any new information and thus you must approach with caution.

Blinking eyes when they talk – This means that there is a level of deception involved. Perhaps the client is trying to show you up as a charlatan and is purposely feeding you incorrect information to see how you react to it.

Not looking directly into your eyes – This may mean that the client is a little ashamed of something and you may have to coax it from them in order to help the client. In this case, try to be gentle and reassure the client so that the client is prepared to confide in you.

Playing with their hands – This denotes that the client is nervous, and it may help to sooth the client so that you are able to make him/her feel more at ease with you. Remember that trust plays a huge part when someone consults a psychic. You need to establish sufficient trust to take away any doubts that the client may have and help him/her to feel at ease.

Other Behaviors to Observe

If a client shows belligerence, the chances are that the client feels on unsafe ground. The reason that people show this type of behavior is that they feel a sense of insecurity. Perhaps they have never experienced psychic readings before and are a little ill at ease and use this bravado to hide the fact that they are insecure.

You also need to be able to recognize the following, in order to feel empathy for the client and this empathy is all important when it comes to making yourself believable:

- *Nervousness*
- *Unhappiness*
- *Fear*
- *Anger*
- *Jealousy*
- *Hopelessness*
- *Loss of faith*

These feelings could be derived from the situation in which the client finds him/herself and your empathy is very important. If, for example, a woman wants you to talk about her dead husband, it would be unprofessional not to pick up on her feelings of desperation or to exploit them. You need to be able to show empathy and to step into her shoes and if this means questioning her a little about the relationship, this will help your powers of observation.

Increasing Your Knowledge

If you are lacking in general knowledge, you can't put yourself over as astutely as someone whose knowledge is vast. Thus, one of the activities that is suggested for people who want to develop their psychic abilities is reading. Read a wide variety of which will give you an insight into human behavior and even if you limit this to good quality fiction, this will help you to be able to empathize with clients who have been through experiences that you would otherwise not be able to imagine.

The wider your knowledge base, the better able you are to draw from it. I recommend that you choose a variety of – both factual and fiction – because reading opens your mind and helps you to experience all kinds of emotions that you may never touch upon in your life and that will be helpful to you in your work.

Concentration Exercises

To develop and hone this part of your psychic ability, you need to have activities that improve your concentration levels. Art can do this if you are artistically inclined. If you like computers, why not try homing in on your concentrative powers by using something such as a program like Luminosity. You have to concentrate because you are given certain questions to answer within a given time. They call it "exercise for the brain" but as far as a psychic goes, it's really and truly great concentration for the mind. That's part and parcel of what you need to develop so if you can find programs that require total concentration, then these are good for you and will help your concentration levels to improve.

Other games that are fun are turning a pack of cards face downward onto a table and trying to establish pairs by turning two cards over at a time. You need to concentrate because you need to remember where certain cards are and, with practice, will find that you improve your concentration. This is vital for the psychic because it's easy to allow outside influence to get in the way when you are trying to give a client a reading. If you have learned concentration through meditation this helps to hone the mind, body and spirit into that moment. However, card games such as this also help your powers of observation and when working with people, that's vital to success.

Sociability – Learning to mix with all kinds of people opens up your understanding of different character types. It is important that you have a fair share of work and play and try to meet plenty of people in your life. Many people who develop psychic abilities find that having a great social life improves the way that they can read people's problems because they also become aware of different mannerisms and the approach that different people have toward their problems. It also helps to work with different age levels. Thus, spend quality time with kids and learn to have a great relationship with older folk.

Chapter 3. Intuition

Many people are familiar with what intuition is, but what exactly is intuition? Some people say that it is the highest form of intelligence. Intuition is the ability to know something even without evidence or analysis. It is about understanding. Sometimes, when the phone rings, you know who is calling.

The truth is that intuition is widespread. Unfortunately, today, people do not recognize it. Many people do not notice the messages from their intuition and only rely on logic or the use of reasons. Hence, they fail to listen to what the intuition tells them. Once they get used to shutting down their intuition, then they reach the point where they can no longer hear or notice it. The good news is that it was never too late to learn to listen to your intuition again.

How to Develop Your Intuition?

The third eye is the base of intuition. It is the key to the power of clairvoyance, also known as clear seeing. The third eye or Ajna chakra is probably the most common chakra that many people are familiar with. It is what will allow you to see into the world of spirits. Remember that the exact location of the third eye is right between your eyebrows.

The good news is that everyone has a third eye. It is just a matter of developing it, and this is something that you can do. Once you create your third eye, you will have powerful intuition, and you will even be able to access the Akashic records. It will depend on how you make use of it. Another compelling reason to develop the third eye is to be able to see prana more clearly. Many can associate many things with the third eye, but the most common of all is intuition.

Every person has some level of intuition. For example, have you experienced knowing who is calling your phone even without looking at it? This is a classic example of the use of intuition. Of course, there are many other practical uses, such as avoiding danger or simply knowing the proper course of action to take in a difficult situation. Indeed, developing intuition can be very helpful.

The best way to develop intuition is simply by using it. If you have not paid attention to your intuition for too long, then now is the time for you to make some changes and start listening to your intuition again. Learn to listen to how you feel. A good approach is to recognize your emotion or "gut feeling" and then use reasons to justify it instead of relying on reasons alone.

It is also worth noting that meditation is a natural and effective way to develop intuition. Here is another exciting exercise that can enhance your intuition:

Use your intuition in your daily life. For example, when the phone rings, try to "guess" who is calling. When you are at the supermarket or when driving, visualize the first person you will see before taking a turn. There are many other ways to put your intuition into work. The important thing is to make use of it regularly. Do not be discouraged if you commit mistakes. The more times that you use your intuition, the more you will get good at it.

There are lots of different ways to improve your intuition. Since your third eye is your center of wisdom and vision, it helps you know your dreams and what they mean. You may even want to try out lucid dreaming or try reading tarot cards. Find different ways to use your intuition during your day.

Since your third eye is where your higher perception levels live, it helps to be more tuned in to your intuition. You don't have to be perfect at impulse. All you need to do is be curious and learn more about intuitive techniques. After some practice, these techniques will become familiar, and you will be confident in your abilities.

The great thing is, there's no need to be serious about it. You can have fun and explore something so that you can keep your chakras open to wonder.

Here are some of the great ways to improve your intuition and energy:

- *Grow psychic awareness*
- *Practice contemplation*
- *Work with your spirit guides*
- *Connect with nature and the elemental energies*
- *Cultivate curiosity about symbols*
- *Focus on the space "in-between" things*
- *Allow your imagination freedom*
- *Guided meditation*
- *Visualization*
- *Dream interpretation and lucid dreaming*
- *Practice divination*
- *Strengthen your root and throat chakra*
- *Allow yourself to be comfortable in silence*
- *Mediate under the moon*
- *Practice intuition*

Intuition is an underrated psychic gift, for it truly is an example of precognition. Anyone whose intuition was right essentially received a momentary glimpse into the future, so the next time your intuition is correct, be proud for your unlocking psychic gifts as you live and breathe!

The third eye is also called the pineal gland. It is a small endocrine system that regulates the wake-sleep pattern. When you talk about the pineal gland, you also refer to the third eye in spirituality.

Activate and Decalcify Your Pineal Gland

The pineal gland or your third eye holds remarkable power. However, only a few people can tap into this power and use it effectively. Many people have an underdeveloped third eye. Even so, the good news is there are exercises that you can do to strengthen your third eye so you can start using and enjoying its immense power. Let us talk about them one by one:

Who is it?

This is something that you can do every time your phone rings or beeps. Ask yourself, "Who is it?" Pay attention to what you see in your mind's eye. Do you see any images or impressions? Be open to receiving messages. This is how you can connect to your intuition. It would be best to realize that you have a strong instinct and only have to learn to connect to it. Of course, this is a technique that is not limited to calls or texts on your phone. You can also adjust it a bit and use it in other ways. For example, if you hear a knock or any sound at night, you can ask, "What is it?" and pay attention to any messages you get from your intuition. The important thing is to start connecting to your intuition once again.

Forehead press

This technique is becoming popular these days. This, however, does not work on everyone, but it is still worth trying. This will allow you some specks of prana in the air. They usually appear as tiny dots or any form of white light. The steps are as follows:

Place your index finger in the part between the eyebrows where the Ajna chakra is. Press it gently and maintain pressure for about 50 seconds. Slowly remove your finger, blink your eyes around five times, and look at a blank wall. Just focus lightly and try to see with your peripheral vision. Do you see tiny dots or any specks of white light? This is prana in the air.

To help you see the energy, you might want to do this in a dimly lit room. Look at a wall with a neutral background. This is an excellent way to use your third eye to see energy, but it is not recommended to strengthen the Ajna chakra. Still, this is worth trying, especially if you want to see prana.

Visual screen

This is an excellent technique to use for visualization exercises. To locate the visual screen, close your eyes and look slightly upward. With eyes shut, look at the area of the Ajna chakra. This is your visible screen. You can project anything that you like to this screen, especially images. You can consider this as some form of the internal magic mirror.

The primary purpose of this visual screen is for your visualization exercises. Here is a simple exercise you can do to increase your concentration and willpower:

Assume a meditative posture and relax. Now, look at your visual screen. Imagine that there is an apple floating in front of you. Now, focus on this apple and do not entertain any other thoughts. This is just like breathing meditation. However, instead of focusing on your breath, focus on the apple in your visual screen.

When you are ready to end this meditation, visualized the apple slowly fade away and gently open your eyes.

You are also welcomed to use any other object for this meditation. If you do not want to use an apple, you can visualize an orange or even an elephant. The important thing is to have a point of visual focus for this meditation.

Charging with the fire element

Remember that intuition is associated with the pineal gland. In the pineal gland is the third eye chakra. Now, this third eye chakra is related to the fire element. Therefore, you can empower your third eye chakra by charging it with the part of the fire. This is a powerful technique, so be sure to use it carefully. The steps are as follows:

Assume a meditative posture and relax. Close your eyes. Now, visualize the brilliant and powerful sun above you. This powerful sun is full of the element of fire. As you inhale, see and feel that you are drawing the energy from the sun. Let the power charge your third eye chakra and empower it.

Do this with every inhalation. The more you change your third eye, the more it lights up and becomes more powerful. Have faith that with every inhalation, you become more and more intuitive.

Keep in mind that this is a powerful technique. If you are starting, it is suggested that you only do up to 10 inhalations in the beginning. You can then add one or two more inhalations every week. You will know if you can execute this technique properly because you will feel pressure on your forehead in your third eye chakra area. Take note that you should not just visualize your third eye chakra getting more robust, but you should also be conscious that your intuition becomes more powerful the more that you change your third eye. Your intention should accompany the power of visualization.

Note

It should note that the Ajna chakra and crown chakra are closely connected. If you want to improve your intuition, it only fits that you also work on your crown chakra. Indeed, this does not mean that you should ignore your other chakras. Again, the whole chakra system is essential to your spiritual development and the awakening of the kundalini.

One of the most hotly debated topics within the psychic community, as well as within the scientific community, is that of auras. Mystics and spiritual traditions have promoted the existence of auras for millennia, covering just about every culture across the globe. Despite the widespread belief in auras, many still dismiss their existence because most people cannot see them. Recent scientific studies have revealed that auras can, in fact, exist, giving credence to the ancient traditions. However, despite their findings, many scientists still debate the nature of auras and the significance they hold. Regardless of this ongoing debate, many people crave the ability to see and interpret the auras of people around them. This will provide the tools needed for seeing auras, as well as insights regarding the true nature of auras and the meaning behind the different forms and colors they can take.

A Basic Overview of Auras

In most spiritual traditions, the nature and appearance of auras are largely the same. A person's aura is the energy that surrounds their body, forming a sort of envelope or bubble of pulsating, glowing energy that reflects their physical, emotional, and mental state of being. Sick people, for example, will have darker, less vibrant auras, some of which even seem incomplete with holes or areas missing. In contrast, healthy, happy people will have brighter auras, usually yellow or white, extending as far as three or four feet from their body, creating a virtual bubble of energy that shields them from negative energy in their surroundings.

Although the basic elements of an aura are largely agreed upon in terms of their size, their vibrancy, and the impact of positive and negative forces upon them, there are a few debates within psychic circles regarding the meaning of their colors. Some schools of thought claim that auras can contain the same colors as chakras with each meaning something similar if not exactly the same as their chakra counterpart. However, other traditions hold that there are fewer colors and that these colors hold a completely different meaning. A perfect example is the color red. While some traditions claim that red indicates sexuality, assertiveness, and a competitive nature, others suggest that it reflects anger or high levels of stress. Subsequently, context is all-important when it comes to interpreting the colors of auras as red may indicate that the individual is strong-willed, or rage-driven, and thus should be kept at a safe distance.

As already mentioned, numerous scientific studies have concluded that auras do, in fact, exist. However, these studies do little to support the idea that different colors represent different psychic abilities or spiritual qualities. Instead, the basic belief within the scientific community is that auras are nothing more than the electromagnetic field surrounding a living being. This is what is referred to as the Bio-Energetic Field within the scientific community. The different functions of the human body, such as circulation, digestion, and respiration, all create electrical impulses that travel throughout the body. Furthermore, these impulses create electrochemical reactions throughout the nervous system. Subsequently, when a person is in peak health, where all of these functions are operating at their highest levels, then there is a tremendous amount of electrical activity taking place all through the body, creating a halo effect around the individual. The healthier and more vibrant the individual is the brighter their bio-energetic field. When a person is ill or has suffered trauma, this field is reduced, both in size and intensity.

While science believes that an aura is largely one layer of energy produced by the electrochemical activities within the body, certain spiritual traditions believe that there are as many as seven separate layers of an aura, each representing a unique quality or condition of the individual. These seven layers of the aura are as follows:

- **Layer one: Etheric**. This layer is the one closest to the body and is usually the easiest to see. Associated with the root chakra, it represents a person's physical health and wellbeing and is bright blue when the individual is in good health. Physically active people tend to have the brightest etheric layers.
- **Layer two: Emotional.** The emotional layer surrounds the etheric layer and is connected to a person's emotional wellbeing. Associated with the solar plexus chakra, it can be any color in appearance—the brighter the color, the healthier the person. When the colors are dark or muted, it represents stress, fatigue, or generally poor emotional health.
- **Layer three: Mental.** The mental layer is the third from the body and is associated with a person's mental health and wellbeing. Associated with the sacral chakra, this layer is bright yellow when in good health. Due to the mental nature of this level, it is easiest to see around the head and neck area and is most vibrant in creative people and intellects.
- **Layer four: Astral.** This level is the fourth from the body and is associated with the heart chakra. Representing the interpersonal relationships of an individual, it is pink or rosy, red, most vibrant among those with loving personalities, whereas it can be subtle or even absent in introverts or those suffering heartbreak or depression.
- **Layer five: Etheric Double**. The etheric double layer is associated with the throat chakra and is the layer that represents your true self. This is another layer that can contain any color, depending on the qualities of the individual. When a person is living a life per their true nature, this level will be most vibrant; however, someone who is disconnected from their true identity will have a muted fifth layer.
- **Layer six: Celestial**. Representing unconditional love and connection with all living things, this level is pearl-white and associated with the third eye chakra. Psychics and other spiritually minded individuals display strong celestial layers.
- **Layer seven: Ketheric Template**. As the last layer, this is the one furthest from a person's physical body, reaching an estimated three feet. Associated with the crown chakra, this layer is gold in color and has the highest frequency vibration. It is considered the embodiment of a person's immortal soul; thus, it reflects the wellbeing of the individual across all incarnations. It also reflects the strength of a person's connection to the divine source.

Interpreting the Different Colors

As already mentioned, there are two main schools regarding the different colors of the aura and their meaning. For this book, the more common interpretation will be used, specifically that associated with the colors of the chakras. The following are the colors of the aura and their meanings:

- **Dark red:** Someone with a dark red aura will generally be hardworking, energetic, and active.
- Bright red: A bright red aura points to someone who has a highly competitive spirit, strives to win at whatever they do and is usually sexually assertive, harnessing raw, primal energy.
- **Orange:** A person with an orange aura is usually very business-minded, capable of handling facts and figures, as well as being good with people. They can also prove adventurous in nature, such as an entrepreneur.
- **Bright orange/yellow orange:** This color points to someone with an academic nature, given to logic and deep thinking.

- **Yellow:** As the color might suggest, a yellow aura represents someone bright and sunny in disposition, spontaneous and expressive.
- **Bright Green:** People with bright green auras are generally social, given to community activities and occupations, such as teaching or daycare.
- **Dark Green:** A dark green aura suggests someone who is good at organizing and being goal-oriented.
- **Blue:** This color signifies a person who is sensitive to others and is a loyal and caring friend.
- **Indigo:** A person with an indigo aura is usually more introverted, preferring solitude and tranquility. As a result, they are usually calm and clearheaded, often showing artistic qualities.
- **Violet:** A violet aura can be found in people who are charismatic, often with a sensual personality, and who can easily make connections with others.
- **Lavender:** Highly sensitive, even to the point of being fragile, lavender aura people are very imaginative and in touch with higher levels of consciousness.
- **White:** This is the highest color, representing transcendence, spirituality, and a unity of body and mind.

One of the main things to look for, in addition to the color itself, is the brightness of the aura. When a person is healthy, happy, and in tune with their inner, true nature, their aura will be brighter and more vibrant. In contrast, someone who is depressed, ill, or suffering inner conflict will have a muted aura, sometimes even brown, representing the dark, dreary condition of their energy.

Chakras and Cleansing Techniques

Although chakras are separate from auras, they are closely related, influencing the strength and clarity of the aura itself. When chakras are balanced and unblocked, flowing naturally and strongly, a person's aura will be more vibrant and balanced. Alternatively, when chakras are blocked or out of balance, the aura will suffer, becoming smaller and more muted in appearance. Fortunately, by understanding chakras, their meanings, and how to manage them, you will maintain good chakra health, thus promoting a strong and healthy aura. The following is a list of the seven chakras, revealing their significance and the location of each within the physical body:

- **Root Chakra:** This is the lowest of the seven chakras, located at the base of the spine. Its color is red, and it represents being down to earth, raw energy, and physical activity.
- **Sacral Chakra:** The second of the chakras, located just below the navel, is orange. It is associated with creativity and procreation, giving life in all forms.
- **Solar Plexus Chakra:** Yellow in color, this chakra represents a person's ability to assimilate to new conditions. It also points to motivation and being goal oriented. Located in the stomach region, it also affects healthy digestion.
- **Heart Chakra:** Located in the center of the chest, this chakra is green and represents love, relationships, and the awareness of one's soul.
- **Throat Chakra:** As the name suggests, this chakra is located in the base of the throat. Blue in color, it affects communication, specifically verbal communication.
- **Third Eye Chakra:** The most commonly known of all chakras, the third eye chakra is located in the forehead, just above the level of the physical eyes. Indigo in color, this chakra represents intuition and insight.

- **Crown Chakra:** The last and highest of the chakras, the crown chakra is associated with peace, wisdom, and spirituality. Violet in color, it is located at the top of the head, just above the crown.

When balanced, each of the seven chakras serves to create, attract, or direct energy to different parts of the body. However, even when balanced and healthy, some chakras will tend to be stronger and more pronounced within an individual, creating specific characteristics that define the person. Someone with a strong throat chakra, for example, will be more adept at giving speeches or just verbal communication in general. The extra strong nature of the throat chakra may affect the overall color of their aura, giving it a blue hue reflecting the nature of the energy itself.

Chapter 5. Telepathy

What Is Telepathy?

Telepathy is the exchange of information through means other than your known physical senses. Often, it involves mental communication using the power of your mind, but other extrasensory factors are possible, as well. The result is a successful transmission of thoughts and ideas between the participants without the use of their ordinary five senses.

Types of Telepathy

You are a human being who possesses some form of psychic energy around you. This energy is what you refer to as your aura. Communication between humans can occur through this field of power, and that exchange of thoughts or information constitutes telepathy. It does not involve any of the known usual physical senses that you use every day to communicate. Telepathy, being a form of non-physical communication, takes various formats. Currently, you have three primary types of Extrasensory Perception (ESP). These forms are:

1.   Instinctual telepathy - a form of communication that depends on your feelings, i.e., your instincts
2.   Mental (mind-based) telepathy - information exchange involving communication between your mental faculties, i.e., mind to mind communication
3.   Spiritual telepathy is a form of communication between yourself and your higher being, i.e., soul to soul communication
Instinctual Telepathy

First, you need to realize that you share this type of telepathy with animals and that it is of the lowest kind. You engage in the extrasensory exchange of information based on your feelings at a particular time. You typically carry out this communication through the usage of your center of emotions and instincts. This specific focal point forms your solar plexus.

Various cultures utilize their solar plexus to attain this telepathy by recognizing the feelings of other people located at a different location. Since it depends on your instincts, this telepathy may take the reference of your sixth sense or your gut feeling. Ideally, this definition means that you can experience someone else's emotional needs in spite of your physical separation by a significant distance.

In one form descriptive of spiritual telepathy, your solar plexus reaches out with a length of a cord-like substance. Your cord extends outwards to link up to another person's extended cable. This link connects each of your solar plexus. Your two ties intertwine with each other and form a telepathic bond between the two of you. This bond is how the transfer of thoughts to your mind occurs.

From your mind, the thought flows into your higher auric planes, such as the brain and implants itself. Your brain registers the specific thought from which it can decipher the relevant information. Finally, your conscious self makes sense of this information and responds appropriately in your physical form. This description is the common comprehension available for your instinctual telepathy.

Examples of cultural communities that use instinctual methods for their communication include certain African Bushmen from the Kalahari region, the Australian aboriginals, and the inhabitants of the Hawaiian Islands. In addition, you can find instinctual telepathy in a family setting. It occurs between parents and their children as well as between lovers in a relationship. When these groups of people report getting a hunch or gut feeling, you know that what they are describing arises from their instinctual focal point, i.e., solar plexus.

Animals exhibit their instinctual telepathy through their mass migrations during different climatic seasons. Besides, your pet animals can distinguish your moods from each other and start behaving like they can read your mind. The attainment of this animal response to your emotional state is via instinctual telepathy. All of these cases exemplify how you share instinctual communication with animals and express why it is your lowest level of telepathy.

Mental (Mind-Based) Telepathy

You have exchange and transfer of thoughts between discrete minds. All your mental faculties need to focus on a specific center of attention to enable this communication to take place. This type of connection is intensely concentrative in practice. Besides, it makes use of your throat level within the much lower planes in your psychic energy field. Mental (mind-based) telepathy is shared among the Buddhist communities and especially with their Tibetan monks.

These gurus typically participate in mental communication of specific Buddhist teachings to their masters known as treasure finders. As earlier mentioned, mental (mind-based) telepathy takes place in the astral plane of the human energy field. This form of telepathy is the way Buddhists often carry out their communication. Besides, its utilization allows for the passage of essential teachings down through generations of Buddhist lineages. The following are the various exercises with which you can carry out and demonstrate mental (mind-based) telepathy:

1.   Mental radio
You and the sender are in two different rooms. The sender sketches an image on a piece of paper and encloses it in an envelope. You tune in (hence the radio reference) using your mind and try to identify the drawn image. Eventually, if successful, you sketch the same model as well. Your image needs to be similar to the one in the envelope contained in the other room.

2.   Extrasensory perception (ESP) card test
Once again, you and the sender are in two different rooms. The sender shuffles a deck of cards containing various symbols and draws out one of the cards. He then tries to communicate the logo to you located in the other room mentally. You need to identify the correct card that your sender had picked out to consider this test a success.

3.   Dream telepathy experiment
You spend a night sleeping in an electronically shielded room, and the sender located in another place. Once you reach your dreaming phase, i.e., rapid eye movement, the sender tries to use his mind to communicate to you a randomly selected image. You wake up at this point and describe your most recent dream. You repeat this process regularly through the night.

Eventually, you carry out a comparison between your descriptions and the original images from the sender. Draw your appropriate conclusions based on the extent to which any set of two parallel images correspond to each other.

4.   Ganzfeld telepathy experiment

In this telepathic exercise, you get into a profoundly peaceful and calm state akin to deep meditation. Your brain shuts out all elements from your physical surroundings or environment. You wear headphones that are playing white noise and simultaneously cover your eyes while you are in a separate room from the sender.

The sender attempts to use his mind to relay a series of mental images to you. In the end, you get to compare the pictures and look for any similarities between the sender's representations and your results. This particular practice is a derivative of the Germans, and it encompasses your whole field of psychic energy.

Spiritual Telepathy

In this type of communication, you need to attain the unification of your mind, soul, and brain. Spiritual telepathy involves a connection between different souls. As the highest telepathic form, spiritual communication utilizes the top-level planes of your auric field. When performing this exercise, you act as a link between the physical and the religious spheres.

The alignment of your brain and soul allows for the implantation of relevant information and messages from a higher being. Your upper master can only form interactions with your soul and is incapable of a direct physical manifestation. Therefore, it is now upon you to disseminate the implanted information from your brain to the general masses. Using your mind, you can spread your message via thought processes straight to the people in the society. Remember that spiritual telepathy requires that your physical, emotional, and mental states are all in harmony.

In preparation, cleanse your physical form of impurities since the presence of any injuries obstructs the complex information flow. Attaining peaceful mental and emotional states are necessary as well. These requisite conditions serve to clear a path for the smooth flow of ideas and messages from your soul to your brain. Once your mind fully acquires the specific information, you can share it with other people through mental transference.

You must note that this form of telepathy is common among people who serve a higher purpose, such as religious and political leaders. They represent a large group of people and can influence their collective mentality. Hence, individual leaders utilize spiritual telepathy to achieve ethical and moral guidance that they can share with their followers.

This telepathy affects a broad spectrum of humanity and its typical lifestyle. Exceptional scientists and gifted artists are sometimes thanks to a higher being for their endowment while not realizing that what they experience is a form of telepathy on a spiritual level. It involves having some additional ability that goes beyond both your general acquired knowledge and your base intelligence. When you attain the highest level of this spiritual telepathy, you experience a state of clear, intuitive recognition and realization known as illumination.

Various religions consider their prophets as illuminated people who can communicate with the highest being. These prophets, in turn, convey the specific message and its relevance to the community. With time and by sharing, this information spreads throughout society. Eventually, this particular message and its associated practices undergo adoption by that specific religion.

Steps to Developing Telepathy

Before dismissing this form of communication as a false entity or a pseudo-reality, you can take some time off to attempt a couple of exercises known to create a sense of telepathy within your auric self. These activities do not guarantee success, but you will notice some significant effects afterward.

Ideally, to achieve telepathy, you need a focused mind and maintain a state of relaxation within yourself. You will need a second person to act as your telepathic receiver. Both you and the receiver should be in separate rooms or different locations. Remember that with your regular repetition and practice, you eventually become better at telepathy.

Developing your telepathy consists of three primary steps, which in turn contain smaller procedures that you can follow to attain your non-physical communication objective. The three main steps are:

1.	*Focus on all of your thoughts*
2.	*Send your telepathic message*
3.	*Practice with your partner*

Chapter 6. Dream Interpretation

Dreams

Dreams can be a way for the universe, your spirit guides, or even your own subconscious to reveal important messages to you. Anyone can receive meaningful dreams, but you'll notice the more you become in tune with your psychic abilities and the universe, the more you will receive these messages. The interpretation of dreams has been practiced for centuries in all manner of ancient societies, and it is still used frequently today.

How to Interpret It?

So how do you tell if your dream is trying to tell you something or if it's important at all? Well, usually, some element or elements stand out clearly and vividly and make an impression on you while you're in the dream, and that you remember when you wake up. If you forget the dream, the chances are it wasn't important. Sometimes there will be a figure that will directly tell you something that you will remember when you wake up. Often, however, it is not so clear. There may be a series of events that happen or an overall feeling throughout the dream that may be associated with some aspect of the dream, or maybe there are people or animals or anything symbolic that you see or interact with. These can all be interpreted and ascribed to your waking life. Remember that if anything in your dream really stands out to you, there's probably something to learn from it.

If there is a figure in your dream telling you something, how they appear to you may be just as symbolic and important as the message they delivered. If in your dream you are led by a deer from the darkness of the woods into a bright and sunny clearing, the message here is easily interpreted to mean you are very stressed and in need of peace of mind (or you are about to enter a metaphorical "eye of the storm" in your life). But the deer has significance too. If you were led by the person, you were in love with or a bird or your childhood pet, these could all put a different spin on the dream's meaning and how you interpret it. If your partner led you, this might signify that if you keep moving through this rough patch, you will be rewarded—you are on a path to this haven together. A bird may signify anxiety or restlessness, a need for freedom. A childhood pet leading you may make the clearing mean your past/your childhood that you have a deep nostalgia and longing for at this time in your life. The steadiness and silence of the deer, as well as its innocent (non-predator) nature and instinctive knowledge of the forest, may be telling you to keep your head up and keep calm and you'll get there. Of course, there are many ways to interpret these things and it also depends on the other context in the dream as well as your life. However, as you've probably noticed, there are many similarities between interpreting dreams and interpreting premonitions.

An important thing to remember when interpreting your dream is to try to do it without bias. This will create the most accurate interpretation, and the most honest. It's also best not to use outside sources like dream dictionaries or dream a-z websites or books unless you're really stuck. If you do feel like you're not getting the full picture, you can describe your dream to someone you know. Even if they have no psychic interest or have never interpreted a dream before, they may see the picture clearly. Say, for example, you dreamt of a bear fishing by the river with her cubs. The cubs fall into the river and are swept away, but the mother doesn't try to save them. Then the dream switches to the cubs back safe and sound with the mother bear. You just can't figure it out, so you ask your friend, and they ask if you've felt distanced or disconnected from your mother recently? Or (if you're a mother) if you've felt that you haven't been taking care of your children and feel inadequate? Right away these clicks for you, and you wonder why you didn't see it before. Always go to a friend or family member for helping interpret if you're stuck BEFORE turning to a dream dictionary, as dream dictionaries don't know all the details of your dream, often providing a vague interpretation of one-word symbols, and they don't know the context of your life.

It is a good practice to keep a journal of your dreams. Writing down a dream as soon as you wake up helps you remember and lock in details that would otherwise be forgotten soon after waking, and even if you do forget, you can go back and reread it and, hopefully, it will evoke the memory of the dream again. As well as helping to remember, it will also allow you to keep track of any patterns that crop up in your dreams and analyze them. If you think a dream is important, always write it down in as much detail as you can remember—everything counts. You can even add a little sketch if you can't put something into words fully.

Another way to start analyzing your dream is by questioning it. Why did I see that person in that context? Why were buffalo present throughout my dream? Why was there a feeling of uneasiness and discordance even though my dream was peaceful? What was the setting of my dream? What was I trying to do? Who was I in the dream? Why was the bright red bird that appeared briefly so vivid? These are a few examples, but feel free to ask any questions you think are relevant to your dream.

One common theme in dreams that people fear is death. Whether it be their own or the death of a loved one, but don't worry—dreaming of death isn't predicting it. Dreams are rarely premonitions and are more commonly reflections of your emotional state and metaphors for what is going on in your life and what you need to deal with. If you dream of death, this may signify massive change or emotional/spiritual rebirth on your horizon. Maybe you're moving, or taking a trip, finishing school, experiencing a breakup, etc. It may also mean a part of you has symbolically died and that inner transformation is in the works. Death is often a symbol of change in our lives. In fact, in tarot, readers often tell the client whom they are reading for not to take the death card literally. Take a look at who or what is dying in your dream and ask yourself why. Why is this person dying, and what do they represent or symbolize as a part of my life? How does this death fit into the context of my life? Even if the person who dies is someone you know, this can still be a representation of a part of yourself or your relationship with them. It could also more literally indicate a fear of losing this person. There are many ways of interpreting death dreams, and almost none of them mean that someone is literally going to die, so put your mind at ease and do some introspection or prepare for some big changes ahead.

Another common dream theme is being chased, stalked, or attacked. Often, the dreamer will feel as if they are trying to move but can't or can only move in slow motion. It can be any villain, creature, or animal chasing or attacking you, or you may not know what is chasing you, but you can sense yourself being pursued throughout your dream. Often dreams like this are closer to nightmares and can cause extreme fear and anxiety for the sleeping person, especially if you know your assailant plans to harm or kill you (or they are already doing so if the dream involves you being attacked). This may represent anxiety or fear you have in your day-to-day life. It can be very literal, such as being attacked by a dog, and you are scared of dogs or being chased by someone who has caused you harm in the past. However, it can also be symbolic, such as being chased by your boss whom you are intimidated by in real life and fear will fire you soon. Or being chased/attacked by an animal whose traits represent things you fear—for example, being chased by an owl may not seem like a very frightful situation, but owls are silent, solitary, and adept hunters so this could represent communication issues or relationship issues or a fear of being alone. Try to hold it up to the context of your life, and really question and dig deep into why that specific entity was pursuing and attacking with the intention of harming you. Attacking dreams specifically can show vulnerability and a feeling of loss of control in your life. Pursuit and attack dreams may not represent outside forces at all and could be showing you that you need to take some time for introspection—your feelings could be what is really "attacking" or "chasing" you, and inner turmoil may be at the root of these disturbing dreams.

Being naked or just in your underpants/inappropriate clothes is another classic theme to dream about. The most obvious interpretation we can get from this is a feeling of vulnerability, feeling too exposed, and metaphorically naked. It can also be linked to a feeling of loss of control and anxiety, or it could point to a need to be liked and a fear that not everyone likes you, that you are judged by others (whether this is true or not). Something else to consider is: if you are hiding anything or have any secrets, this dream may reflect that you feel everyone knows. The bottom line is these dreams are known to indicate insecurity of some sort, so take a look at what is happening in your dream or who is in the dream and seeing you naked or not seeing you. This is likely a reflection of who or what makes you insecure in your waking life. If it isn't obvious just take a look straight away at your life and think of areas where you are insecure. Maybe you quite literally are insecure about your body and enjoy the safety of hiding it beneath layers of clothes. There may be areas that you haven't even thought about. These are spots where you need to work on and build up your confidence—a message which a dream of this sort was trying to convey to you. On the other hand, if you felt good and positive about being naked or semi-naked, then this is a good sign! You are likely feeling very confident and empowered in your life at the current moment and feel free as though nothing can stop you. Again, one literal meaning of this dream could be that you are very comfortable and confident with your body and are not insecure about its appearance. It can indicate that you are happy with yourself as a person and don't feel the need to seek validation from others.

What Are Spirit Guides?

Spirit guides are souls on the other side that have either been assigned or have volunteered to help a person in the physical realm. There are several types of guides.

Ascended Masters

Ascended Masters are super charged spiritual beings. They once walked a spiritual path on earth but have now transcended to the point of no longer needing to reincarnate to the earth plane to learn karmic lessons. Ascended Masters still have a purpose to teach, heal and become spiritual guides to many. They are represented as gods, saints and religious and spiritual symbols we honor today in art, sculpture, scripture, music, and more. Some examples of known Ascended Masters are Jesus Christ, Buddha, Mother Theresa, Saint Germain, Krishna, just to name a few.

Master Guides

Master Guides are assigned to you at birth. When you come into the physical world your master guide is already there with you. You may not have met your master guide in either this physical world or in a past life. They are generally not your relative but have had enough experience to help and guide you on your life's journey. They still reincarnate yet they are old souls, and their main purpose is to guide you on your life's lesson and offer guidance as you embark on your spiritual path.

Task Guides

Other guides are more like task guides. They are assigned for a specific reason. A task guide steps in around a particular area or during a specific time in your life when you may need more specialized assistance. They sometimes step in around a particular impending decision. For example, what career is best for you? What is your purpose? They may show up when you're switching careers or when there's a major transition. Perhaps you're having a medical issue, therefore a guide will step in that specializes in that to help with an illness, diagnosis or to find the best treatment. They may simply step in to offer you support in a time of need.

Maybe you are inventing or creating something. There may be a special guide that steps in for that. For these task guides, they move on once their assignment is complete.

Gatekeeper

Then there is the **gatekeeper**. You can think of them as the bouncer at the night club. The gatekeeper is the threshold to allowing certain spirits to step through and communicate with you and which spirits are forbidden access. If you set an intention with your gatekeeper to only allow the highest vibrational spirits to step through, your gatekeeper will honor those intentions. This allows them to discern "who gets through" to communicate with you.

Family Members

Your loved ones may also be on the other side guiding you. They may be there to support you or to help you open up your medium gifts. Grandparents, Aunts, Uncles, Friends, Parents, Siblings, etc. There are no limits as to who on the other say may step forward to offer love and support. Some of your family guides may be either generational or karmic. They may even be family members that go back several generations and are with you to help clear karmic links in this lifetime.

Having a connection and a relationship with your guides is a very important part of your spiritual growth. If you build a connection with your guides, you can communicate with them more clearly and effectively. You will find that your guides will help to direct you, inspire you, and help you to stay on track.

The relationship you build with your guides provides you with the resources to lean on your spirit tribe. Your spirit tribe always has your back.

Release the need to have names and expectations when you are starting out. It's more about trusting that your guides are there and believing, trusting and surrendering to the power of the guides. Whether you feel that it's your imagination or not, through the practice of meditation and raising your vibration you will begin to experience these guides around you. Be patient as it does take practice and commitment. You want to develop the ability to blend with those guides so that you're not pushing or trying too hard to make that connection. If you push, you will simply lock into your logical mind which results in naturally lowering your vibration.

When you allow yourself to relax with your guides, you may begin to receive more information. For example, your guides may give you their name using a symbol or object. Let's say you see a word or image on a billboard. In that moment, if a thought or feeling pops in "oh, that's the name" or "this is a message", this is when trusting it is most important.

They serve as a reminder that you don't have to keep it all to yourself and that you do have someone to connect and communicate with that wants to see you succeed.

Honorable Mention: Angels

Angels are different than other guides but deserve recognition. Angels have never incarnated into the physical world and come in with unconditional love to offer support, protection and to watch over us. Guardian angels are assigned to help to keep you safe.

Chapter 8. Guided meditation

This meditation session uses guided imagery to help relax the mind, open the potential of your inner spirit and bring a sense of calm to your life. Use it anytime you need a pick-me-up, and on a regular basis to maintain good mental and spiritual health. Let's begin.

Find a seated, comfortable position in a quiet room. Settle in, relaxing your hip flexors, back, and shoulders. Roll your shoulders and neck gently back and forth, releasing any tension that may have built up. Close your eyes.

Take a deep breath in and out, pushing your anxieties out with your exhale. Take a few breaths to clear yourself of all of your negativity. It is now gone, and you now have space to accept calm, positive thoughts.

Imagine that you are perched comfortably on a smooth, dark rock by the side of a large pond. The rock is almost soft to the touch, and the curve of the rock gently cradles your bottom and legs. The warmth from the day's sun warms your body as it comes in contact with the rock. Feel the warmth on both hands as you rest them on the rock.

Now, look out onto the pond, clear and deep in the middle. It is so pristine that you can see every rock and branch that specks the floor. You see a few fish here and there, milling around, also soaking in the mid-day sun.

A light breeze touches your skin with the warm air and causes the very surface of the water to gently sparkle. You are the only one sitting by this pond, and there are only the sounds of the water trickling in from the nearby spring, and the birds chirping in the trees around you. Look up to see the tips of branches reaching out from the forest, harnessing the energy of the sun, the life-giving force.

See the light, transparent through the round, oblong leaves. They rustle lightly in the warm breeze. You take a deep breath, soaking in the smell of fresh air, and the earthy aroma of the forest.

Across the pond is a grove of pine trees, whose silhouettes remind you of pipe cleaners, almost fluffy looking. The light shines through the needles, creating a soft glow. You see a single bird, flitting about the branches of one of the trees, likely searching for a mid-afternoon snack. It flaps its wings, effortlessly hopping from branch to branch. The energy in this tiny bird is envious, something you hope for.

Yet, at this moment, you are soaking in all of the energy you could need. The warm sun bombards you with positivity, and the gentle breeze brushes negativity away from your spirit. There is a sense of calm here unlike any other.

At this moment there is peace and quiet, no responsibilities or worries. It energizes you to your very core, creating a sense of urgency to feel this way forever. You imagine your life looking and feeling like every day. You vow no matter where you are in life, to imagine in your mind that you are here, at this moment, relaxed as can be. You see the green water, feel the warm, smooth rock, feel the sun kiss your face. In every moment going forward, there is only this feeling.

Open your eyes and carry this image with you. Now is the time to live your best life, go forth with the energy given by the sun. It is eternal and never-ending. Simply harness this image any time you need a little pick-me-up.

Chapter 9. Astral Travels

The very idea that humans can exit their bodies while sleeping is ancient. Countless people believe it is possible to communicate with cosmic beings by vivid dreams and visions that are experienced by astral travel.

Between eight and twenty percent of people say they have had something similar to an out of body experience at one point in their lives. A sensation that their consciousness, or spirit is leaving their body. Many experience this during sleep or while hypnotized; some can do it while just relaxing.

The astral plane is one in the fifth dimension. This is where dreams take place. Where mystical teachings are given and where the dead go. You might get lucky enough to meet spiritual beings there. You can discover what happens when you die, your purpose in life, receive guidance, have premonitions about your future, have an awakening, learn wisdom about death, learn your inner defects, see your spiritual obstacles, learn what you don't know about yourself, and discover secret knowledge. You will find yourself in another world that exists outside this world. You can fly, walk through objects and walls, meet new people and travel to distant lands. It is a wonderful experience.

The reality is made by thoughts projecting consciousness into the physical realm. When your astral project, the conscious mind will leave the physical body and move into the astral body for the experience. You stay attached to your physical self through a silver cord. Some might see this cord when they astral project. To be able to astral project, you must feel completely relaxed, wear comfortable clothing, and be lying down. Put a comforter over you since the physical body might get cold when your spirit travels out of it.

You will stay aware of everything you experienced when you were not in your physical body.

Some people can do this naturally, while others are a little afraid to remove their consciousness from the physical body, so they choose not to learn.

Astral travel can be achieved either awake or through deep meditation or lucid dreaming. People who have experienced astral projection say their spirit left their physical body and moved into the spirit world. This concept dates back to ancient China and has been around for thousands of years.

Psychics say the mind that dreams hold the astral body, and this causes sudden jerks that wake you up or falling dreams. Many dreams aren't remembered and thus causes astral travel to be a subject of individuality. Those who believe in astral travel will often mention that ghost sightings are typically described as transparent apparitions that walk along the earth.

It isn't clear if every object has an astral counterpart or if the spirit just incarnates into a body, and this results in astral travel. The phenomena might be something entirely different. Astral travel deals a little about life and the things that happen after death.

There are two different thoughts on the nature of astral travel. A broad definition of these would be a phasing model and mystical model.

The Phasing Model believes that it's possible to leave your body. The astral plane and the physical world are both areas of our conscious spectrum. When someone chooses to project, they are phasing into a different area of consciousness and the locations there. You can compare this to changing the radio station. This viewpoint is seen as the external reality is only a state that is created internally.

The Mystical Mode has many astral maps and belief systems, but are connected to the beliefs that Astral travel happens outside the physical body. An energy body is thought to carry the consciousness out of the physical body. Higher planes are reached by progressive projections of subtle energy bodies from other projected bodies. This body is connected to the physical one through an energetic connection that looks like a silver cord some refer to as an umbilical cord.

There are hundreds possibly thousands of techniques to help your astral travel. Everybody is different, so something works for one may not work for another. Try one and if it doesn't work for you, move to a different one.

The Rope Technique

The main object in this technique is to picture a rope hanging off the ceiling. The point of this rope is to provide pressure at a certain area on the astral body so that it will separate itself from your physical one

Reach out with your imagined hands and pull on yourself. Pull yourself hand over hand up the rope that is above you. You may experience dizziness. This sensation will become stronger the farther up the rope you go.

Continue to climb and you will start to feel the vibration. Your entire body will feel like it is vibrating and you may end up feeling paralyzed. Focus completely on the climb and don't stop.

This is where you feel yourself being freed from your body. Your astral body will leave the physical in the rope's direction. You will now notice that you are hovering above your body. Now your free.

Watch Yourself Sleep

Lie down and make sure you're comfortable on your back, look towards the ceiling. Completely relax and allow your mind to let go of unwanted thoughts.

Let yourself know that you are going to watch yourself fall asleep. You will have to be clear about your intents. Let the body sleep while your mind stays alerted. Tell yourself to keep consciousness while your body is going into a trance.

Once you completely relax, you will need to become familiar with the sensations that your body has as you fall asleep. You need to be aware while this happens. You will feel your body feels numb and heavy.

Pay attention to your body's sensations. You might feel like you are floating or swaying. You might feel tingling sensations in certain areas. You could even feel vibrations surging through your entire body. You may even have buzzing in your ears. Whatever you feel, don't panic as these are signals that you are on the right path.

You need to visualize you are rising from your bed and float to the ceiling. How will it feel if you did float? Make this experience as real as you can. Hold this image. If everything works, you will notice that you are floating above your body.

The Monroe Technique

An important part of this is that you completely relax.

Now try to get yourself to go to sleep without falling asleep. Keep an awareness of being between awake and asleep. This is what they refer to as a hypnagogic state. Let this state deepen and release all of you bad thoughts. Now peer through your eyelids into the blackness.

Now relax deeper. Bring vibrations into your body and make them become more intense. You need to continue to control and grow these more. During this time is when the astral body will leave your physical body. Then roll yourself over, and you will see the physical body below you.

Out of Body Experiences from Lucid Dreams

Lucid dreams are where the dreamer is aware of dreaming. In a lucid dream, the person is already outside their body.

To achieve astral travel from lucid dreams, you need to become obsessed with out of body experiences, and you have to desire it. It's important that you read as much about it as you can. You need to think about it constantly.

When your mind is ridden with thoughts of out of body experiences, you need affirmations and triggers so you can have lucid dreams. All day long think about having a lucid dream. Ask yourself if you are dreaming now.

Once you're in one of these dreams, and you aware of it, you will notice that you are no longer in your body. You will be able to make yourself to see your bedroom. When you do this, your dream world will disappear, and you will find yourself floating about your body.

Displaced Awareness Technique

Shut your eyes and let yourself enter a trance state. Notice your room. Feel yourself about your shoulders and see all around. Don't acknowledge anything directly.

Now picture the astral body rotating. When you have finished the mental rotation, your astral head will be where your physical feet are. The astral feet should be where the physical head is positioned. Now that you have this, picture the room from this perspective.

Let go of where you are located and get rid of your sense of direction. This is what you want

When you're comfortable, imagine floating toward the ceiling. Make this feel as real as you can. During this you will suddenly find that you have left your physical body.

The Jump Technique

When this technique is performed correctly, you will awaken from your dreams, and they will become lucid. This has to be done well.

Ask yourself repeatedly throughout the day if you're dreaming or not. It is important to do this because you need to know where you are. You have to make yourself doubt that you are in the physical world. For proof, jump just like you are flying. If you are really in your physical body, your feet will hit the ground. If you're in a dream when you jump, you will begin to float

After a few days of this, you will notice that you start to jump in your dreams to see whether or not you are dreaming. When you jump, you will be floating.

The Stretch Out Technique

Lay down, close your eyes, and relax. Imagine your feet stretching and getting longer by an inch or so. When you have this in your mind, let your feet shrink back to normal. Repeat with the head. Now alternate between your feet and head until they stretch about two feet. Now stretch them together. This starts the vibrations and will cause you to feel dizzy.

After you have practiced this a little, you will feel like you are floating and can command yourself to rise to the ceiling.

The Hammock Technique

Imagine that you are stretched out on a white hammock connected between palm trees at the beach. Picture yourself moving with the wind. Try to recreate this sensation while you picture yourself swaying back and forth. Continue this until you feel the vibrations begin to grow. Once the vibrations start, let your astral body roll out of the physical.

Do That Relaxing Thing

Let your body relax until you can't feel it. Continue to repeat this notion in your head and stay focused. Don't allow yourself to give up. Say it out loud slowly if that helps.

"I will have an out of body experience. I will let myself go to sleep, but I will take this waking consciousness everywhere I go. I will leave my body with complete awareness."

Continue repeating this even after you become tired, and all you want to do is roll over.

Chapter 10. Psychic Games

Psychic games are a good way to have fun as you learn and develop your psychic abilities. You do not need to be so serious when you enhance your abilities. In fact, you will notice that you are more effective when you are having fun. When you are having fun, you are charged with positive energy, which is the best state to make use of your psychic abilities. Here are the notable psychic games that you can try:

Red or Black

For this game, you only need to use a deck of ordinary playing cards. Playing cards have two colors: red and black. You just have to guess the color of the cards. To do this, you can rely on your intuition, divination, or even micro kinesis. Use whatever ability would apply and the one that you want to develop.

Shuffle the cards then put it face down on the table in front of you. Now, predict or divine the color of the top card. Is it red or black? Say your answer aloud and then check if you got it right. Since a deck of cards only have a limited number pertaining to each color, it is advised that you reshuffle the whole deck after every two or three guesses/attempts. Again, you can use any ability of your choice. For example, if you want to apply psychometry, then you might want to touch the top card and try to get some sense impressions to help you predict its color correctly.

Dancing Candle

This is a game to help you develop your ability to project energy. For this exercise, you need to use a candle. Light the candle and focus on it. You need to make the flame lean in the direction of your choice by projecting energy to it. The idea here is to push it with energy. So, gather energy on the palm of your hand. Once you feel that you have enough energy, you should position your hand towards the candle with the palm facing outward.

Now, slowly move your hand to the flame and push it with the accumulated energy. The flame should lean/bend as you push it with energy. Remember not to put your hand close to the candle flame. If you need an advanced version, then you can simply project energy directly to the flame without accumulating it in your hand.

Pendulum Swing

This game presents many opportunities as it can be used to develop different psychic abilities. But first, what is a pendulum? A pendulum is any weighted object that is suspended on a chain or string. You can buy many beautifully designed pendulums from metaphysical and occult stores, as well as online. You can also create your own pendulum. It is easy to make your own pendulum. For a basic pendulum, you can use a thread and a needle. The needle will act as the bob of the pendulum. Hold the end of the thread with your hand and allow the pendulum to hang freely. It should be still before you use it. This pendulum is very sensitive to energy, so be careful not to move it. Another option that you have is to tie the end of the thread to something so that you would not have to hold it anymore. However, if you are using it for divination, then it is advised that you hold the string of the pendulum in your hand.

If you want to use it for divination, then you can ask the pendulum questions that are answerable by yes or no. However, the first thing that you need to do is find out how the pendulum responds to say yes, as well as how it moves to signify a no. This is easy to do.

As you hold the pendulum and have it hanging still, say, "Show me yes." The pendulum will move. Take note of how it moves. Is it in a clockwise, counterclockwise, or any other pattern of movement? Once you have the movement for a yes, you can ask her it would move for a now, "Show me no." Again, take note of how it moves. Once you understand how it moves for yes and for no, then you can start to ask it questions. This is a simple kind of divination with a pendulum, which can be very effective if you practice it long enough.

You can also use the pendulum to develop your other abilities. For example, you can to the end of the thread somewhere and have the bob hanging still. Now, you can project energy or even use telekinesis to make the bob (needle) move. Use whatever ability you want to make it move.

Projection

This is a good game to play with a friend. This will help you learn to project prana more effectively. The first thing that you should do is to identify who will be the sender and who will be the receiver. The receiver should close their eyes as the sender projects energy to them. The receiver should tell which part of their body the energy is projected. When you want to take it one step more, you can also add a certain quality to the energy, and the receiver should be able to identify it. This game can develop your skill in projecting energy (sender), as well as in increasing your awareness of energy (receiver).

If you ever make use of negative energy, be sure to do some cleansing afterward. It is not good to keep any negative energy in your system. When you play this game, it is important that you and the other person are very honest with each other, as you need to know if you are able to send and receive energy properly. If nothing appears to occur on your first few tries, do not be discouraged. Just keep on practicing.

To take it a step further, you can try merging your energy and projecting it to someone or something, and see what happens. If you ever do this, it is advised that you only make use of positive energy, as it is never a good idea to send out any negativity to anyone.

Shielding

You can ask the sender to project negative energy to you. However, before that, you should first surround yourself with a shield. This way, you can test just how effective your shield it. So, how do you create a shield? There are many ways to make a shield. The most common shield is known as the bubble shield.

To create this shield, simply imagine a strong bubble of light surrounding your body. Be fully convinced that it will protect you from all psychic attacks and negative energies. Charge it with energy as much as you can. Take note that the lifetime of a shield is only as good as the energy that you feed it. Therefore, if you feel like your shield is getting weak, you should recharge it again with energy. Normally, a regular shield lasts for about three to five hours before it will need to be recharged. You can also switch roles with your friend so you can also try to project another against their shield.

Chapter 11. Out of Body Experiences from Lucid Dreams Tips

The key to understanding out of body experiences from lucid dreams is in understanding what really happens during them. With careful research and experimentation, advances are being made in how we view our universe. It's been proven that information can be transferred from one person's brain to another through simple thought alone. It's possible that information and thoughts can travel 30 feet or more!

It is the physics of our brain that are limiting in the types of experiences we can have. Any attempt to circumvent this limitation will allow for larger and faster experiences.

I'm going to go out on a limb here and suggest a few things that you should do to prepare yourself for experiencing out of body dreams from lucid dreams.

Think!

Have you ever tried thinking about your body being in another place? Most people have, but haven't really thought about all the possibilities involved. Picture yourself being in another place right now. Try moving your body as you do this. Feel where you are but do it without actually moving. How close is your perception to how you really are? Can you get the feeling of what actually being there physically would be like?

If you can, then you may have already had an out of body experience from a lucid dream! If not try again, and then again, until finally nothing else seems to work. You'll soon understand how the brain and the physical body interact in this way.

Think Further!

There is more than one way to use pure thought to get out of your body and into another place that isn't physical plane location specific.

As I mentioned above, thoughts can travel a long way. It's been suggested that thoughts travel at least 30 feet and probably even further. So, you could imagine your body being in another place and still be at your physical location. Make a movie in your mind of being in another place then imagine waking up to find yourself there!

Play Around with The Possibilities of Your Perceptions!

A friend of mine told me that she was thinking about how it would feel if her body were in another place as she was laying down ready to go to sleep one night. She said that she thought to herself, "If I were here right now it would feel ____", then felt her perception change. She said that she felt like she was actually there. She was physically laying in her bed but felt like she was floating there. She then focused on how it would feel if she were in the place her perception showed her and again this resulted in a change of how she perceived herself to be located. This went on for at least 5-10 minutes before the sensations faded away.

My friend works as a hypnotherapist and finds that this type of work is best done with clients who are laying down or sitting up while being hypnotized. The position in which the subject is placed seems to have some sort of influence on how deep the hypnotic state is induced and maintained.

Be Open to The Possibilities!

Once you begin to experiment and learn what out of body experiences from lucid dreams are really all about, you will find that there is almost endless exploration involved. The more you think about it, the more you will discover just how unlimited your awareness really is. You'll start thinking that everyone else must be out of their minds to believe in such things!

It's actually thought by some researchers that out of body experiences from lucid dreams are incredibly common and almost everyone has had them at least once!

Sleep in A Comfortable Position!

It's thought by some researchers that our ability to be aware when we are asleep is limited by the way we sleep. When we sleep on our backs our heads tend to go down into our necks, so it's thought that this is what limits us from being aware while in a dream state.

It's also been shown that there seems to be a correlation between how relaxed someone is during sleep and their ability to have active and lucid dreams. Research has shown that people who are naturally lazy, or just plain out of it during the day tend to have better dreams.

Control Your Environment!

The better you feel about the environment you are in while dreaming, the better chance you have of having an out of body experience from a lucid dream. If you want to focus on leaving your body, then make sure everything else is just right.

If you can't move around freely and explore, then pretend that it's ok! Start thinking that you are free to roam around and do whatever comes naturally. If you are in a virtual world, then just imagine that there is no limit on what can be done!

Chapter 12. What is an Empath

Do you know someone who can tell you exactly how someone else is feeling? This person might be an empath.

Empath

Empaths are people who are highly sensitive to other people's emotions, and they often experience them in a physical manner. They live in a perpetual state of empathy – experiencing the entire world as if it were happening to them. When we're born, we all have natural empathy—we feel for our friends when they're hurt or happy for their successes. But as we get older, our empathy often changes. We become more social and less empathetic. However, many empaths as they grow up are left with feelings of guilt and shame for being overwhelmed by the emotions of others. Some may even deny that they are sensitive to other people's feelings and experiences. All this can lead to them living a life of isolation and loneliness, and leave them feeling unhappy with their lives. Empaths who have negative associations with their empathic feelings can develop anxiety, depression, or even suicidal thoughts at some point in their lives.

How Do Empaths Feel?

Empaths often feel things more deeply than most people do. The emotions of others become their own emotions. If someone around them is happy, they may feel joy. If someone is angry, they may feel rage. Empaths also experience what's known as emotional contagion, which means they will catch and spread emotions to others around them – sometimes these are positive feelings and sometimes not.

What Causes Empathy?

There isn't a universal cause of empathy, but studies have indicated that genetics can play a role in determining if you're an empath or not. When you are born, your genes dictate whether or not you're sensitive to other people's emotions. However, the majority of empaths probably aren't born this way—they develop after being exposed to uncontrollable stressful situations throughout their lives. These situations can range from being bullied at school, to watching their family members suffer from mental illness, or even surviving a natural disaster such as a hurricane or earthquake. Children who are born prematurely or have health conditions may also have high empathy.

How Can an Empath Live with Themselves?

For most empaths, being an empathic person has brought them a lot of pain and suffering. We all have the internal voice, the conscience, which tells us when we're doing something wrong. However, for those with high levels of empathy (and even many who don't), their conscience isn't so clear. They're constantly bombarded with emotional messages. These messages can tell them to lash out at others, withdraw from the world, or even take their own life. Empaths are constantly battling with these internal voices and often find themselves in a life of silence and isolation.

What is also very common with empaths is that they cannot clearly differentiate between what is real and what is not. They may have an entire episode of being overwhelmed by their emotions because someone cut them off in traffic when there was no one else around, but they can't tell if what happened was real or not. In fact, they may even attribute their feelings to other people's actions and speak badly about them. Sometimes, the more they try to understand what is happening to them, the worse they feel—which can lead them to withdraw even further from others.

Empaths May Become Selfish

There are some who believe that being an empath means that you're a horrible person – that you don't love or care about anyone else in the world, and you only care about yourself. This isn't so; most empaths are caring people who just have difficulty separating themselves from the emotions of others. Most of the time, empaths just want to help others and be good friends – but they don't always know how. Thankfully, some empaths have learned to cope with these emotions and live happy, healthy lives.

Chapter 13. Are you an Empath?

How Do You Know If You're an Empath?

Empaths are extremely sensitive, carefully tuned instruments when it comes to feelings. They feel anything, sometimes to an extreme, and are less apt to intellectualize sensations. Instinct is the filter through which they experience the world. Empaths are naturally providing, spiritually attuned, and good listeners. If you want a heart, empaths have got it. Through thick and thin, they are there for you, world-class nurturers.

The trademark of empaths is that they understand where you're coming from. Some can do this without handling people's feelings. However, like myself and many of my clients, others can end up being angst-sucking sponges for much better or worse. This frequently overrides the superb capability to absorb favorable feelings and all that is beautiful. Their bodies take in these and grow if empaths are around peace and love. Negativity, though, often feels assaultive, stressful. Thus, they're especially easy marks for emotional vampires, whose worry or rage can damage empaths. As a subliminal defense, they may gain weight as a buffer. When thin, they are more vulnerable to negativeness. A missing out on the reason for overindulging. Plus, an empath's level of sensitivity can be frustrating in romantic relationships. Many remain single, considering that they have not found how out to negotiate their unique cohabitation needs a partner.

When empaths soak up the impact of stressful emotions, it can activate an anxiety attack, depression, drug, food, and sex binges, and a myriad of physical signs that defy traditional medical diagnosis from tiredness to agoraphobia. Because I am an empath, I want to help all my empath-patients cultivate this capacity and be comfortable.

Empathy doesn't need to make you feel too much all the time. Now that I can align myself and refrain from taking on society's discontents, empathy continues to make me freer, sparking my compassion, vitality, and sense of the miraculous. To identify whether you're an emotional empath, take the following quiz.

You Can Ask Yourself:

- *Have I been described as "too emotional" or overly sensitive?*
- *If a friend is troubled, do I begin feeling it too?*
- *Are my feelings easily hurt?*
- *Am I emotionally depleted by crowds, requiring time alone to restore?*
- *Do my nerves get rattled by sound, smells, or extreme talk?*
- *Do I choose to take my car to locations so that I can leave when I please?*
- *Do I overeat to handle emotional stress?*
- *Am I scared of ending up being swallowed up by intimate relationships?*

If your answer is "yes" to 1-3 of these questions, you're at least part empath. Reacting "yes" to more than three indicates that you have found your emotional type.

Acknowledging that you are an empath is the first step in taking charge of your emotions instead of continuously drowning in them. Remaining on top of empathy will enhance your self-care and relationships.

Signs That You Are an Empath

If you are fascinated to find out what exactly defines an empath and have natural emphatic abilities, here are some qualities and signs that you may identify with.

- **Your empathy is inherent.**

It is the skill that makes you understand others' experiences and emotions beyond your point of view.

Say your buddy just lost their canine of 15 years. Empathy is what permits you to understand the level of pain she's going through, even if you have never lost a precious animal.

But as an empath, you take things a step further. You pick up and feel feelings as if they belong to your own experience. Somebody else's discomfort or joy becomes your discomfort or happiness.

- **Intimacy overwhelms.**

Empaths often find frequent close contact hard, which can make romantic relationships challenging.

You wish to connect and develop a lasting relationship. However, spending excessive time with someone results in stress, overwhelm, or stress over losing yourself in the relationship.

You might likewise discover sensory overload or a "torn nerve" feeling from excessive talking or touching. When you try to reveal your requirement for time alone, you absorb your partner's hurt feelings and feel even more distressed.

Setting healthy, clear boundaries can help minimize distress for the empath. Safeguarding your mental and emotional health should also be vital to you, otherwise, energy will be drained from you.

- **You have the right instinct.**

Ever felt like you have a strong inclination that things are not, right? Or maybe you can sense that someone cheated, or something is good or bad instinctively? Your empathy is present in this situation.

Empaths tend to detect subtle insights on others' ideas, like telling if a person is truthful or not.

As an empath, you might put a great deal of faith in your instincts when making decisions. While others may consider you spontaneous, the truth is that you are only trusting your intuition to guide you to the right choice for you.

- **You enjoy nature.**

Anybody can gain from spending time in a natural environment. Empaths might feel even more drawn to nature, and remote locations since natural areas offer a soothing space to rest from overwhelming feelings, sounds, and emotions.

You might feel totally at peace when hiking alone in a sunlit forest or viewing waves crash against the shore. Even a peaceful walk through a garden or an hour sitting under trees might lift your spirits, relieve overstimulation, and help you to unwind.

- **You don't thrive in crowded spaces.**

According to researchers, empaths can soak up unfavorable or favorable energy by merely being in someone's company. In crowded or busy places, this sensitivity might appear magnified to the point of being almost intolerable.

Empaths feel everything more intensely as compared to an ordinary person. If you can quickly sense how others feel, you'll likely have a tough time handling the emotional "sound" from a crowd, or perhaps a smaller sized group of people, for an extended amount of time.

When you're picking up on negative feelings, energy, or even physical distress from people around you, you may become overloaded or physically unwell. As a result, you may tend to become solitary or limit the company to a few.

- **You can NOT care.**

An empath does not just feel for somebody-- they feel with somebody. Taking in others' feelings so profoundly can make you want to do something about them. Empaths feel obligated to help in any way. In situations where an empath is not able to help the other person, he feels dissatisfied.

Empaths find it hard to have fun when someone is in pain or is struggling, thus, he will act upon his natural inclination to assist in alleviating their distress, even if that implies absorbing it himself.

Being concerned for others' welfare is not bad, but it may sometimes lead to ignoring your own needs. Overly caring for others can lead to fatigue and burnout, so it's important to conserve some energy.

- **People easily confide in you.**

Sensitive, compassionate individuals tend to be great sounding boards. Other people, especially your loved ones, may feel comforted by your assistance and connect to you first whenever they experience difficulties or troubles.

Because of too much caring for others, empaths have difficulty distinguishing that they are nearly overwhelmed. Therefore, finding a balance is essential. Without limits, unattended generosity and level of sensitivity can pave the way for "emotion dumps" that may be excessive for you to manage at an instant.

Because of their trusting nature, empaths are prone to ploys, abuse, or manipulations. Your earnest desire to assist individuals in distress can leave you unaware of indications of malice or evil.

Since you can sense pain, you better understand the discomfort due to habits and wish to assist. Nevertheless, it is not always up to you if the other person is not ready for your assistance.

- **You have increased sensitivity to noises, smells, or feelings.**

An empath's oversensitivity does not just associate with his emotions. It is not very easy to distinguish between empaths and overly sensitive people, but you may discover that the empath is more sensitive to the world around you.

The signs may include:

- Odors and fragrances affect you more highly.
- Jarring sounds and physical sensations may affect you more strongly.

- You choose to listen to media at low volumes or get information by reading.
- Specific sounds may trigger an emotional response.

You require time to recharge.

Oversensitive persons are easily drained and get fatigued from their exposure to another person's pains and struggles. Even an overload of positive sensations might tire you, so it is essential to put in the time you require to reset.

If you do not shield yourself from negativity, you will likely get burnt out, which may significantly impact your life and health.

Requiring time alone doesn't always imply you're an introvert. Empaths can likewise be extroverts or fall anywhere on the spectrum. Perhaps individuals energize you-- until you reach that point of overwhelmingness.

Extroverted empaths may require extra care to strike the ideal balance between hanging out with others and restoring their emotional reserves.

- **You dislike conflict.**
You likely dread or actively avoid dispute if you're an empath.

Non-caring people easily hurt oversensitive persons. The slightest criticism, whether intentional or unintentional, will cut into an empath's heart.

Fights and arguments can likewise cause more distress, given that you're not just handling your feelings and reactions. You're also absorbing the feelings of the others included. However, when you wish to attend to everybody's pain, do not understand how even minor disagreements can end up being harder to manage.

- **You always feel like the odd man out.**
Despite being highly attuned to others' sensations, lots of empaths find it challenging to associate with others.

Others may not understand why you become exhausted and worried so easily. You might have difficulty understanding the feelings and emotions you feel or absorb like you are always different from others, leading to the empath keeping to himself. You might avoid speaking about your sensitivities and sharing your intuitions, so you feel less out of place.

The world should understand that it is never easy to feel that you do not belong, yet you care deeply for others. The empath is a special gift to the world. It is uncommon, yes, but it is an essential part of your personality.

- **You tend to be alone.**
Isolation is an empath's sanctuary to allow him to recuperate from the confusing and painful feelings. But taking time out too long can also be damaging to an empath's psychological health. There are various kinds of isolation, and some might provide more therapeutic benefits than others.

Attempt to take your time alone outdoors, when possible, practice meditation in a quiet park, walk in the rain, take a picturesque drive, or garden.

Think about adding an animal to your life if individuals drain you quickly. Empaths might connect to animals more extremely and draw deep comfort from this bond.

Benefits of Being an Empath

Most of what we see as advantages of identifying as empath lies behind those inconsistencies. Although an empath would possibly consider itself an introvert, many of its gifts often lie in being a people person. Since empaths are able to absorb other people's feelings and energies around them, they are naturally very good at reading people. This also means they have good intuition and instincts in general, which can prove to be a very practical life ability. This is useful in that they are excellent at selecting who is trustworthy and who is dishonest.

Although these abilities can often seem daunting, being a strong character judge is certainly a big help for empaths. This insight and character judgment cannot come as naturally with non-empaths who have issues connected to other individuals, which can trigger problems. Empaths can also tell when a person is lying to them, which can prove to be an important skill in contemporary society. In various careers that work with other individuals, these talents also help them succeed. Empaths also make excellent teachers, therapists, health care professionals, businesspeople, and every other position requiring a deep understanding of individuals. Being a good human behavior predictor is one of the strongest qualities of an empath.

Empaths are also excellent at defending themselves and others from intimidating individuals because they have sound judgment and instincts. Did you ever meet someone you felt was just a little off? Perhaps it was the new significant other of your friend who had dubious motives, and you proved right. This is a basic functional capacity that an empath possesses, and that possibly goes back to empath's evolutionary origins. The capacity of empaths to experience energy and feelings helps them recognize threats quickly and defend themselves and those around them. Another advantage of their gift of deep and precise insight is this. If you think you have strong instincts and your first instinct is typically right, but your abilities have not been completely established, then you might still be an empath. Many empaths have intuition, but since they have not formed it, it is dormant. In addition, this powerful insight, such as manifestation or lucid dreaming, can be used for several different gifts.

Empaths are normally very innovative people as well. This is one of the gifts that come with an empathic personality that can be built and honed, but usually, empaths feel that they naturally come to creativity. They can turn these feelings into artistic expressions, such as art, because empaths are so in contact with emotions and sensitive to different emotions. Although individuals who are closed off and disconnected from their feelings can have trouble with creative blocks, empaths can normally channel and convey their feelings naturally. Not only can they do so by tapping into their own emotions, but because they can so quickly absorb other people's emotions, they can even transmit other people's emotions.

This imagination, such as painting, literature, or even different spiritual practices, can translate into many distinct forms. Channeling the emotions of others makes empaths understanding to the point of expression, which is a creative asset. Moreover, this imagination will allow empaths to better explore the energy that flows inside and without humans. Empaths can better understand their own inner energies through artistic writing, which can improve both the self-expression and self-understanding. By consuming and channeling the emotions of other cultures, empaths will, in fact, become more in tune with their own thoughts and feelings.

The capacity to heal others is another gift that empaths possess. Since they can recognize, understand, experience, and act upon other people's feelings, this makes them really able to determine how to support people. This is one of the attributes that makes such strong therapists and doctors feel empathic. Empath, though, also makes perfect holistic doctors and energy healers, because they are so much in tune with the energy that others are projecting. Empaths may also feel as if they are curing themselves by curing others. If you identify as empath, then in several group settings, you probably find yourself taking on the role of mediator.

Do you find yourself feeling happier as a result when you support friends or family? This is because, when there's a problem, you internalize the negative energy. If your friends are battling, even if you are not directly involved, as a consequence of all the negativity and misery swirling around you, you can feel irritated and nervous. However, by acting as a mediator, you can heal the energy which negatively affects both your friends and you. This also benefits you, in a way, as you boost the vibrations that surround you, helping you to internalize more positive emotions.

This is a major reason why empaths use their healing gift, so they can heal themselves by healing others too. This shows the altruistic nature of empath. Empaths want to assist others because they feel better because of it. This is also why in professions where they support people, such as in nursing or therapy, empaths are also able to feel incredibly fulfilled.

Empaths also have the unusual ability to build deep bonds with other people and cultivate them. This can be incredibly rewarding, as they find that in their lives, they have the potential to develop very close relationships with people. Interestingly enough, in addition to humans, the empath may also shape those deep bonds with animals. They are able to perceive the feelings of other species, and they have a deep connection with nature as well. As it offers satisfaction, this caring capacity to build relationships with various individuals and even animals are a gift to empath. Though introverted, Empaths ultimately desire communication. Since they are so capable of consuming energy and feelings, they can create these bonds quickly, which contributes to emotional fulfillment. This makes good partners, friends, and family members feel empathetic.

Ultimately, possessing these powerful emotional skills and the ability to build strong emotional connections helps empaths to draw tons of love and positivity into their lives. In addition, while experiencing the pain and sorrow of others can seem like a downside of being an empath, they still feel the pleasure and affection of other people. Essentially, they feel it in a heightened way as empaths feel joy, which is one of their greatest gifts. These are all gifts that allow empaths with other people to build powerful and unique emotional connections. These connections also enable them to excel in various aspects of their lives, especially in interpersonal situations. Empaths are very well-liked in general, making them good friends, partners, co-workers, etc. In social settings, this helps them feel relaxed and valued, which can in turn put them more at ease in the case of overstimulation. This is one of the greatest gifts that come with being an empath, and these strong bonds are also reinforced by some of the setbacks that empath could face.

Challenges of Being an Empath and How to Overcome Them

Although becoming an empath is definitely a gift valued by many people, it does come with its fair share of challenges. If you identify as empath, then you may be faced with all of these problems even if you have not officially classified or even identified them. Whether or not you feel that you are susceptible to any of the characteristics mentioned, acknowledging them is important to understand how to cope with some of the external difficulties resulting from being an empath. In addition, you might see an overlap between some of these common challenges and many of the gifts we just went through that you have.

This is because, depending on the setting, many of the characteristics the empath possesses may be positive or bad. In the past, you would not have given this much thought. But you can recognize how they both negatively and positively impact your life by identifying these attributes now, and how you can become more in tune with yourself. As an empath, you are possibly very attuned to other people's emotions and resources.

But this book will help you become more in tune with yourself by teaching you about what makes you. Overstimulation is a common challenge faced by empath, as already stated as a characteristic of empath. Since their brains are basically hypersensitive to distinct stimuli, in situations where they are surrounded by a lot of people and/or movement, empaths may quickly become overwhelmed and exhausted. Particularly in circumstances, empaths can experience this even with people they are close to, simply because they need time to recharge alone. This may have been experienced in a school or workplace environment. Has a friend ever asked you to grab dinner after work but after 8 hours of intense stimulation, you just couldn't imagine spending any more time with other people? This is nothing to be ashamed of—it just means you're recharging by spending time on your own.

There are some steps you should take to prevent the consequences of overstimulation if you are in a career or living condition that allows you to be constantly surrounded by other individuals. Self-care is extremely necessary, particularly for empaths, to ensure that we allow ourselves to recover from over-stimulation and burnout. Another thing empath may do to integrate some time alone to recover is to take breaks or maintain some kind of distance. If you live with roommates, and feel like you're constantly surrounded by people, locking yourself in your room for some time alone is perfect. As no one wants to spend time with someone who is obviously tired and not themselves, people are normally really understanding.

The overload of negative energy is another problem that empathizers often face in their daily lives. This can be in any situation, but if you're surrounded by negative people who can't stop moaning, or you're also getting irritated after checking out the news, it's probably a sign that you need some self-care. Since empaths are so easily able to absorb even the subtlest energy around them, they could find themselves exhausted or emotionally distracted as a consequence if they are around many negative people. It is very important to practice self-care, energy healing, and solitary activities to prevent the overwhelming feeling.

You will also find that you need to spend less time with the people who drain your energy from you or make you feel negative feelings while you are around them. This is also a form of self-care—it is important to cut constantly negative people out of your life, particularly for empath, to protect and ensure your own happiness. This is better said than done, of course, and another obstacle posed by an empath is that they appear to attract these negative individuals. This is the book for you if you feel as if you are constantly pulling adverse energy into your life and have no idea how to stop, particularly in social situations. The first step is to recognize that you might be sensitive to these traits.

Chapter 15. The Potentials of your Energy

If you're sensitive to other people's energies, it's important that you understand the potential of your energy as an empath. Learn about the different levels of empathic sensitivity and how they can impact your day-to-day life, as well as tips on how to manage your sensitivities.

Empaths are highly sensitive people who absorb or pick up on other people's emotions, thoughts, physical state, and energy. This is sometimes called "The Empath Effect."

What is the "Empath Effect"?

The "Empath Effect" is a term coined by Andrew Johnson to describe how sensitive people feel the emotions of others. In other words, they feel other people's emotions more than they have emotions of their own. One way that empaths show this difference is through the "externalizing" of their own feelings instead of bottling them up inside.

Another way that empaths show this difference is through their behavior. Empaths are very empathic and therefore are more apt to act in a manner that reflects another person's emotions, actions, or intentions. This is sometimes called "mirroring."

Empaths can read other people's emotions and energy, and they are able to feel what the other person feels. Empaths will respond to others' energies by taking them on. This can cause empaths to feel drained or overwhelmed.

Here we'll be talking about the potential of an empath's energy by giving a rundown of each level of empathic sensitivity.

There are three primary levels:

Level 1: Generalized Empathy

This is what we'll call the "blank slate" level of sensitivity. At this level, empaths feel the emotions of others but don't feel their own. They're not sensitive to the energy of others and don't really know how to manage it.

Level 2: Body Sensing

This is where most people start out as empaths. At this level, empaths can feel other people's emotions and absorb them like a sponge. Usually only a few people can handle Level 2 energies. And Field-Managers are often placed here because they're "on the field" as in they feel other people's emotions (field) and are highly intuitive (manager).

At this level, empaths will often use their imagination to picture what other people are feeling in order to identify the emotion. Sometimes empaths will feel another person's discomfort or pain.

Level 3: Sensitivity to Other People's Energy

This is where empaths can start to sense energy. It's where they can start feeling the physical state of other people such as their hair standing up, goosebumps, and energy pulsing from them.

At this level empath can store and re-channel energy with ease. In addition, empaths also have an easier time with psychic abilities at this level because they're able to sense and decipher these things within themselves easily.

Level 3 empaths will also be able to see auras and feel other people's emotions. They will also be able to tell when someone is lying.

Level 4: Psychic and Energy Sensitivity

Once empaths reach this level they can start seeing and feeling the emotions of everyone in their vicinity, not just one person. Some of these empaths may overextend themselves in a crowd because at this level, they'll feel or sense every single emotion. At this level, empaths can't help but take on the energy of others because it gets "poured" onto them from all sides. In addition, some empaths may even do "energy dumps" in order to release the energy that has been forced onto them by others.

Level 4 empaths can also feel the energy and intentions of other people, and they can also feel more acutely what someone is intending to do or maybe even think about doing.

Level 5: Psychic and Energy Vulnerability

At this level empath will be able to see others' future actions, or at least sense them. This means that even if an empath doesn't know what another person is thinking right now, he or she may be able to sense that this person will take certain actions in the future.

At this level of empathy, it's not uncommon for empaths to have prophetic dreams about another person's past, present, or future. They might also receive psychic messages from other people through their dreams as well.

At this level, empaths will feel what other people are feeling and occasionally they will feel what others intend to do. Level 5 empaths tend to be the most emotionally sensitive of all empaths.

Level 6: Psychic Attacks

A psychic attack can be defined as an act of violence on an empathic person without physical contact. When a psychic attack takes place, emotions like anger or hate are being directed toward the empath via telepathy or any other means of communication. An empath who is attacked may end up feeling ill, psychically ill, and even physically ill as a result.

Level 6 empaths are able to heal themselves quickly, but others may not be so fortunate.

Level 7: Psychic Vulnerabilities

This is where empaths start feeling the energy of people around them and they may sometimes feel what those people intend to do. They will also suffer from a physical ailment in order to keep other empaths safe from harm. The high level of emotional intervention at this level stems from the understanding that everyone around an empath plays a key role in his or her life, and therefore it's absolutely necessary for that person to stay happy and healthy so that the empath will too. If an empath doesn't have good health, then he or she won't be in a position to help others out on a daily basis.

Level 7 empaths are able to see the energy of living things, such as plants, animals, and humans. In addition, some empaths will have a very hard time paying attention to anything else while they're engaged in this level of psychic activity; basically, they will be completely tuned into another person's energy.

Level 8: Psychic Vulnerability to Another Person

This is where empathic people feel another person's emotions at all times no matter who they're with. At this level an empath can physically feel what others are feeling including the emotions that others may be experiencing even when the empath is far away from another person. Empaths do not have to make physical contact in order for them to sense what another person is experiencing. They are able to feel what the person is feeling even if they're in another country.

Level 9: Psychically Reaching Out to Others

At this level empath may find themselves being inside of other people's bodies. Empaths who reach out to others may actually touch or hug other people, and those people will sense that someone is touching them. It's difficult for an empath to reach out to another person without making physical contact with that person, but it's not impossible.

Level 10: Psychic Acceptance of Self and Others

This level of psychic activity cannot be achieved unless an empath has reached a certain level of self-understanding as well as the understanding of others around him or her. Even though this level of empathic activity is the highest anyone can achieve it will go away if the empath doesn't grasp what it means to be an empath.

Chapter 16. Stop Absorbing Stress and Energy

The Empath will always work hard to help and heal others, but what about them? Who is taking care of the Empath? This question comes up a lot for people who are working hard to live their lives as giving and compassionate people, especially if they are highly empathic and are more likely to help you before they help themselves. Sound familiar? You know this story all too well.

The health of the Empath can get compromised easily, especially if you are not doing anything to protect your energy and take time to recuperate after challenging experiences. At this point in your life, you are probably so used to dealing with everyone else's feelings, it just feels normal, and it doesn't occur to you to take a different approach.

The process of recovery for an Empath differs widely from person to person, but overall, it can feel like an endless cycle of ups and downs if you are not preventing yourself from getting too caught up in another person's distress. Here's some of the ways the Empath's emotional and physical health can be compromised:

- Feelings of grief, melancholy, and depression
- Tender and achy muscles, joints, and limbs
- Common cold and allergy symptoms
- Weakened immune system
- Chronic neck, shoulder, and back pain
- Insomnia
- Undiagnosed physical or emotional pain that is the result of absorbing too many people's toxic or negative energy
- Symptoms similar to chronic fatigue and autoimmune disorders
- Paranoia
- Anxiety and worry, sometimes chronically
- Tiredness and exhaustion
- Low self-esteem or low self-worth
- Difficulty maintaining a healthy weight
- Dysfunctional emotional bonds with other people that are repetitive and habitual
- Alcohol or drug abuse
- Addictions to food, substances, or entertainment, such as television or gambling
- Difficulty letting go of personal problems
- General feelings of fear about life; lack of security

And more…

It might be hard to be certain of that being an Empath could lead to all of these problems and issues. The issue is not about being an Empath; the issue is about not understanding your gift and learning the best methods for taking good care of your own energy.

All too often, Empaths are left without recourse and end up feeling one or several of the symptoms listed above. If you are able to understand the way our energy works, then you can understand why other people's feelings have such a volatile impact on an Empath.

The human heart is electrical. It has energy radiating out from its center as far as 3 feet outside of your chest. Is that amazing?! Your heart is always emitting a force field of energy that can literally be affected by anyone you come into contact with. So, imagine that you are feeling happy, joyful, relaxed and affectionate and then all of a sudden you come within two feet of someone who is angry, frustrated, rejected and emotionally wounded. All of that energy is radiating out of their heart 2-3 feet outside of their body and coming into your sphere of energy.

A lot of people will not notice this energy, but an Empath picks it up like a radio signal. Empaths have an antenna for these types of energies and pull them in like a tractor beam. And it's not just the energy at the heart level. Your body has multiple energy centers like the heart that are all working together to keep your emotional, physical, and mental energy in balance.

The Empath may not be aware that it is happening when it does, but as soon as they come into contact with enough of those low emotions and negative feelings, they have just collected a whole lot of other people's distress, sorrow, and misfortune, sometimes without even talking to them.

When you have enough negative energy circulating in your own universe of vibration and frequency, you disrupt your own balance and end up dealing with a variety of symptoms that can lead to or look like the list from above. Some of the more chronic issues build up slowly over time and many of them are the result of toxic partnerships and environmental conditions.

It helps to understand this idea and imagery so that you can be aware of how to protect yourself from other people's energy spheres. The more you collect, the harder it is to maintain good health. The more you learn to protect your energy and stop absorbing the energy of other people around you, the easier it becomes to stay balanced emotionally and physically.

The following techniques are designed to help you remain true to your empathic heart while connecting to your own energy and staying grounded so that you don't absorb other people's emotional distress and baggage.

Grounding and Protecting Meditation

Grounding is a method that helps you connect your energy to the earth below your feet. Even if you are wearing shoes and you are on the 25th floor of a skyscraper, you can still ground your energy.

For people, who are also electrical current and vibrating frequencies, grounding is basically the same concept, allowing you to redirect your focus and energy to a more balanced state of affairs. If you are an Empath and you are in the midst of a lot of emotional energy, you can easily lose your footing and become ungrounded, leaving you vulnerable to the energies of others. The idea is that you maintain grounding as a way of protecting your energy from taking on too much anyone or anything else's.

The rules of grounding are simple:

1.   Keep your focus on your own energy.
2.   Center yourself.
3.   Maintain.
4.

The energy of yourself can get lost in the dynamic forces of what's happening around you. Self-awareness isn't selfish, it's healthy and responsible. In order for you to stay grounded, you have to be aware of yourself. Centering yourself means holding that awareness and being able to freely exist in that nature. You don't have to be a statue.

You can move and enjoy your expressiveness and personality. Centering means you get to practice being yourself while you remain grounded. Then, all you have to do is maintain that balance within yourself so that you can stay open and heartfelt with the people around you.

The following meditation is something you can perform in the morning before you leave the house, in the bathroom at a restaurant, in your parked car, wherever you need it at the moment.

1.   Begin by closing your eyes and taking a deep breath in. Inhale through the nose. Try to inhale for a count of 5 to 10.
2.   Slowly exhale through the mouth for the same count as you inhaled.
3.   Bring your hands together, either in your lap or in front of your heart. They can be palm to palm, or just touching- whatever works for the environment that you are in.
4.   Take another deep inhale followed by an exhale.
5.   With your feet on the ground, wherever you are, imagine a shaft of light coming out of the bottom of each foot, like the roots of a tree.
6.   Picture the light getting long and going through the Earth's crust, pavement, or whatever floor of the skyscraper you are on so that it goes all the way to the center of the Earth (If you don't make it all the way to the center, that's okay, as long as the light roots from your feet are going deep into the ground).
7.   They can be a color or they can simply be golden or white depending on your personal preferences.
8.   With your visual of these light roots penetrating the Earth, now see the energy of that light coming back from the Earth, up through your feet and into your body, through your heart, and out of the crown of your head. You still want to see light connecting deeply into the Earth.
9.   Sit in this posture for several inhales and exhales. See all of your being connected deeply to the Earth and feel that earth energy coming back up through you and filling your body.
10.   When you feel grounded and protected, you can open your eyes and move forward with your day.
This meditation is very simple and only takes a few minutes of your time. It can really help you rebalance yourself after a distressing moment or an intense conversation with a difficult person. When you connect to your own energy and ground it to the Earth, you are giving yourself permission to exist, take up space, and return to your center so that you don't lose yourself in the sea of other people's energies.

I have personally used this before a business meeting and after, during an airplane ride (and the beams of light from my feet had to go all the way down from 30,000 feet in the air to connect to the planet), and in a hospital before a procedure. I have heard of others using this meditation in their cars in parking lots after getting out of a busy shopping center, in the bathroom at an office party, and during childbirth.

It is a very simple and versatile tool and uses creative visualization to help you connect with your own energy through your connection to the Earth. I highly recommend using this technique before a challenging conversation, but you can also picture this while you are involved in the conversation. As with the Listening Bubble or the Energy Magnet, you can practice seeing yourself grounded in this way with your eyes open so that you can easily maintain that grounded and protected feeling the whole time.

Affirmation of Empowerment

Affirmations are an excellent tool to help with so many different processes. An affirmation is basically a mental program and here is how it works. If you have the same pattern of thought repeated over and over again, it becomes a significant neural pathway that your brain automatically uses without you having to think about it. It is the same way habits are formed, both good and bad, and can contribute to how you think, believe, and feel about the world.

Chapter 17. Coping with Hypersensitivity

It's upsetting enough to feel like you're being watched 24/7 by an unknown force. But when spiritual hypersensitivity is paired with religious beliefs, the intensity only compounds. Now, you're not just anxious and paranoid —you also believe that someone out there wants to hurt you and undermine your values because of your faith.

Here are best ways to cope with spiritual hypersensitivity:

1) Get Some Perspective

Have a friend or loved one who doesn't share your beliefs give you a neutral opinion on what is going on in your life. This could be anything from what they think about the situation at hand, to how they perceive the general state of things for you right now. Their perspective may be the perfect tonic for your own way of looking at it.

2) Make One Change

Look for one thing that has changed in your life, and then try to focus on that for a while before changing whatever else is going on around you again. For example, if a loved one dies and it makes you angry and upset, make a note that something has changed and focus on that till it feels better again. Once you start to feel better, let go of it and move on to something else.

3) Observe the Patterns

Take note of how a new change in one area of your life leads to another change in another area. Sometimes these things happen quite quickly, like when something stressful happens at work and then you fight with your spouse later in the evening. Other times, the changes might not happen right away, but they can still be tracked with some careful observation.

4) Look for Reassurance

While this will only temporarily alleviate the anxiety, it is still important to get reassurance about what is going on in your life when changes like this are happening. Make a list of all the things you know about and downplay the possible reasons for what you are feeling.

5) Clarify Your Values

Take some time to collectively decide on the things that are most important to you. This could be as simple as writing out a list of your five favorite hobbies or five favorite movies about each topic and then adding them up together, or it could be as complex as polling family members for consensus. The point is to make sure that not only are your values being honored in your actions, but they are also being put in position where they will have an impact on others around you.

Don't overlook the importance of your basic values, either. They can be the basis for some of the more difficult religious topics you are experiencing. For example, if vengeful spirits are plaguing you, it's possible they want to punish you for your good deeds toward others.

6) Set Boundaries

If you have any beliefs in afterlife for instance or life after death, it may be helpful to set up some boundaries. This could be with thoughts and ideas about what will happen after death, or even with how long you will actually remember someone who has passed away before their memory is officially gone.

Chapter 18. How to Protect yourself from Energy Vampires and Narcissist

Energy vampires are individuals who—here and there—purposefully channel your enthusiastic energy. They feed on your eagerness to tune in and care for them, leaving you depleted and overpowered.

Energy vampires can be anyplace and anybody. They can be your mate or your closest companion. They can be your work area mate or your neighbor.

Figuring out how to identify and react to this poisonous conduct can assist you with safeguarding your energy and shield yourself from a lot of enthusiastic—and physical—trouble.

Peruse on to get familiar with how an energy vampire acts and what you can do straightaway.

They don't take responsibility.

Energy vampires are often magnetic. They may sneak in the clear when issues emerge because of this appeal.

They're sly and may nail issues to another person in pretty much every circumstance.

They never acknowledge culpability for their job in any contradiction or issue. You're often left holding the blame—and conceivably the fault.

For instance:

- "I can't accept nobody could get this right. What a shame!"
- "I just stayed there. He continued blowing up at me; despite everything, I don't have the foggiest idea what I did."

They're Constantly Associated with a Show

Energy vampires consistently wind up in the center of a fiasco, thrashing from focus to focus with their enthusiastic and sensational conduct.

When they've arrived on you, they toss this show onto you in trusts you'll retain it, fix it, and right their boat.

For instance:

- "For what reason am I generally the one everybody gets frantic at? I don't merit this."
- "I can't take this any longer. I didn't do anything to Ellen. However, she's quit conversing with me. For what reason can't everybody be as kind as you?"

They Generally One-Up You

An energy vampire never prefers to be beaten, and they aren't quick to share the spotlight. This is one of their numerous narcissistic propensities.

They battle to feel certified satisfaction for someone else. Rather, they want to pull energy to take care of their passionate requests.

For instance:

- "That is great news. I really went after another position today, as well, and I truly need some assistance with my resume. Do you mind looking it over?"
- "So glad for you! Just three additional certifications to go to find me!"

They Decrease Your Issues and Play up Their Own

Energy vampires feed off your enthusiastic energy. Also, if you're pitiful or disturbed, your energy supplies are lessening.

To empty the most energy out of you, energy vampires will shift the consideration of the conversation to themselves, transforming your consternation into their passionate smorgasbord.

For instance:

- "I realize your activity doesn't pay well, however in any event your activity is entertaining. You need to assist me in finding another one."
- "You're super overwhelmed at work, and I get it, yet I incredibly need to converse with you today around evening time about this issue with Mark."

They Act Like a Saint

Energy vampires place their issues decisively on the shoulders of others. They assume no liability for their commitments to their difficulties.

What they're looking for is enthusiastic help to support their confidence.

For instance:

- "He's generally so irrational. I do as well as can be expected, however, it's sufficiently never."
- "This day began terribly, and it just deteriorated."

They Utilize Your Amiable Attitude Against You

Individuals who are delicate and humane are practical objectives for energy vampires. You offer a listening ear, a benevolent heart, and interminable energy.

In that manner, energy vampires utilize your very nature against you, depleting you of your essentialness.

For instance:

- They hoard your time at each social event so they can have as a lot of your energy as possible get.
- They realize you'll feel regretful turning them down for espresso or a supper date, so they ask normally.

They're Mutually Dependent

Codependency is a sort of relationship where each activity is intended to inspire a specific response from the other person.

It's an endless loop of conduct, yet energy vampires once in a while perceive that they're in them.

They utilize these connections—often sentimental ones—to keep turning a pattern of dramatization and passionate need.

For instance:

- "I realize this is certainly not a decent relationship, yet it's such a great amount of superior to attempting to get over him and figure out how to date once more."
- "If I simply overlook him for a couple of days, he'll thoroughly ask for pardoning and return slithering."

They Reprimand or Menace

At their center, energy vampires are often shaky. They may utilize dehumanizing strategies and reactions to keep their "prey" shaky, as well.

In this state, you sense that you owe them your consideration and should keep on attempting to stop the unjustifiable assaults.

For instance:

- "I was too inept to even consider expecting better from you. Every other person deals with me like trash, so why not you?"
- "You were in a tight spot from the earliest starting point, and I disclosed to you that."

They Use Guilt Outings or Ultimatums

Energy vampires often depend on guilt outings to get what they need. They realize disgrace is an incredible weapon against individuals who are humane and mindful.

Similarly, ultimatums are a compelling method to catch an individual's consideration and pressure them into accomplishing something they in any case might not have any desire to do.

For instance:

- "I don't have the foggiest idea how you anticipate that I should make it without you. I'll self-destruct."
- "If you truly care for me, you'll call him and disclose to him the amount I love him."

They Scare

One stage expelled from censuring or tormenting you, terrorizing is a device some energy vampires go to when they have to work up some passionate grub.

Dread is a forceful enthusiastic response. If an energy vampire can agitate you, they can reinforce their personality.

For instance:

- "I won't reveal to you this over and over."
- "You don't merit advancement. You don't show that you even truly need it."
- Why it makes a difference and what to do.

Energy vampires request a great deal from the individuals they target.

This persistent channel on your assets can noticeably affect your prosperity. After some time, abundance stress can prompt nervousness, wretchedness, coronary illness, and that's only the tip of the iceberg.

That is the reason, it's imperative to perceive the practices and afterward work to expel them.

This may include setting up dividers to ensure against an energy vampire's endeavors—or expelling the individual from your life.

The thoughts beneath may not work for everybody. Attempt them and form your methodology as you go until you're ready to feel in charge and secure.

Set Up Limits

In spite of the fact that this might be actually quite difficult from the start, you can and ought to create aspects of your life where you won't permit an energy vampire to enter.

Try not to consent to get-togethers like supper or espresso dates. Maintain a strategic distance from the end of the week trips and other broadened occasions where they'll be in participation.

At work, you can restrain communications among you by not consenting to snacks and not halting by their work area to talk.

You may need to begin little, concentrating on a couple of territories, and afterward extend.

Modify Your Desires

You can't fix an energy vampire; however, you can reshape your assumptions regarding them.

This may include stopping your passionate valve and not offering exhortation when they vent their issues to you.

This may likewise mean you can't utilize them as an enthusiastic delivery either. They'll need to respond.

Try Not to Offer Them a Bit of Leeway

If the energy vampire calls, stops by or messages, don't give them the room.

Offer a reason—"I'm excessively worn out" or "I'm excessively occupied" will do. You could state that you have designs or don't feel well.

When they keep interfacing with pardons and not getting the enthusiastic energy they need, they'll look somewhere else.

Gatekeeper Your Passionate Limit

Energy vampires utilize nonverbal prompts to know when they have somebody on the snare. Your outward appearance, the manner in which you lean, by the way, you fasten your hands—an energy vampire can take these as indications of your venture.

If you rather offer stone-confronted reactions and just offer short articulation to their inquiries, you won't free yourself up to their requests, and you can save your energy for you.

Cut Them Out Altogether

Much of the time, you have the opportunity to extract this individual from your life totally. This may appear to be emotional, however, you need to recall that you're ensuring yourself at long last.

A few people carry unforeseen softness and solace to your life. They pop with energy, for all intents and purposes electrify you with their essence. And afterward, there are the individuals who forget about you feeling pushed. Or on the other hand blameworthy. Or on the other hand, depleted down to your absolute last atom. I call them energy vampires, and repulsive or submissive, they come in all structures. The wail sister, for one, generally sees herself as the person in question. The world is consistently against her, and she'll relate each shocking thing that has happened to her, floundering in each apparent slight. The charmer is a steady talker or joke-teller who must be the focal point of consideration. The blamer, then again, gives out unlimited servings of blame. And afterward, there's the busybody, the associate who claims she nearly kicked the bucket from a high fever or the neighbor who lives in limits of feeling—life is unimaginably acceptable or horrifically terrible. Regardless of which sort of energy vampire you're managing, you're permitted to leave. A large number of us discover this extremely difficult to do. We're apprehensive about being thought of as inconsiderate; we would prefer not to insult individuals. In any case, there are a lot of approaches to expel yourself from a slaughtering discussion. When leaving isn't a choice, you can in any case keep up your energy level by making a couple of minor changes.

Perceive the Signs

One of the principal activities is to perceive when you're being depleted, and that starts with checking out your physical responses. Is there a fixing in your chest when someone, in particular, enters the discussion? Do you feel tired when you hang up the telephone in the wake of talking with somebody? Does your cerebral pain or do you feel what I call "smeared" when another visitor at a mixed drink party begins conversing with you?

Take a Deep Breath

The second you feel destroyed—or trimmed in or worried—I suggest calmly inhaling. Breathing is a great method to focus yourself. Simply follow the breath and disclose to yourself that you realize what's going on and you can manage it. It's essential to recall our individual force. I know from working with patients that we can lose it without any problem. The moment someone comes in who's bossy or accusing, we fondle reduced and tense. If we can concentrate on the breath or on a picture of a striking nightfall or a view from a peak, the pressure will drift away.

Chapter 19. Empaths Love Differently

Empaths love differently. This is because, as the name suggests, an empath is someone who picks up on the emotions of others. As such, they are more sensitive to emotional energy and tend also to be more emotionally reactive than other people.

The empath will take on different feelings and moods around them so that they can feel what other people feel. This can even lead to an empath feeling deeply about something or someone that is not themselves, such as a stranger.

Empaths are sometimes people who make great therapists because they can actually feel the emotions of their clients. It is like they have an ability to walk a mile in another person's shoes, and this is useful in counseling.

Empaths Love Deeply

Because empaths have the ability to sense others feelings and take on these feelings as their own, they also love deeply. Their love for another can run deep, especially if that other person opens up to them and allows themselves to be vulnerable with the empath.

Empaths can absorb another's pain and suffer with them. This means that if an empath has an accident, the empath may be in pain physically and emotionally at the same time. Empaths will experience a very real physical and emotional reaction to something like this, which is understandable.

Empaths are sometimes labeled as "tortured souls" who are unable to love others as deeply as they would like because they feel so much pain themselves. Other empaths have even been called "soul vampires" because they steal another's joy and pain to feel better about themselves. This is a common misconception, though.

Empaths Love Slowly

Empaths love differently because they are more in touch with their emotions. This means that an empath is very unlikely to fall in love quickly and intensely. They may have a number of relationships that are on-again-off-again because they will not commit unless they are sure how the other person feels about them. Empaths are often the type to take a lot of time to really get to know someone. They need to get to know a person's past, their fears and insecurities, their hopes and dreams, their family history- everything. This process can take months or even years, but it is completely worth it if they find the right person. An empath who is sure of themselves will not fall for someone until they feel ready.

Empaths Love Vulnerability

The empath often fears rejection because they are more aware of other people's feelings. This can lead an empath to reject vulnerability, which is something that they truly need when it comes to love. The feeling of rejection for an empath can be more intense than for another type of person because the empath is so sensitive in the first place.

Empaths know how important vulnerability is when it comes to love and relationships, though, and they do their best to allow themselves to be vulnerable with other people. This can build strong relationships because they will be able to feel close to another person in a way that another person cannot feel close to them. There are some special types of relationships that an empath may be more likely to enjoy than others. For example, an empath may find the best part of dating is the "getting to know you" stage, where they do not make a big deal out of getting physical. This stage is also when an empath will fall most in love with someone else, seeing this new person as their true love.

Empaths Love Intensely

Once an empath is in love with someone else, they will turn that love on full blast. They will shower their new partner with gifts, affection, and words of love and praise. This is because they finally feel like they have found someone that will love them for who they are.An empath may be very controlling in a relationship, especially if it does not feel very equal to them.

Chapter 20. What is a Psychic Empath?

Understanding psychic empaths is not an easy task. You must first understand what it means to be a psychic empath, and once you have done that, then you need to learn how to protect yourself from them. Psychic empaths are people who have the ability to feel other people's emotions and energy in their own body. For example, if someone is having a really bad day at work because they just got fired, some of the feeling of anger and sadness could leak into the psychic empath's body even though they are far away from what is happening.

Not every person who has this ability knows what they are doing or how it will affect them in the long run. Therefore, it is important for you as a psychic empath to learn more about what you are going through and how to control your ability. An article was written by HowStuffWorks that provides an in-depth description of psychic empaths and how they work.

A psychic empath feels other people's emotions unconsciously. This is a very disturbing experience for the person who is feeling these emotions and can take away their ability to function properly in society. There are steps you can take to help curb these feelings of suddenly becoming overwhelmed with emotion, but there are also ways that this trait can be helpful in your life. A few examples of how you can use this ability to your advantage are:

First, you must understand how an empath works. Empaths are very in tune with the energy all around them. This is because they have a very strong connection and a natural bond with nature. They can even feel the energy around other people and animals, whether it is good or bad energy. When these feelings are sensed by the empath, they become just as affected by it as if they were to physically feel it themselves.

Psychic empaths can experience a wide variety of feelings when becoming overwhelmed with others' emotions. These feelings can include feeling:

This is why it is so hard for an empath to be around other people. They are not malicious or evil, they just don't know how to handle the onslaught of emotions that are being shot their way. Even if the person with whom they are dealing does not feel any negativity toward them, it deeply effects the empath. The stronger the emotion felt by another person is, the more affected that psychic empath will become. This could be a simple touch or a deep connection with someone which allows them to sometimes see into their loved one's thoughts and even allow some limited amount of feeling to transfer from one person to another.

Now it is time to discuss ways that an empath can protect themselves from this natural ability. First, psychic empaths must recognize their ability. It is very important for them to know that they have the power to feel other people's emotions because that will help them control how much they absorb from another person. It will also prevent them from being overwhelmed by strong emotions and possibly feeling helpless if they sense a lot of negative energy.

Another stage that must be understood is the difference between empathizing and projecting. Empathizing is an activity that psychic empaths do unconsciously, but projecting can be done by simply concentrating on a certain emotion one wishes to create in another person.

It is very important for an empath to understand the stages of protection because it will make them more aware of what they are doing to their bodies when they become exposed to other people's emotions.

One way is if you have already recognized your ability, then you can remain calm in the midst of chaos around you and allow your energy to remain centered on yourself instead of others. Move your energy away from the negativity and think about what you want to do to help yourself feel better.

Another way to protect yourself is to keep your heart open at all times. An empath cannot connect with people who have closed hearts or who don't understand how much they can affect other people through their emotions. Keeping an open heart will allow for connections with like-minded individuals, and it will also prevent the chance of someone using your gift against you.

There are many people who become overwhelmed by the presence of another psychic empath. These people are known as:

Psychic empaths must always exercise caution when around others experiencing strong emotions in order for them to stay safe. It is best for an empath to sit down and take some time to understand their own abilities and how they work. If this is your first encounter with a psychic empath, then you must proceed with caution in your mind because they may have already been affected by the energy of another person and may not know what their reaction will be.

The more you understand your psychic abilities, the better you will be able to control them. It is vital for an empath to learn how to disconnect from those around them and not allow others' emotions to invade their own energy field. They must also learn self-protection techniques so that they can remain safe at all times.

Being psychic isn't just about feeling other people's feelings, it is also about trying to keep your own feelings grounded and balanced in a world full of other people who aren't doing as good with their emotion control. The more time you spend alone through the day with your own thoughts, the better off you will be with keeping a level head. Sometimes people get so consumed with other people's energy that they forget that there is a whole world of feelings and emotions inside their own body.

A psychic empath can also protect themselves by surrounding themselves with the right people and by making sure they know who those people are. It is important for an empath to learn how to identify those who are hurting because it will allow them to be careful around them and make sure they are prepared if their feelings start getting hard to manage. If you find it hard to control your emotions, then you should realize you are only human and not a machine. If you find your energy is draining so much that you need a break, then take some time to recharge.

If you fall victim to an angry person, and if they are someone who doesn't understand what they are doing, then walk away. If they are someone who is aware of their own abilities, then it may be useful to try to talk with them and explain how their negative emotions affect those around them. It is best for an empath not to allow other people's negativity to affect them if they can help it. They should also beware of trying too hard to change another person or help them learn from the past--it will only make things worse for everyone involved.

Chapter 21. Meditation tools for empaths

It is difficult for a non-empath to grasp the concept of feeling people's emotions. Imagine feeling happy, sad, anxious and fearful all at the same time. And these are just some of the emotions that could be going through an empath at any given time.

Meditation is recommended for anyone but highly recommended for empaths. Your ability to absorb foreign emotions and energies make you susceptible to anxiety and stress, which make your life difficult.

Meditation seeks to quieten the mind for a moment and give it a break from the dozen competing emotions seeking to occupy it. Empathy is a gift that can make things easier at the workplace, but it can also make things difficult. If you cannot control the dozens of emotions, you are dealing with, you will be overwhelmed and your work performance will suffer. That moment of silence and calm gives your mind clear so you can go through your day without being overcome by emotions. These are just some of the many ways in which meditation will enhance your day:

Improve Concentration

You achieve more when you focus on one task at a time as opposed to multitasking. Sounds like an irony, right? Shouldn't attending multiple tasks at a time get more work done? In making this assumption, we assume that the brain can focus on multiple things at a time. However, research shows that the brain cannot multitask. It only rapidly switches back and forth between the tasks, losing details in the process.

Our affinity for multitasking can be seen on the way we work on the computer. How many tabs do you open at a time? Some have as many as 10 tabs, sometimes even more. You are answering emails, working on a report, downloading a song, watching a sport rerun, listening to a podcast and so on; all at once. Or rather switching rapidly from one to the other.

Try to open one tab at a time. You can only open another one if the content is directly related to the first one. For instance, you may open an email that has data that you need for your report. Basically, attend to one task at a time. After the report is done, you can then proceed to answer emails. Tick as you go along. Check out how much you manage to get done by the end of the day, compared to when multitasking. The difference is clear; single tasking achieves more.

Why is multitasking so common if it does not achieve much? People gravitate towards multitasking by habit. We are so used to attending to multiple activities at work and everywhere else. It makes us feel busy, even when busy is not equal to productive. This habit is not easy to break. You try to concentrate on a particular activity, and then just a few minutes later your mind wanders to something else.

Meditation teaches your brain to shut out the distractions. You can consciously keep yourself from being distracted by the other things fighting for your attention. You will find that you are able to give one task your full concentration, thereby attending to every detail. After that, you proceed to the next with similar diligence. At the end of the day, you will be consistently productive at your job.

Enhance Working Relationships

Meditation makes you a happier, more positive person, and this reflects in your relationship with others. At the workplace, positive interactions with colleagues lead to higher productivity. In companies where employees participate in meditation training, the teamwork improves significantly.

The manner in which colleagues relate to each other plays a significant part in the efficiency of the entire company. Work issues aside, think of each of those workers as a separate individual, with their personal issues ranging from family, relationships, finances, health and so on. They come to work on the backdrop of these issues. Add to these the dynamics of the job. You have a lot that is potentially fatigued and stressed.

With such emotions, the relation suffers. Arguments, disagreements, and frustrations will be common. Eventually, you have a batch of disgruntled workers and declining productivity. Here, meditation comes in handy both at an individual and institutional level. When people meditate, they are calmer and more grounded. They respond to the issues of their lives more positively. At work, they interact well with their colleagues and form a strong, efficient team, boosting productivity.

Reduce Stress

Stress originates from your body's reaction to threats and demands. The danger here may be real or imagined. Your mind goes into overdrive; the common 'fight or flight'

Response. Meditation may not affect the issues causing you stress, but it will change your reaction towards them.

Meditation helps you achieve moments of total peace and relaxation. Some will describe it as that moment when you think about nothing. Your mind is blank, and pleasantly so. You actually deflect all thoughts so that your mind is quiet for a moment.

Whether your stress is coming from work-related issues or from personal ones, it is bound to affect your productivity. A stressed mind has a horde of thoughts constantly going in and out, trying to find a solution. If your mind had a sound, you would be hearing multiple voices shouting back and forth at no particular order. The thoughts keep you from focusing on any particular task. You will have your mind racing all day long, yet nothing productive to show for it.

Meditation teaches your mind to be silent. Every time the thoughts seem to overwhelm you, you can quieten your mind and regain clarity. It only takes a few minutes, and the positive effects will be felt for hours.

Meditation does not mean that you ignore the issues stressing you. It means that you do not allow these thoughts to cloud your entire day and disrupt your focus. By meditating often, you can remain productive even as you seek out solutions.

Improves Creativity

Meditation declutters the mind. Just as it is difficult to find your way around a room littered with clutter, so it is trying to work with a cluttered mind. Picture yourself trying to work on a cluttered desk. The tones of items keep attracting your attention, distracting you from the task at hand. You decide to take a moment and clean it all up. You remove everything from your desk. From there, you decide what comes back to the desk, what comes back to a different position, and what stays away. You can also decide to add some new items that you find necessary.

The same applies to your mind. When trying to create a concept, too many thoughts can disrupt the process. Take a moment of mindful meditation and clear your mind. From there, you can rearrange your thoughts. You can disallow those you did not find helpful and invite new ones. Whenever you feel your mind lagging, you can regain clarity by meditating and ensure that you remain productive all day.

Better Sleep

Stress and anxiety often disrupt sleep. The thoughts racing through your mind deny you any meaningful sleep. You will be in bed for an average of 8 hours or so, yet morning will find you still tired. You spent the better part of the night tossing and turning, whether consciously or subconsciously. Poor sleep leads to fatigue, which in turn affects your productivity.

Meditation works great in inducing sleep. Try the simplest meditation technique of all; mindful breathing. Just lie on your bed and listen to your breathing. Inhale and exhale consciously. If you find it hard to concentrate, try counting your breaths. Should any thoughts try to intrude, let them float by? Do not dwell on them. Just keep breathing.

If you have had a particularly negative period, you can try to add a positive affirmation to your breathing. Repeat words such as 'I am healthy and whole' as you breathe. The words will draw in positivity and you will drift off to sleep in a better mood.

After a good night's sleep, you wake up fresh and vibrant. You will make decisions with clarity and will definitely be more productive.

Greater Emotional Control

Meditation helps you gain greater control of your emotions. You're less likely to react in anger or frustration. Such reactions are often sources of conflict in the workplace. Once a company introduces the concept of meditation, you have workers who have better control of their emotions and are less likely to get into wrangles.

Once you feel a negative emotion threatening to overwhelm you, take a moment of meditation. Calm down and breathe. Let the moment pass. That will keep you from overreacting, which could have far-reaching consequences.

If you are a leader, emotional control is even more crucial. You will be faced with emotionally charged situations where everybody will be looking up to you for direction. How do you keep your calm when everybody else is going over the top? You can take a moment to meditate. Better still, you can lead the entire team into meditation. Let everybody keep quiet, sit up and breathe. They should concentrate only on their breathing; nothing else.

Within a few minutes, the entire team will be calmer. They will look back and wonder what the bickering was all about. They bring their issues to the table peacefully and participate in looking for solutions. Should a similar incidence arise in the future, even in your absence, they know exactly what to do? When peace prevails, the team is bound to be more productive.

The Meditation Process

Can you train your mind to be quiet? Can you calm your mind enough to concentrate only on the present moment and nothing else? Can you block out emotions? As an empath, you are probably so accustomed to multiple emotions that the idea of having a clear mind seems unattainable.

Think about it; how many things are on your mind at any given time? Let us say you are sitting at your desk at work editing a document. You have multiple tabs open. The first one is your email, so you can check out any new one that comes in. Remember they are also those you are yet to reply to. On a different tab, you are antagonizing over some sports rerun, noticing how badly your team is doing. You are also half-listening to a conversation your colleagues are having about that finance meeting last week. Oh, you also have your eye on the clock. Is it lunchtime yet? You have to check out that restaurant in the new mall 2 blocks away. Oh, and there's a gym there too. You need to stay in shape.

All these items fighting for space in your mind. How many are these; like 7? Sounds like such a high number when you stop to count, yet this is nothing unusual. Our minds are constantly burdened with information going in and out. No wonder fatigue and anxiety have become the order of the day. Unfortunately, even with all this activity on your mind, you are hardly productive. You are like the proverbial rocking chair; activity without much progress.

Chapter 22. Guided meditation

How we can calm our fears, heighten our psychic awareness and develop the gift of empathy

This article is about guided meditation for developing psychic and empath abilities. In these times where fear seems to dominate most thoughts, it can be tough to tame our own shadows.

Let us look at a few different types of meditation and how they can work to enhance your psychic abilities. I know that these topics can be very overwhelming because there have been many books written on this subject, however it is my goal to write about the basics that everyone should know. Examples of such books include: The Gifted Child, Gifts of the Spirit, Emotional Intelligence by Daniel Goleman, Mindsight by Mohali Csikszentmihalyi and The Wisdom of the Dream by Carl Jung.

Guided Imagery is a powerful tool that may help you to heal and grow. It is an extremely effective and creative form of visualization technique. This type of meditation can be used to develop and enhance psychic abilities in those who use it properly. It can also be used for healing, one example being the witnessing of a crime scene, which allows us to see the evidence on a level that we cannot normally see because our minds are not trained to do so.

You may have heard of the terms "guided meditation" or "guided visualization" before. When you read through this article, it will become clear why these terms are sometimes interchangeable with certain types of meditation. They all come from a spiritual point of view and therefore, can be categorized as a type of psychic meditation, but there are also differences in how they are done. The main purpose of guided meditation is to loosen the grip of fear or any other negative emotion and to develop psychic awareness and empathy.

There are three main types: Visualization, Object Meditation and Internal Image Meditation.

Visualization is used for developing psychic abilities in beginners or those who need a gentle approach in learning how to use this kind of meditation. This technique is best for those who are interested in developing their intuition, as well as heightened awareness. You may visualize a certain object and then meditate on it. This will help you to see the object more clearly in your mind. You may use this technique for developing empathic skills so that you can understand others better by using your own intuition.

Object Meditation is another type of guided meditation that can be used to develop psychic abilities. If you have a special object, like a club or a wand, then you can use it as the focus for your meditation. You might want to say prayers or affirmations while focusing on the object. This helps to put more energy into your meditation as well as your psychic development.

Internal Image Meditation is the most advanced type of guided meditation and can be used by advanced practitioners. This is the type that has been used by those who have done extensive studies on psychic development and intuition. The advantage of using this meditation is that you can become very in tune with your body so that you can achieve a deeper level of awareness. You can create an image of your body and then meditate on different parts of it. This helps you to become more in touch with your body, which is a huge step towards developing psychic abilities. It should also be noted that there is a certain amount of risk when using this type of meditation because you may gain access to information that you had not wanted to know about.

Chapter 23. Tips for Raising an Empath Child

Empath children are special and unique, but to a parent who doesn't understand the gift, it doesn't come across that way. You may think your child is needy, emotional, and oversensitive. You may have even punished your son or daughter because they tend to act out in ways you don't understand. You want them to be happy but don't think that encouraging their sensitivities will help them in the long run. You may have accused your child of being too emotional (this is especially true for boys) and told them that they will need to grow a thicker skin if they are going to make it in this world.

You have been to counseling, therapy, spoken to friends and family, but you just can't seem to figure it out. The thing is that you love your child and you refuse to give up on them, so you continue seeking answers and fate has led you to this book.

Signs That Your Child is an Empath

Always feeling unwell: Does your child always have an upset stomach, a headache, or a sore throat? Are they constantly complaining that they are in pain? Do you walk into grocery stores and your child is fine, then five minutes later they are complaining that something is wrong? Most parents chalk this behavior up to attention seeking, and some doctors have even labeled children as hypochondriacs. However, the reality is that highly sensitive people pick up on other people's illnesses, and they can become so in tune with the other person that they actually start feeling their pain.

Although it can get quite frustrating having a child who is always sick, you should never take it out on them. Now that you know that they are not attention seeking, showing your child that you are concerned, you care, and are there to support them is the most effective way to handle this trait.

Extremely sensitive to the emotions in their environment: Empath children will tap into every emotion that is around them. If you and your husband have had an argument and you are trying to hide your anger from the kids, your empath child will pick up on it. Emotionally, there is nothing you can hide from them. Empath children latch onto things such as energy, atmosphere, and body language.

There is no sense in hiding your emotions from an empath child because they will pick up on them immediately. What you can do is be as open and honest with them as you possibly can. Obviously, there are some things that children don't need to know. In these circumstances, let them know that there is a problem, and you are trying to resolve it, but try not to avoid telling them because they are too young to understand. With everything else, you will make things easier for you and your child if you tell them the truth.

Very responsible: While you might think that your child just enjoys being helpful, it runs a lot deeper than that. Empaths feel as if other people's happiness is their responsibility, so much so that they will abandon their own needs to go above and beyond the call of duty to help someone. If they can't, they get very upset with themselves. An empath child might take on worries and responsibilities that they are too young to handle. You may have already experienced this, but don't be surprised if you are ever struggling with the bills and your child gets upset because they are too young to go out and get a job to help.

Let your kid distinguish that you are thankful for their help but that they are too young to intervene in adult affairs and mommy and daddy have it all under control. Encourage your child to relax and have fun and continue to reinforce that it is not their responsibility to make other people happy. Once you can get your son or daughter to understand this, it will free them to enjoy their childhood without having the burden of feeling they are responsible for other people's problems.

Difficulty sleeping: Are there times when your child finds it difficult to sleep at night? Empath children can become exhausted and anxious if they are overstimulated, including having too many things to do throughout the day without taking enough breaks, multi-tasking, and no alone time. They then find it difficult to wind down at night because they are still feeling the stimulation in their system from earlier in the day.

Empath parents are not the only people who struggle to get their kids into bed on time—it is a common problem. The only difference is that empath children are not being defiant when they don't want to go to bed, they simply find it difficult to go to sleep. Here are some tips to help you with this.

Establish a Night time Routine. Children need structure; it provides them with a sense of security and safety when they know what's coming next. A bedtime routine will help your child develop sleep associations to let them know that it's time to go to bed. A good routine might include:

- *Taking a bath*
- *Brushing their teeth*
- *Putting on pajamas*
- *Getting into bed*
- *Reading a story*
- *Goodnight hugs and kisses*

You can change the routine depending on what works best for your child. It's important to remember that it's not what you do during the routine, but how consistent you are with it.

Avoid stimulating drinks. One of the main ingredients in soda is caffeine, and if you allow your child to drink a can of soda, make sure you give it to them early on in the day so that it doesn't affect their ability to sleep.

Turn off electronics. Kids love gadgets just as much and if not more so than adults. If allowed to, they will continue to play with them right up until bedtime. The light emitted from the screen emulates daylight and tricks the brain into thinking that you should be awake. All electronic devices such as games, laptops, and televisions should be switched off and locked or removed from the room an hour before bedtime.

Provide a good sleeping environment. Your child's room should be conducive to sleep. Soft playing nighttime music will also help your child fall asleep as well as drown out any of the other sounds in the house.

They find it difficult to tolerate noise: Are you getting frustrated because your son doesn't like going to the game with you? This isn't because he doesn't like sports, but because he is unable to tolerate crowds, clapping, cheering, booing, and loud music. Basically, noise is a huge irritant to empath children.

Short of keeping your child locked up in the house, there is no way to avoid exposing your child to loud noise.

Let them wear earmuffs or earplugs. Earmuffs are great for blocking out sound, and there are plenty of fun looking earmuffs and earplugs that your child will enjoy wearing.

Encourage your child to take breaks. When taking your child to a noisy event such as a family gathering, as well as wearing earplugs, you can also take him or her outside for a break when it appears that things are getting a bit too much. This will help them settle down so they can go back and enjoy the rest of the event.

Disliking people or being in certain environments: You might think that your child is rude because there are some people that they are just not able to tolerate. This may come in the form of them refusing to say hello or running from them when they come to the house. Do you dread taking your son or daughter to certain places because you know they are going to start acting up? That's because they don't like the environment because there is negative energy and bad vibes that they are unable to handle.

Empaths have very strong intuition, and they automatically know when something is not right. If they don't like one of your friends or a family member, trust their judgment and distance yourself from the person. It will probably save you from problems in the future.

If your child doesn't like being in certain environments, don't force them to go there. It will only make your kid anxious and depressed, and you wouldn't want to be responsible for upsetting them.

Chapter 24. Build Your Self Confidence

Building self-confidence is an ongoing process that needs determination and energy. Here are some steps to think about when you are trying to build yours:

Step Out of Your Comfort Zone

You have to stir up that urge burning within you to be extraordinary.

Perhaps you have a brilliant idea that your belief could benefit your company, but you do not know how to share that with your boss. Perhaps you have a crush that you never dared to approach.

The problem that comes with not acting on these desires is that you will stagnate right where you are. Truth is, when you fail to explore new experiences, you are letting fear take away your sunshine. You are simply digging deeper into your zone of comfort. The hole that you have been sitting in for several decades now.

Yes, it may be intimidating to make the first approach into the unknown, risking being embarrassed by failures. But if you think about it, it's just 'FEAR' – False Evidence Appearing Real. What is the worst that could happen? Often times, you are just overthinking. Stepping out of your comfort zone can be so daunting, but it is important if you wish to fulfill your life's purpose and have unshakeable confidence. This could be the way you can finally prove to yourself that you can achieve anything you set your mind to.

After all, what is the worst that can happen? You can share with your boss and steer the company to success, or the boss simply turns it down. You could ask that girl or boy out, and they could say either yes or no – You also get your answer without wasting too much time guessing. Either way, it is a win-win situation.

The secret to having solid confidence starts with you!

One thing that I will tell you for sure is that to get out of your comfort zone; you have to start by setting micro-goals that will all eventually add up to the bigger picture. Micro-goals simply refer to small pieces of the larger goal you have. When you break your bigger goals into chunks, accomplishing them becomes quite easy, and you will have so much fun while you're at it. This will also build up your momentum to keep pushing until you have reached your target.

So, we suppose that you have a business idea or strategy that you would like to share with your boss but haven't gotten the courage to do it. What you can do instead is break your major outcome into smaller goals that eventually yield similar outcomes. Take small steps to get started, no matter how small it is. Instead of taking the big leap and feeling overwhelmed, starting small will take the pressure off you. When you do this, you simply make things quite easy to digest and make follow-ups easy.

So, you like that girl or boy and have no courage to tell them how. But he or she may not be single in the first place. So, your micro goal should be to establish a rapport with them first before you dive into the deepest end of things. Even before you ask them out on a date, get to know who they are by just initiating a short conversation with her/him. Isn't that better? This does not sound like you are stalking them.

That said, you have to appreciate that when you set micro-goals, it allows you to step out of your comfort zone. As you achieve your micro-goals one after the other, you will realize that every small win can help you get the confidence you need to move forward. Challenge yourself that you are going to do something out of the ordinary every day and see how that grows your confidence.

Know Your Worth

Did you know that people with rock solid confidence are often very decisive? One thing that is pretty admirable with successful people is that they do not take too much time trying to make small decisions. They simply do not overanalyze things. The reason why they can make fast decisions is that they already know their big picture, the ultimate outcome.

But how can you define what you want?

The very first step is for you to define your values. According to Tony Robbins, an author, there are two major distinct values; end values and means values. These two types of values are linked to the emotional state you desire: happiness, sense of security, and fulfillment among others.

Means Values

These simply refer to ways in which you can trigger the emotion you desire. A very good example is money, which often serves as a mean, not an end. It is one thing that will offer you financial freedom, something that you want and hence is a means value.

Ends Values

This refers to emotions that you are looking for, like love, happiness, and a sense of security. They are simply the things that your means values offer. For instance, the money will give you security and financial stability.

In other words, the means value is the things that you think you desire for you to finally get the end values. The most important thing is for you to have clarity on what you value so that you can make informed decisions much faster. This, in turn, will give you a strong sense of identity, and that is where you draw everlasting confidence from.

One way you can do that is ensuring that you define your end values. You can start by dedicating at least an hour or two each week to write down what your end values are. To get there, start by stating what your values are that you'd like to hone to get to your dream life.

Some of the questions that might help you put things into perspective include:

- What are some of the things that matter most in your life?
- Are there things that you do not care about in your life?
- If you were to make a tough decision, what are some of the values that you will stand by and what are those that you will disregard?
- If you have or had kids, what are some of the values you will instill in them?

Create Your Own Happiness

Happiness is a choice, and also the best obstacles are self-generated constraints like thinking that you're unworthy of happiness.

If you do not feel worthy of joy, then you also don't believe you deserve the good things in life, the things that make you happy and that'll be precisely what keeps you from being happy.

You can be happier. It is dependent upon your selection of what you focus on. Thus, choose happiness.

Happiness is not something happens to you. It is a choice, but it takes effort. Don't wait for somebody else to make you happy because that may be an eternal wait. No external person or circumstance can make you happy.

Happiness is an inside emotion. External circumstances are responsible for just 10 percent of your happiness. The other 90% is how you behave in the face of those conditions and which attitude you adopt. The scientific recipe for happiness is external conditions 10%, genes 50 percent and intentional activities - that is where the learning and the exercises come in - 40%. Some people are born happier than others, but if you're born unhappier and practice the exercises, you will end up happier than somebody who had been born more joyful and does not do them. What both equations have in common is that the minimal influence of outside conditions on our happiness.

We usually assume that our situation has a much greater impact on our happiness. The interesting thing is that happiness is often found when you quit searching for it. Enjoy each and every moment. Expect miracles and opportunities at each corner, and sooner or you will run into them. Whatever you focus on, you may see more of. Pick to concentrate on opportunities, decide to focus on the good, and choose to focus on happiness. Make your own happiness.

Be Ready to Embrace Change

Have you ever found yourself obsessing about the future or the past? This is something that many of us find ourselves doing. However, here is the thing; the person you were five years ago or will be five years from now is very different from who you are right now.

You will notice that five years ago, your taste, interests, and friends were different from what they are today, and chances are that they will be different five years from now. The point is that it is critical when you embrace who you are today and know that you are an active evolution.

According to research conducted by Carol Dweck, it is clear that children do well at school once they adopt a growth mindset. In fact, with the growth mindset, they believe that they can do well in a certain subject. This is quite the opposite of what children with a fixed mindset experience because they believe that what they are and all that they have is permanent. Therefore, having the notion that you cannot grow only limits your confidence.

What you should do to embrace all that you are is stopping self-judgment. Most of the time, we are out their judging people by what they say, how they say it, what they wear, and their actions. In the same way, we judge ourselves in our heads comparing our past and present self.

For you to develop a strong sense of confidence, it is important that you start by beating the habit of self-judgment and negative criticism. Yes, this is something that can be difficult at first, but when you start to practice it, you realize how retrogressive that was.

You can start by choosing at least one or two days every week when you avoid making any judgment at all. If you have got nothing good to say, don't say it. If there is a negative thought that crosses your mind, you replace it with a positive one.

Gradually, your mind will start priming to a state of no judgment, and it will soon become your natural state of mind. This will not only help you embrace others but also accept yourself for who you truly are.

Be Present

Sounds simple, right? It is important and necessary that you build your confidence. By being present, you are simply allowing your mind, body, and soul to be engaged in the task at hand.

Let us imagine speaking to someone that is not listening to what you are saying. This is something that has probably happened to a good number of us. How did you feel? On the other hand, imagine speaking to someone, and you feel like you were the only person in the room. Feels pretty special, huh?

Chapter 25. General Types of Empaths

While art is fundamentally about self-expression there are many forms that it takes, such as painting, sculpture, dance and the like. The same can be said for empaths. Although the fundamental reality of being an empath remains fairly the same, there are several different types of empath that a person can be.

Emotional Empath

Emotional empaths are the most common type of empath, and the most basic. This is the variation that most people identify with when they think of the term 'empath.' As an emotional empath you will be able to sense the emotions of those around you, thereby knowing what a person is feeling regardless of their outward appearance. The ease with which you can sense the emotions of others can be both a blessing and a curse. Although it can be a good thing to know what another person is truly feeling, the truth is that you can sense the emotions of others as easily as you sense your own feelings. This can make it difficult to differentiate between the two at times, causing a fair amount of emotional confusion as a result.

To say that you can sense other people's emotions may actually be understating your experience somewhat. The fact is that you cannot only sense how others are feeling, but you can share in those feelings as well. Again, this can cause significant confusion with regard to your actual emotional state. You will probably experience mood swings as a result of how others are feeling, and this can make you seem unstable in extreme cases. Subsequently, it is important to develop the ability to differentiate between the emotions of others and your own feelings. This will help you to stay true to your emotional state regardless of the environment you are in. Additionally, by remaining detached you can prove more beneficial when helping those around you since you aren't allowing your own energies to be altered or drained by their emotional experience.

Physical/Medical Empath

The second type of empath is the physical/medical empath. If you possess this type of empathy, you will be able to sense another person's physical health and wellbeing. Essentially, the experience is the same as with an emotional empath, however, instead of being able to tap into another person's emotional state you are able to tap into their physiological state. One way this takes shape is that you get an image or a sense of something that is wrong. For example, if someone has a chronic illness, such as diabetes, the word 'diabetes' might appear in your mind, seemingly out of nowhere. Alternatively, you might actually be able to feel the symptoms of another person the same way an emotional empath can feel another person's emotions. This can be very distressing if you don't know what is going on since you may experience numerous symptoms throughout any given day, even though you are in perfect health yourself.

Some physical/medical empaths can actually see issues in another person's energy, such as blockages, imbalances and the like. This is where practices such as Reiki can prove a very beneficial profession, as such an empath could use their abilities to detect and help correct a person's energy issues. For the most part, people in this category choose medical professions where they can use their intuition to help diagnose and cure the patients they see. Needless to say, the same detachment that can benefit emotional empaths can go a long way to benefiting physical/medical empaths as well. After all, you can't be of much use to others if you think the symptoms, you feel are yours rather than theirs!

Geomantic Empath

Geomantic empaths are those who can sense the energy of a place, landscape or environment. If you have ever experienced a solid emotional retort to being in a place you might be a geomantic empath. However, this is only true in the case that the environment is relatively free of people. After all, if there are many people in an area you might actually be picking up on their energies, which is what an emotional empath would do. Geomantic empaths, in contrast, feel the energy of an environment that is relatively deserted, meaning they are feeling the energy of the place, not of other people.

As a geomantic empath you will feel a deeper sadness anytime you witness trees being cut down or patches of natural land being developed for human use. The sorrow you feel for such an event would be similar to the sorrow an average person would feel for a tragedy in which numerous lives were lost. Essentially, as a geomantic empath you identify all life as equally sacred and the fact that you feel the energy of natural environments only strengthens that fact.

There is another form of experience for geomantic empaths, one that involves 'energy fingerprints.' Anytime you feel extremely sad, frightened, happy or angry when you are in a place it could point to the energy imprint left by countless people who had specific experiences in that place. For example, an old jail might make you feel depressed and sad, whereas an old theater might make you feel happy and excited. This is the result of the emotional fingerprint left by those who were there when the place was active. All in all, if you are a geomantic empath, it is important that you leave places that make you feel uncomfortable and spend time in places that bring you peace and joy, such as forests, beaches and other natural environments.

Plant Empath

One of the things that most empaths discover at some point in their lives is that the energy that flows through humans is very much the same as the energy that flows through all of nature. Therefore, it will be no surprise to discover that there is an actual form of empathy that specifically focuses on plants. If this form describes you then you are a plant empath. Like a physical/medical empath you are able to sense and identify the physical wellbeing of those around you. However, in this case instead of people it's all about the plants around you. This means you have an intuitive green thumb!

As a plant empath you can feel the actual needs of the plants you come into contact with. To the outsider this can seem as though you are keenly observant, capable of discerning a plant's health by even the subtlest of signs. However, the truth is that you only find those signs because you know what to look for. This can make you very capable working in such places as parks, nurseries, or for any type of landscaping company. Not only will you be able to detect problems early on, but you will also know intuitively how to address those problems, using techniques that most others wouldn't even have thought of.

If you are a plant empath you probably have numerous plants in and around your home. This is because healthy plants give off energy that is rejuvenating to an empath, regardless of type. By nurturing plants to their optimum health, you are actually helping to create an environment that benefits you as much as you benefit the plants. Although some might scoff when you talk to your plants or hug your trees you know that such actions are as natural as when two people talk to each other or engage in an embrace.

Animal Empath

Most empaths feel a closer bond to nature, resulting in them having more plants and animals in their lives. However, an animal empath takes this bond to a whole new level. Much like a plant empath, animal empaths are able to sense the condition and needs of any animal they come into contact with. One of the main differences between plants and animals, however, is the depth of communication that can occur between animals and animal empaths. While plants can communicate needs and conditions, animals can communicate feelings, thoughts and even desires. Make no mistake, just because an animal can't express their thoughts with the spoken word doesn't mean that those thoughts don't exist.

As a result, animal empaths make the best veterinarians, pet sitters and animal psychologists. Most actively seek out jobs in such areas since helping animals is a very real part of an animal empath's design. Furthermore, like physical/medical empaths, animal empaths can detect illnesses in an animal, making it possible to treat animals more quickly and effectively as a result. The only downside is that most animal empaths will become fairly antisocial, choosing to spend their lives with animals over people due to the connection they have with the animal kingdom.

Claircognizant/Intuitive Empath

Finally, there is the type of empath known as the claircognizant/intuitive empath. These empaths are capable of not only sensing the emotions of other people, but of actually perceiving other people on an intuitive level. This means they can receive information from another person just by being around them. Scientific studies have demonstrated the possibility of this phenomenon, specifically as it relates to the actual nature of thoughts. It turns out that thoughts are comprised of energy, making it possible for them to be perceived much the same way that emotions are. The single difference is that claircognizant/intuitive empaths seem to pick up on energies of a more conscious nature, such as thoughts, intentions and personality traits.

The main advantage that claircognizant/intuitive empaths have is that they can perceive a person's true identity quickly and easily. This means that they know what a person is like regardless of outward appearance or even their emotional state. Subsequently, they are able to get the most accurate first impressions of a person. In more extreme cases claircognizant/intuitive empaths can all but read another person's mind, making them virtually telepathic. Unfortunately, this level of perception can easily lead to sensory overload. It is recommended, therefore, that claircognizant/intuitive empaths develop the ability to 'turn off' their abilities at will in order to allow them the ability to recharge their batteries. Additionally, it is advised that they carefully choose the company they keep, ensuring that they spend time with people they can trust and feel comfortable around.

Chapter 26. Best Careers for Empath

Empaths thrive in a low-stress environment. Therefore, it can be challenging to come up with an ideal form of employment for an empath. Traditionally, they tend to excel in small companies, solo jobs, and other low-stress arenas. Working full- or part-time from home is an ideal situation where the emphasis is away from the frenzy of office politics, toxic coworkers, and constant interaction with others. A job where you can plan your schedule and breaks according to your needs and requirements is ideal. An empath's natural inclination toward healing and helping others opens up a variety of career options. Creating a career by using one of your strengths is a great way to harness your empathy and create a livelihood. This looks at career choices that allow you to use your gift to help others.

Psychologist

Empaths make brilliant psychologists because they have a keen awareness of human nature and emotions. They are capable of understanding what others feel and can sense the reasons for these feelings. Mental health is as important as physical health. A mental health issue is as debilitating as a physical illness. These days, there is a growing demand for mental health specialists, and an empath is well suited to this role. Their inherent understanding of emotional suffering, coupled with the ability to help others, works brilliantly well in this field. They are also good at listening and offering helpful advice.

Nurse

Empaths are natural healers and caregivers. They are automatically drawn to anyone who is in pain. In fact, empaths often go out of their way to alleviate any suffering others are experiencing. Because of this natural desire to help others who are not well or ill, becoming a nurse is a good career option. A nurse is a healer, and it helps channel your empathy to reduce a patient's anguish. Working in nursing homes, hospitals, or even private houses allows you to use your empathy to comfort and soothe others.

Veterinarian

Empaths have an affinity toward animals. They feel deeply for nature and all its creatures, which is not just limited to human beings. It might seem surprising, but empaths are quite good at understanding what animals feel. You might have heard the term "horse whisperer" or an "animal whisperer." Well, that deep connection with nature allows an empath to understand the pain and suffering of other beings who cannot communicate as people do. It makes empaths feel deeply for them. Empaths make excellent vets because of their natural desire to heal and comfort sick pets.

Writer

Empaths are extremely creative. If you have a passion or a flair for writing, consider turning it into a full-time employment opportunity. Writing is a creative outlet to channel your feelings. Usually, empaths experience a variety of emotions foreign to them, and these emotions can trigger your creative juices and help you write. You can become an author, a freelance writer, or even a blogger. Allow your inner storyteller to come to the forefront and lose yourself in the journey. Writing can be a great escape from the world and is an excellent way for an empath to spend time alone.

Musician

As with writers, musicians are extremely emotional beings. If you have a knack for music and are an empath, consider turning it into a career opportunity. From writing songs or poetry to singing and even playing an instrument, there are different things you can consider. Beautiful music is composed by those who understand pain. Since an empath's heart naturally goes out to others, their understanding of pain and suffering is more heightened than others. In a way, you are using your strength as an empath to carve a career for yourself.

Artist

Empaths make excellent artists due to their boundless creativity. Writing can be used as a medium for an empath to express themselves, and art does the same. An empath's energy and imagination can be channeled through art using multiple media. It can be a video channel on YouTube showcasing your creativity, working as a freelancer, or even selling your artwork through online and offline portals. An empath's soul is attuned to the constant ebb and flow of human emotional currents, and creating art becomes meaningful to them.

Teacher

A teacher's primary role is to guide their students toward success. Teachers inspire and push their disciples to excel in life and work toward their goals. Since empaths are all about uplifting the human spirit and collective progress, teaching becomes a good option. Their loving hearts, coupled with helping hands, make them an ideal candidate for this profession. Proper support and motivation can work wonders in one's life. A teacher is able to offer these things to their students, especially to those who do not get this at home.

Life Coach

Empaths thrive when happy people surround them. They are not jealous of others' success and, in fact, rejoice in this feeling. They also like helping others. Since they are excellent listeners and problem solvers, becoming a life coach is a great option. Since you always have the best interests of others at heart, being a coach will come naturally to you. If you have noticed most of your loved ones or acquaintances depend on you in their times of need for advice, it is all because of empathy and compassion.

Guidance Counselor

Just like teachers, even guidance counselors have the power to shape the life of a young adult. Guidance counselors act as mentors. Since empaths are great listeners and problem solvers, they often come up with brilliant advice. This is precisely the kind of advice a young adult needs during the formative years of their life. Also, this is a truly rewarding and fulfilling experience for the empath. As a counselor, you will be assisting pupils while working toward their endeavors, making sure they stay on the right track and pursue their goals. You will be required to offer them encouragement and motivation to explore opportunities that come their way. All these things come naturally to an empath, and it is a great way to channel your superpowers. Since empaths are good at understanding what others need—even if they do not understand themselves—working as a guidance counselor will be a fulfilling experience.

Social Service

Empaths like helping others and often go out of their way to do it. Since the world desperately needs empathy and compassion, social work is one avenue you must not overlook. It is personally rewarding, fulfilling, and uplifting. These are three things an empath always seeks in life. Whether you decide to become a social worker or work with a non-profit organization, there are different things you can do that will help you give back to society.

Empaths make a wonderful difference in every life they touch, and social work is a natural fit for you in this world. However, when it comes to social work, you need to be cautious. Empaths thrive on happiness and generally feel better about themselves if others are happy. If the story does not end well or things don't turn out for the better, it can take a toll on an empath's wellbeing. When you work with some of the worst-hit members of society or negative elements, you have to take care of your energy levels. If you take things too personally and let it consume you, your job will quickly overwhelm you.

Hospice Worker

As with nurses and anyone else involved in the medical profession, becoming a hospice worker is another role to consider. Offering comfort and solace to dying patients and their family members will put your empathy to good use. Facing a life-threatening illness is seldom easy. It takes motivation and courage to work with such individuals. Hospice work involves elements of spirituality and social work. This work is quite appealing to an empath because it is not rigid and does not limit their abilities. It helps channel your empathy to elevate grief.

Self-Employment Opportunities

Any form of self-employment is a good idea for an empath. If you are self-employed, it means you do not have to depend on others for your livelihood. You are your boss and can set your work schedule according to your needs and requirements. It gives you complete control and autonomy over your business operations. It also reduces any interactions with others, which are common in a typical corporate setting. Self-employment gives you a chance to explore your creative side and turn one of your passions into a paying form of employment. The tech-dominated world you live in has opened up new doors for self-employment opportunities. From drop shipping niche stores and online businesses, there are several avenues you can explore. Most of these businesses can be conducted from the comfort of your own home. Well, what more could an empath want?

Now that you know the different job opportunities available to you that will help harness your energy, certain jobs are not ideal for empaths. To enhance your empathic abilities, it is best to avoid jobs that drain your energy. For instance, any job where you constantly deal with others or the public, in general, can be extremely stressful. Some obvious jobs that are not suited for an empath include sales where you deal with customers or offer technical support, advertising, selling products, or marketing. Even being a cashier can feel overwhelming. If you are constantly in touch with others, you absorb their energy, feelings, and physical symptoms. Other career options that are not ideal for an empath include anything related to politics, public relationships, human resource management, and executives responsible for managing big teams. Becoming a trial lawyer will be emotionally exhausting too. However, certain branches of law will work well for an empath that requires the emotional maturity to deal with trying matters such as domestic violence or abuse. Any career that doesn't stimulate your creativity or imagination and requires an extroverted nature is not advisable. Generally, the conventional corporate setup might not be the best choice either.

Chapter 27. Understanding Empaths from a Scientific View

There have been many things in life that appeared to be magically until we were able to figure out how they worked and understood the process it tool. Unfortunately, the research on empaths is still being performed. But one is that has been studying is the concept of mirror neurons and it is casting a bit of light on a possible explanation as to why empaths are able to experience the emotions of others.

Mirror neurons are described as a neurophysiological mechanism involved in the way that people are able to understand another person's actions and learn to imitate them. In some of the first studies about the context of motor skills discovered that these neurons fired when monkeys watched another person perform an action. This created the hypothesis that watching a person will trigger some form of an internal response to help us mimic what we are seeing. This act of watching people experience something activates neurons in the brain even when we are not performing an action.

Marco Iacoboni, Professor of the Faculty of Medicine at the University of Califonia, Los Angeles, believed that mirror neurons could be the physiological basis for morality and empathy since they affect how we interpret and perceive the experiences of people that are around us. In the simplest form of the neuron, they are triggered through the observation of some type of physical gesture in other people that fires the same neurons in the person that is watching. The amazing part of this is that it will happen consistently even though the person that is observing the action is not actually moving anything. It is simply an internal version of the action instead of physical imitation.

Let us say that you are at a football game. Neurons that are activated in the quarterback when he snaps the ball are fired in you as you watch. This same thing happens when you are watching a person experience some type of physical pain or if you notice a facial expression of worry or anger. The brain is able to interpret the meaning of these different situations by experiencing things through mirror neurons. There are many different ways to trigger these neurons, such as seeing a ball get to throw, hearing the sound of the ball being caught, or when you say the word throw.

The actual firing pattern of these mirror neurons is actually very sophisticated as well. In fact, the firing pattern depends on the context or meaning of what is being observed. Both of the actions will involve all of the same muscles, but they do not necessarily have the same intentions behind it, so they are going to end up triggering different mirror neuron pathways.

This is the reason Iacoboni thought that the neuron's firing patterns were so complex that they would let people know the intent behind a person's actions depending on the context. The importance of the process becomes very apart once you start to think about how understanding and relating to other people is important in how we make it through society. This is supported through several bodies of research on the theory of emotional contagion.

Emotional Contagion

Emotional contagion is when a group or a single person is able to influence the actions of other groups of people through a conscious or unconscious induction of attitudes and emotional states. This process is very deeply rooted in the human psyche. There are studies that have discovered that newborns can imitate the facial expressions of people after a couple of minutes of life.

There are even adults who unconsciously imitate the demeanor of other people. This mimicry passes emotion on from one person to another and plays a large role in social relationships. In fact, people tend to like others who imitate them. The reason for this is likely that mimicry helps us to feel connected to others. It provides us with a positive emotional experience as well. Emotional contagion, basically, comes from basic mimicry as we try to feel loved by people around us. From the moment we are born, we start to register and then try to reproduce non-verbal language.

Even though science has managed to make it this far, the experience of an empath still seems to show that there is another human process where humans are able to innately sense the emotions of other people that aren't totally controlled by their conscious mind. Empaths probably would not have a problem with being able to turn off their abilities from time to time so that they can simply feel their own emotions. However, their experience is unconscious, and it takes a lot to control it. Many empaths have reported feeling overwhelmed by the emotions of others.

Typically, when a person is interested in improving a skill, they will make a conscious decision to do so, and they follow this by some type of practice and learning experience. Some people are better at doing this than others, so their need for practice may be shorter than others. For empaths, the physical manifestation is the first to happen. They start feeling the emotions of others, and they are unable to realize what is happening. Only after this are they able to start working on their quest of understanding what is going on. The first thought of many empaths is, "How do I stop this?"

Being empath never shows up as a learned skill. It is not something that a young child can hope to have and start to develop throughout the years with the practice. The initial trigger is typically a physiological one that will lead them to an emotional experience and then it leads to conscious awareness. They are going to feel first, and then they will learn to understand their gift later on. Many empaths say that they are not able to control the process. Very little of the population actually has the ability to be an empath. Everybody is able to perceive the emotions of other people, but only an empath has the unusual sensitivity to feel the emotional cues around them.

Electromagnetic Fields

The findings behind electromagnetic fields are because the brain and heart create an electromagnetic field. HeartMath Institute says that these fields send information surrounding person thoughts and emotions. Empaths are very sensitive to all of this input and tend to find that they are overwhelmed by it. Empaths tend to have a stronger physical and emotional response to changes that happen within the electromagnetic fields of the Earth and Sun. Empaths are able to understand that everything that occurs to the Earth and Sun is going to have some sort of impact on their own energy and their mind.

Heightened Sensitivity to Dopamine

Dopamine is the neurotransmitter that increases neuron activity and it connected to the pleasure response. Studies have found that the introverted empath tends to be more sensitive to dopamine than extroverts are. This means that they do not need as much dopamine to be happy. This could also be the reason why they tend to be content with simple meditation, time alone, and reading. They do not have to have external stimulation from social gatherings. Extroverts need to have a rush of dopamine from those types of events. Extroverts just cannot seem to get enough dopamine.

Synesthesia

Synesthesia is a neurological condition where a person has two senses that become paired within the brain. For example, a person is able to see music when they hear a certain piece, or they are able to taste words. Some of the world's most famous synesthetic are Billy Joel, Sir Isaac Newton, and the violinist Itzhak Perlman. However, with mirror-touch synesthesia, a person is able to feel the emotions and sensations of other people within their own body as if it was actually their pain.

Psychological Understanding

Empathy has been a common psychology term for some time that was used to describe the ability to understand what a person could be feeling. This experience is often referred to as, "walking in someone else's shoes." Empathy is a very important part of social interactions. Empathy has the ability to affect the way we act toward other people. In a sense, the glue helps to hold humans together.

Theodor Lipps, German psychologist and philosopher is often said to be the father of the word empathy. He described empathy as the way that we perceived the minds of people around us through a simple process of inner imitation. This process takes part in several areas of the brain, such as the cortex, endocrine system, autonomic nervous system, and hypothalamic-pituitary-adrenal axis.

While there are some people who suffer from some type of psychopathologies, such as sociopaths, who exhibit a lack of empathy, the skill is a strong biological foundation. Babies are able to recognize several types of emotions from a very young age and toddlers are even able to create empathy as they age. Young children are able to spot different emotions of people around and they can correctly interpret them.

There are being recent studies who are described two systems that are used in psychological empathy. One, emotion-based contagion, and two, cognitive perspective-taking system. Emotional empathy has been found to activate what is called the inferior frontal gyrus. Cognitive empathy is connected more closely to the motor mirror neuron system. For the well-known American psychologist Rogers, on the other hand, the idea of empaths was more connected to cognitive empathy than to emotional one.

In psychological experiments on empathy, they will often use observation to trigger an empathic response in a person. They make the empath watch a person who is paced into a situation that should create a strong emotion.

Rogers said that empathy has, what called, an "as if" condition. A person may be able to experience empathy when they are able to imagine the way another person may feel. This is not anything like what an empath is feeling. Empaths feel things as if they were their own. It is not something that they have imagined, and neither is it coming from some external stimuli.

Chapter 28. Helping Others

As an empath, your number one purpose in life is to help others. Empaths, as a whole, were born to help the Earth usher into a new, more compassionate existence. You are here to awaken people to the truth of their actions, to protect the Earth from harmful practices and to otherwise work as an energetic and possibly literal activist on the mission of saving the planet.

There are many different ways that this can be done, and it is important that you understand that it is not up to you to do all of the different practices that are meant to help heal the planet. Through this, you are all working together to create a more positive experience on Earth while also saving her from the destruction of humanity. It takes each of us fully committing to doing our unique part to create the entire web of healing energy that is needed to reverse the damage that is being done to our planet and our society.

Helping others can come in many ways, such as helping younger empaths identify their true nature and being a guide who shows them the way. You can also support and protect them as they discover their sensitivities and learn to awaken to the energy that exists all around them while supporting them in understanding their own unique gifts and expressing them to the world around them. Another way that you can support the Earth is by simply having empathy for others and by having compassion for what they are going through. In many ways, this very act will help people heal and experience a more positive existence in their lives. Often, this can be done in a simple manner, such as by showing empathy and compassion for your friends and family and working with them to teach them about the truth of who you are and how you are. This way, your friends and family can stop calling you "just sensitive" and start respecting your gifts and even taking your advice as you offer it.

You can also show up for humanity by identifying your unique passion or purpose and learning how to turn this into a side business or even a full-time business so that you can devote even more time to helping. Some empaths have a hard time doing this because they feel guilty charging money for their gifts, but the truth is that the more you are compensated for your gifts, the more you are able to empower yourself and serve your purpose. Through this, your acts of service become far more potent and you are able to do even more for the world, which means that you can completely change the face of humanity as we know it, alongside other empaths.

To help you get a stronger feel for how you can help others while also helping yourself, we are going to dig deeper into what you can specifically do, without draining yourself and your own energy.

Helping Younger Empaths

Every day, new empaths are being born and raised in a society that still largely struggles to support empathic people. The way our society is built and structured is not ideal for young empaths, as it continues to expose them to massive amounts of trauma and overwhelming energy that can make growing up for them difficult. If you had a difficult upbringing yourself because of your own sensitivities, then you can understand exactly what children are going through on a day-to-day basis. Sadly, younger empaths who are struggling to find their way on this Earth are still being exposed to the same struggles that many adult empaths once faced.

Learning to become someone that can show the way for younger empaths means that you give younger empaths the opportunity to understand themselves and their own gifts at a much earlier age. You also give these children or younger empaths the opportunity to step into their purpose and begin helping with healing the Earth at a younger age, which means that you are able to have a better impact on healing the world around you. Being a guide is a big role those adult empaths take on as they grow to understand their own unique gifts and use them responsibly.

Being a guide to young empaths does not necessarily mean that you need to go out of your way to "recruit" younger empaths or find them so that you can help them, although you can do that if you feel called to do it. If, however, creating resources and support systems for massive numbers of young empaths does not resonate with you, you can easily help by making yourself available and supporting those who cross your path. Supporting your own children, other younger people in your family or even those in your friend's families if the relationship buds naturally is a great opportunity for you to begin helping younger empaths feel more empowered and seen in their lives. This way, you can also educate them on what their gifts are, how they can protect themselves and what they can do to live better lives overall.

It is important that if you want to take on the role of helping younger empaths, you also take on the role of helping and healing yourself. Attempting to guide younger generations through their own struggles and traumas when you are refusing to face your own can be challenging and can lead to you having a hard time really supporting these younger ones. You may also end up passing on conflicting or incomplete information that may lead to unfavorable results, such as younger empaths massively struggling to actually feel empowered because what you informed them about may have been tainted by your own projections.

While this does not mean that you cannot help if you are still struggling or healing yourself, it does mean that you should be mindful of what you are saying and the information that you are passing on to younger empaths. You always want to do your best to be as objective and supportive as you can while giving them the ability to feel seen while also feeling free to explore their gifts.

Helping younger empaths is an incredibly noble purpose to take on, no matter what capacity you choose to take it on. Knowing that your own experiences and knowledge are going to support youth in having a better experience than you did can be incredibly healing. It also helps the world in general as these younger individuals can step into and embrace their power much quicker, which results in them being able to help heal the planet much quicker too. The faster we can wake people up, support our fellow empaths and place power in the right loving and caring hands, the faster we will be able to save our planet and our species from the damage that the world is inflicting on it, overall making a much happier world to live in.

Having Empathy for Others and Helping Others Heal

Many empaths feel as though they have to do something significant and special with their gift because they feel a deep sense of obligation to others. This deep sense of obligation can make it hard for you to know how to help others and can make the act of helping others feel like a huge burden or pressure on your shoulders. You may begin to feel as if there is nothing you can do to live up to this expectation because it is so big and challenging, which means that you are going to have a harder time actually showing up for other people.

This overwhelming burden-like feeling often arises in empaths who feel that they have to heal the world and that they are the only ones for the job. Often, empaths forget that there are millions of others just like them who are doing the same thing and that they are not alone in their task. There is plenty that can be done from just one person, but just one person is not responsible for doing everything to heal the planet. You are allowed to have boundaries and to pick and choose when and where you are going to show up and how you are going to show up when you do choose to show up.

Learning how to show up with boundaries means that you can be present more fully when you do decide that you will do this for people. Rather than feeling like you are only allowed to show up when other people need you to, you can take the pressure off and just focus on showing up this one time.

Believe it or not, compassion and empathy are two wildly undervalued and underserved energies in our world. Many people find themselves struggling to get access to an individual who has the capacity to genuinely experience compassion and empathy for them, which is precisely why they may be so attracted to you. For many, you may be the first person who has willingly shown up compassionately and with the capacity to truly understand them. You may not be aware of this or you may be fully aware of this and this may further lead to you feeling like you are obligated to be "the one" for them.

You need to trust that if you choose not to talk to a person or support a person in need, they will come across another empath who can help them. At this point, they are ready to receive the support, which is precisely why they have found you and why they will go on to find another person if you are unavailable to help them too.

For the moments that you are available to support them, though, make sure that you are entirely present. Focus on just letting yourself feel into the natural empathy, compassion and care that rises from within you. Know that you do not have to "train yourself" to experience these things because you were born with the unique gift of being able to feel these energies even without knowing how. For you, these come as a second nature and they make logical sense. Let yourself lean into that natural balance and trust that you can have a stronger impact on others if you focus more on being present and holding your energy than you do if you let yourself be overwhelmed by the burden you have placed on yourself.

Chapter 29. The Process of Empathy

The process of empathy has six very distinct phases and are said to overlap each other. However, it is good to note that all six phases can be grouped into two categories. The first category is the cognitive level, while the other is the emotional level. Within the scope of the cognitive level, the three major phases include the theory of the mind, cognitive empathy, and perspective-taking. For the emotional level, we have Identification, true empathy, and emotional contagion.

We are going to talk about each facet of the empathetic process in detail. I will also analyze why each phase is considered unique from the others.

The Cognitive Level

1.   Theory of the Mind
The Theory of the Mind is said to be the ability of an individual to attribute mental states, including the intents, beliefs, pretensions, desires, knowledge and the likes either in oneself or those of others.

2.   Perspective Taking
This has been defined as the ability of one to see things from a point of view that is very different than that of one's own. We will be able to find a different number of traits that fit this description.

To begin with, we must first acknowledge the fact that we all have varying perspectives on the same situations and phenomena. So, even if we "agree", it is very likely that we will all have a different perception. This leads to a type of relativism in what we tend to perceive as "reality". As a result, we cannot assume that everyone completely agrees with us especially is the object in questions does not have a clearly defined aspect. For example, love has a plethora of definitions. So, even if there is a consensus on what feeling love entails, there is not clear consensus on a definition of the word. Hence, the perception of love is very personal to every individual. Ultimately, attaining consensus can be a monumental task.

3.   Cognitive Empathy
This term can be defined as having awareness of the needs of others. As such, it is one thing to empathize with others, that is, to feel what others feel, and it is another completely different thing to be aware of what others need. Consider this situation: you are in the care of a sick person. This person is going through pain and discomfort on both a physical and emotional level. So, you empathize with them. You feel that they feel. As a result, empathy takes place, but both parties are not conscious of what is actually occurring.

When cognitive empathy takes place, the empath is fully aware of what they are feeling and will use that to "sense" what the other person is feeling. After a while, the caregiver knows when the other person is in pain or is feeling depressed as a result of their illness.

The Emotional Level

4.   IDENTIFICATION
Identification occurs on a deeper, emotion level. While the cognitive level creates a level of awareness in the empath, the emotional level creates the actual feeling and sensation of empathy. This is a gut-level reaction that occurs any time there is an empathetic reaction. Consequently, the empath is able to absorb what others are feeling. The end result of this

situation is the empath imbibing their surroundings. This is one of the fundamental reasons why empaths tend to become overwhelmed when faced with large groups of people especially in situations of despair and suffering. Imagine yourself, as a finely tuned empath, working as a relief worker in the zone of a natural disaster. The feelings of the affected people will certainly cause you to feel a great sense of despondency. This can lead to a great sense of loss and suffering, as well.

5.　　TRUE EMPATHY

True empathy happens when a person, not just an empath, is able to truly put themselves in the position of someone else. This usually happens when the empath has been through the same, or similar situation. For instance, the empath will pick up on feelings of sadness from someone else as a result of the loss of a loved on. This is empathy. However, true empathy will occur when the empath has also been through the loss of a loved one. This maximizes the empath's ability to fully immerse themselves in the emotions of others.

6.　　Emotional Contagion

As stated earlier, this is when a person, basically anyone, ins influenced by the circumstances surrounding them. For instance, when a person goes to a sporting event, they may be influenced by the reaction of the crowd even if they have little interest in the sporting event itself. Yet, it is the reaction of the collective group of individuals that leads to an emotional response in the individual attending the event.

Also, emotional contagion is very common in the workplace. When the environment in a place of work is tense, this rubs off on even the most of cheerful employees. This is why psychologists strive to understand what motivates employees and what can lead to creating a positive atmosphere within the workspace. While the link between positive workspace atmospheres and high levels of productivity is clear, what is not fully understood is what drives workers as a collective group. Of course, we have a clear understanding of what motivates individuals, but not as a collective group. As such, if a person works in a toxic environment, it is quite probable that they will end up become influenced by this environment to the extent that it affects their life outside of work, as well.

Emotional Contagion vs. Empathy

So, the debate rages on: are emotional contagion and empathy the same thing? The short is answer is no. Emotional contagion is a part of a greater system known as empathy.

Now, the long answer is that emotional contagion is simply a perception of someone else's feelings based on their environment whereas as empathy is the process by which the individual is transported to the same state of others.

Let's consider this example: a caregiver is tending to a terminally ill patient. Emotional contagion would occur when the caregiver is affected by the patient's despondent state, but the caregiver would really care less if the patient died the next day. In fact, they would be glad if they did. This callous and inhuman attitude highlights how emotional contagion is not necessarily the same as empathy.

An empathetic caregiver is not only noticeably affected by the suffering of the patient but is actually in pain along with the patient. Then, when the patient finally passes away, the empathetic caregiver would most like become shattered at the loss.

The Mirror Neuron System

Mirror neurons are a specific class of vasomotor neurons, initially found in territory F5 of the monkey premotor cortex, that release both when the monkey completes a specific activity and when it watches another individual (monkey or human) completing a comparable activity. These cells empower each one to reflect feelings, to sympathize with someone else's torment, dread, or euphoria. Since empaths are thought to have hyper responsive mirror neurons, we profoundly reverberate with other individuals' sentiments.

Furthermore, the mirror neurons have been said to be triggered by external events. For instance, when our spouse gets hurt, we also feel this kind of pain. When we have a happy friend, the same feelings rub off on us, making us happy. As a result, mirror neurons provide us with physiological evidence that allows us to explain the reasons behind empathy. Research has also shown that individuals who have brain lesions in the parts of the brain which house mirror neurons tend to feel a lack of empathy. Since psychopaths are unable to feel empathy, they have no trouble inflicting pain on their victims.

Evidence of this system in the humans emanates from neuroimaging studies and noninvasive neurophysiological investigations. Neuroimaging further brought about an understanding of the two main networks that exists with the mirror properties: one resides in the parietal lobe together with the premotor cortex and the caudal part of the inferior frontal gyrus. The other is formed by the insula and the anterior medial frontal cortex (limbic mirror system). In this type of system, there is the involvement of the recognition of behaviors that can be said to be highly effective.

Mirror-Neuron System and Communication

Gestural Communication

The mirror neurons represent a neural premise of the systems that make the immediate linkage between the message sender and the beneficiary. One study has suggested that the mirror neuron framework speaks to the neurophysiological component from which language developed. Its functioning is comprised of the way that it shows a neurophysiological instrument that makes a typical (equality prerequisite), nonarbitrary, semantic connection between imparting people.

Electromagnetic Fields

Scientists in this field have concluded that the brain and heart have a role to play in this study, considering that they highly generate electromagnetic fields. HeartMath Institute made it clear that these are the fields that are in charge to the role of transmitting information about the humans' thoughts together with the emotions. We get to understand that empathy as well, can be overwhelmed as it is sensitive to the input. Notably, empaths have proved to have a strong physical and emotional response when there are changes in the electromagnetic fields of both the sun and earth. Happening on the earth and sun have a significant effect on the empaths state of mind and energy.

Chapter 30. Empaths and Society

Heading out into society in this day and age can be quite daunting. It is said that there are two types of societies. We will take a look at each, then see how they intertwine with each other.

Community

A communal society is one that everyone benefits from — meaning, there is a balance between what an individual wants and what is best for the community. The community is always the primary recipient in order to maintain peace, harmony, and balance. When there is a communal society, the people within it tend to put their own wants and needs aside for the greater good of that community. The community members are put second in comparison to the community as a whole. Thus, when the community is suffering, the individuals within suffer as well. On the other hand, if the community does well and has many benefits, the individuals in that community will benefit from it as well. Some people may not like that idea because there may be some people who work extremely hard for the community, but there are others who do not lift a finger. This may be difficult for some to handle because everyone will get the same benefits regardless of how much work one does. In order for this to work, everyone needs to be on board.

Individual

In this society, people are able to focus on their own success, identities, and skills. The community as a whole will not be the focus, nor will they have any issues if the individual fails or does not become as successful as they thought. An individual-oriented society will allow individuals to focus on their own goals. This type of society is about the personal development and achievement of each individual. The focus here is not on the peace and well-being of the entire community but the happiness of each individual. Let's just think about a society where someone is wildly successful. They typically end up giving back to the community where they grew up or lived in; thus, the community benefits from the individual's success as well.

Some people actually have a mixture of both societies. When they are both intertwined with each other, it can be difficult to focus on what is better for which. It happens when a person lives in an individualistic mindset but also has empathy toward others. It can be somewhat of a battle if someone has these two ideals intertwined. For example, they want to succeed, but they also want to help everyone else out. Many people who have this internal conflict tend to get anxiety, depression, and/or have low self-esteem. They may feel as if they are unworthy of love or success. They may be depressed, or they may have a combination of all due to low self-esteem. There are plenty of factors, both environmental and societal, that are contributing, along with trauma and past abuse. It is important to recognize and be aware of the different issues that people face when trying to help themselves as well as others.

Since empaths do have both individual and communal goals, it can be hard for them to find their place in society that is satisfying for both aspects.

Social Anxiety and Empaths

Being an empath can be tough, especially when you are expected at social functions of all sorts. Social anxiety is typically common with empaths; however, some may just be describing the feelings that they get when they are around others that are quite toxic. We have to remember that we are all human beings, and we do need a human connection with others. When someone explains and states that they have social anxiety, they may be seen as odd or weird in some way. However, social anxiety does not mean we have something wrong with our character. It may actually indicate that we may be more intelligent. Anxiety puts us on high alert. Those who are mothers and have children typically have more anxiety than others. They want to protect their children, hence why they develop a sense of heightened awareness.

There are five signs that your social anxiety may be an empath sensitivity:

1. It is selective.
2. You were not bullied or abused in childhood.
3. You do not fear rejection; rather, you avoid people who make you uncomfortable.
4. You are a pro at reading people.
5. Crowded places make you feel overwhelmed.
6.

It is selective. If you are just fine at times but tend to become extremely anxious when around certain people, then your anxiety is selective. When you come across some with low vibes, you may tend to heighten your senses, which can be quite overwhelming. This could be when someone makes you uncomfortable. You can typically tell if they have hidden bad feelings toward you, if they have negative emotions, or if they are being passive-aggressive. You will start to notice people's body language when you are around, and you will begin to understand your surroundings, plus the way you may react to it. If you do find that being around someone in particular gives your intense anxiety, try to figure out what it might be about them that is causing this. It could be your gut telling you to get away from that person as they mean harm to you. Just try to be aware of your body and mind when you are in any situation that makes you anxious.

You were not bullied or abused in childhood. Typically, when someone has anxiety, it stems from a traumatic event in childhood, such as being bullied or abused. However, if you did not have any of that happen to you, you may just be able to pick up on other people's vibrations.

You do not fear rejection; rather, you avoid people who make you uncomfortable. It has been said that social anxiety is tied to an overwhelming fear of being rejected. It could be that you are afraid of being laughed at or not fitting in. However, what if you do not have a fear of rejection? It might not actually be that you fear rejection; it could be that you are afraid of other people due to the bad energy that they give off. That bad energy may drain you, so you might not want to be around them. Fear can be tricky at times. You can say that you may be afraid of someone but understanding why and then taking action to avoid them will be the best for your health. In this instance, it is not about the fear of rejection; it is about your dislike for the way that certain people make you feel uncomfortable.

You are a pro at reading people. If there is ever a time when you get a gut feeling when you are in a situation and just cannot put your finger on what it may mean, it may be that you are picking up on someone's ill intent or toxic existence in your presence.

"If you indeed have an empathic ability, most probably, you get this feeling quite often. Whether you ignore or listen to this gut instinct, you are eventually proven right about the people you meet" (Reisch, 2017). If you are repulsed by someone the first time you meet them, then you could be sensing that they have low morals or standards. They could take advantage of you or could potentially harm you in some way. This instinct happens because empaths can sense nuances in behaviors, such as nonverbal cues or body language (e.g., not looking in the eye). These cues will tell the empath when someone is lying to them and will let them sense when someone is up to something that is not authentic. If someone is being inauthentic, lying, or hiding something, you will be able to pick up on that. Always listen to your gut.

Crowded places make you feel overwhelmed. Crowded spaces can be a huge drain of energy for an empath. Thus, you tend to feel depleted when you are surrounded by too many different energies. If you tend to avoid places that are particularly busy during peak hours, such as a grocery store or a mall, because you know it drains the energy from you, you are considered an energy-sensitive empath. There are also ways that this causes physical issues, such as dizziness and weakness. So, if you find yourself with any physical or emotional symptoms while in crowded spaces, it is time to choose your outings wisely in order to save your own energy.

Social anxiety can be seen as a way for empaths to hold close the true connections that they currently have with others, and it is not that they cannot form new connections. Having social anxiety is not necessarily a bad thing, even though people may treat you like it is. When your brain is always active, you are constantly searching and analyzing your surroundings. It is said to be a protection tool, and that, to most, is never a bad thing.

So, what if you do not like how social anxiety tends to take over your life? How does one prevent this from happening? Here are some tips on how to prevent empaths from developing anxiety:

1. Mix it up.
2. Express emotions.
3. Talk to your emotions.
4. Clear your inner self.
5. Ask for help.

Mix it up. However, expressing your emotions will allow you to feel a sense of clarity. Keep yourself busy so your mind does not dwell on certain situations and issues. If you are not busy or cannot mix up your schedule, try to find someone to confide in that you trust. If you are able to get your feelings out, they will not stay bottled up inside.

Chapter 31. The Psychology behind Empath People

The first component of empathy is cognitive empathy, which is the ability to understand what another individual is thinking or feeling. The second component of empathy is emotional empathy, which allows a person to share the same emotional experience as someone else by either mimicking their emotions or through intellectual understanding. The final aspect of empathy includes compassionate empathy when an individual feels sympathy for someone in pain and offers help willingly.

This will outline the basics behind these three components and provide ways for people with high levels of empathy to navigate interactions with others who do not have as much of this trait.

Cognitive Empathy

This is the ability to put yourself in someone else's situation and then make a decision or judgment about how you would feel based on your thoughts and feelings. For example, if you see a person drop and break something they were holding, you might stop and help them pick up the pieces or if you were feeling more emotionally sensitive, you may offer kind words while helping them clean up the mess.

Those who are more cognitively empathetic can also transfer this trait to their writing; this means they can often write from other perspectives by thinking how they might feel in a certain situation. For example, if you wanted to write a story where a man was abused by his stepfather, you might imagine how that would feel if you were the man and how you would feel when someone tries to help you. With this type of writing, it is important to remember that the feelings are not based on real-life experiences, and one should always be sure that what is being written is not morally or legally wrong so as not to offend anyone.

Emotional Empathy

Emotional empathy can be seen as similar to cognitive empathy, but the difference being that emotional empathy requires one empathize with another person's emotions (rather than their thoughts or actions). An individual with high levels of emotional empathy might react in the same way as the person they are empathizing with. For example, if one were to hear a story about a woman who just had a miscarriage and is saddened by the news, an empath person is likely to feel sad as well while someone without this trait may not understand how they could be feeling that way. The best way to understand emotional empathy through writing is to share one's own emotions with the reader rather than forcing them to feel certain emotions.

An example of this would be from Paulo Coelho's "The Alchemist", which describes an alchemist and his role in learning about emotion. He has been given a mysterious book and through these books he is able to learn about the use of love in potions; this allows him to understand the magic that love has and how it can affect others.

Compassionate Empathy

Compassionate empathy is one of the rarest forms of empathy. It has been referred to as "giving a hug" or feeling "the pain" of another person when they are hurting. As with emotional empathy, compassionate empathy is not solely based on emotions; an empath person can also transfer this trait to their writing by learning from another individual's feelings.

An example of this would be rather than focusing on the pain that a character is experiencing, the writer focuses on how they can relieve that pain for the other person. This allows them to share their own emotions with others and feel the things they feel even though they are not actually hurting another person.

People who have highly sensitive personalities (HSP) often display high levels of empathy and tend to seek out relationships with those who also have high levels of empathy.

Most people find it difficult to understand why empaths are so affected by what others are feeling or think about them, but there are ways for both parties to help each other navigate through situations together and enjoy each other's company.

This can be done by trying to find out a bit about the other person, what makes them happy or sad, and then attempting to relay this information back. This will help make the other person feel a bit better as well as allow them to learn more about themselves.

Another option for those with high levels of empathy is to let them know how their actions affect others. An empath may want to help another person by going out of their way to help them in practical ways.

An example would be letting a child know that they are looking through the window and see them eating a cookie before they eat it themselves; empaths often try to avoid people feeling too much pain this way because it makes them feel as though they have caused severe physical damage in others. Other feelings empaths try to avoid sometimes include anger, jealousy, and sadness.

It is also important for an empath not to focus on things that they can't change or will never change; it is better for them to refocus on the things they can change like relationships with other people and situations. By doing this, an empath can gain a better understanding of the things they can change rather than feeling bad about themselves and the way others are feeling.

In conclusion, empaths try to maintain healthy relationships with others because they want to avoid causing them pain. They also look for ways to help others as well as themselves without hurting their feelings or stealing their emotions away from them. While empaths may often be seen as overly emotional, particularly during events such as family gatherings or weddings, knowing how to navigate through feelings together is the best way to maintain a healthy relationship with someone who does not have these traits.

Conclusion

Thank you for making it to the end. Empaths are people who are sensitive to other people's emotions. The term empath (empathy) is used in a variety of contexts, from one who can feel the emotions of others, to one who easily picks up other's thoughts and feelings without the use of psychic abilities.

There are a lot of empaths in this world, and they usually know when something is off with somebody. They sometimes get overwhelmed by other people's energies and may start feeling sick or exhausted.

As an empath you may get tired and feel overwhelmed by people around you. You may want to take a step back from time to time and be alone. This doesn't mean they dislike being around people, but that their energy is drained by others. Empaths deal with people's negativity and their own energy becomes chaotic when they are constantly bombarded with the energies of others. There are times when an empath simply needs to be alone in order to recharge their batteries and become centered again.

It is also important for empaths to surround themselves with loving supportive friends and loved ones because sometimes they can become very confused by other people's negative intentions or thoughts that suddenly pop into their mind. It is hard for an empath to get rid of what other people are thinking or feeling because they have an innate sense of what people around them are feeling.

When dealing with an empath it is useful to remember that their energy is always going to be chaotic because their own emotions and thoughts become mixed up. It can also be helpful to ask empaths how they feel or think in general in order to keep them focused and on track, if this isn't possible the best thing you can do is ask them directly. This brings down the energy levels in the relationship between you and your partner, so try not asking too many questions or giving them your input when they are already overwhelmed by other people's emotions. Empaths may feel a desire to share their true feelings and thoughts, but this can be overwhelming for them when they have already spent too much time dealing with other people's emotions.

It is generally recommended that empaths not tell anyone about their sensitivity because it can be very frustrating to deal with all the different types of energy that comes from people around them. Be sure that you are telling your partner about your sensitivity so that they know how much you can get overwhelmed by the negative energy coming from others.

Take time for yourself and take after your heart. The blessing of being an Empath will continuously direct you within the right course. Let it appear you the way by taking after your instinctual, instinct, and understanding of the world along with your increased faculties. Being an Empath is as it were troublesome if you permit it to be. Take control of your endowments and let the world see how superb you are.

Psychic abilities are no longer the superstitions that people whisper about in the shadows. These powers are not possessed or used for evil and not for just speaking to people that have crossed over. As you have learned, psychic abilities are available to all at birth. These abilities are born in your frontal lobe, growing or dying depending on childhood experiences or support from family members early in life. Depending on your childhood, you may find as you practice these exercises that psychic abilities come naturally to you because you have been able to practice and experience these powers from a very young age. Others will find that, although it may feel different at first, psychic abilities are not impossible to achieve. Through intense concentration and continued practice, one can gain the ability to open one's mind and allow energy to flow in.

Once you have mastered the meditation exercises, you can practice many different forms of psychic powers. One state may come more naturally to you. Once you find your natural shape of psychic abilities, you should embrace that and continue to practice and master the form. Psychics are typically specialists in one or two forms of psychic powers. It is essential to practice all the forms several times to find the ability that it will be meant your mind to perform. You can use this form of psychic power to enhance your life, bring you closer to people in your life, connect with your body and open yourself to the universe around you to feel peace and happiness every day of your life.

BOOK 2

INTRODUCTION

Reiki originated in Japan, and for a long time was an exclusive Japanese technique with the sole aim of reducing stress and increasing relaxation to promote holistic healing of the body and the mind. A person gives reiki to another person, the basis of this is the philosophical premise of Reiki according to which we all have a 'life force' inside us – an energy that cannot be seen, that flows through us and gives us life.

Reiki is administered using hands; by 'laying hands' by one person on another, which allows for the transference and fixing of the 'life force' inside us. Reiki is all about energy and fixing the imbalance of energy that occurs due to the world we live in. It's far more natural and communal than any other form of healing since no artificial substances are used – it's about the connection between human beings using their own energy to fix other people.

The premise of Reiki is that if your 'life force energy' reduces, you are susceptible to contracting illnesses and feeling stressed. If your 'life force energy' is high, it gives you immunity against sickness and contributes to your overall happiness and health.

Reiki itself is a word that is an amalgamation of two different Japanese words – the first is 'Rei' meaning 'The Wisdom of God or a Higher Power' and the second is 'Ki' which is the life force and energy that flows through us. So, if we define Reiki using the definition of these two words, it's the healing of life force energy inside us, guided by spirits or higher wisdom that we cannot see. Reiki is intricately linked to spirituality – treatment by a Reiki master spiritually fulfills and charges you.

Many people talk about how it made their whole-body glow with the radiance of spiritual and deep-seated energy. Reiki doesn't just focus on the physical body, but also on the immaterial aspects of it – emotions, mind, and spirit.

The benefits of Reiki are innumerable from relaxation, security leading to a reduction in anxiety, peace, and wellbeing.

Reiki has been proven to work on many people, and there are numerous accounts of people who could never fix themselves through medicine, but Reiki for them produced miraculous results. Reiki is not as complicated as it seems; it's just based on a different knowledge system to the one that we are used to.

It is natural and therefore, carries far fewer risks than other methods of spiritual healing. If your goal is self-improvement, not just in a physical way, but also a spiritual way, Reiki is undoubtedly going to help you. Reiki can solve every disease that is known to man, and unlike artificial medicine, it ensures that the disease does not just return in a few years. If you don't want to leave other medicinal techniques and practices that you are using, don't worry – Reiki can be used in conjunction with any other therapeutic technique without causing any problem in recovery.

Reiki might seem mystical and complicated, but in reality, it's an easy technique to grasp. Reiki is not taught like how we generally think teaching goes - it's a system of schooling where a master teaches his student by transferring his knowledge of Reiki during a session or class.

Reiki is an ability that has to be acquired from the master in a process known as 'attunement' – this is a process where the student taps into the 'life force energy' of the world through the master to hasten their recovery and wellbeing. Reiki is egalitarian; you don't have to be spiritually enhanced or intellectually brilliant to grasp it. People of any age or background can learn Reiki and have done so over the last hundred years.

Reiki is linked to spirituality and has a spiritual framework, but it cannot be classified as a religion.

Reiki does not have a set of pre-conditions that you must believe in to subscribe to Reiki healing; it's not dogma, and there are no fundamental opinions that you must believe in blindly to be part of the Reiki healing circle.

Reiki also does not ask you to believe in something to see the miracle of it occur; in fact, you don't even have to believe in the healing powers of Reiki for it to work on you. So, even if you come as a skeptic, Reiki will work no matter what you might feel about it personally.

Reiki does have spiritual aspects attached to it, and historically, it has been seen as a way to connect to God. So, while undergoing and learning Reiki, you might feel a connection to God, which will help you understand Reiki on a spiritual level, rather than merely on a rational basis.

Reiki does not promote itself as a religion, but it does ask you to believe in goodness and respect. Reiki's fundamental value is the life force energy that connects us all, so it believes in promoting peace and harmony by letting go of anger and prejudices that we might have.

Along with Reiki, if you want to heal holistically, the founder of Reiki Dr. Mikao Usui, suggests that you practice universal ideas of ethicality to promote social good along with peace and harmony. Dr. Mikao Usui, after developing Reiki, decided to further it by adding a few ideas to his Reiki system. These ideals are based on the five principles that the Meiji emperor of Japan believed in, and who Dr. Usui considered as an inspiration.

The reason for adding these ideas to Reiki was to provide it with a form of spiritual balance where it wasn't just concerned with pure spirituality but also tried to blend itself with changes in the physical world. His goal was to make people realize that you can only make the spirit heal itself if you consciously decide yourself to improve the conditions that you live in.

You can't just hope that everything will fix itself; you have to develop an inner will to fix yourself and your conditions. Reiki healing will always be temporary, unless and until the student actively participates in the process and takes responsibility for their healing.

The Usui system of Reiki is not just limited to the use of Reiki energy; it also requires a commitment from the client. This doesn't mean that you have to blindly believe that Reiki is going to solve all of your problems, but as you gradually learn about it, you have to use it to motivate your own recovery from within.

Once you start believing in the values of grace and dignified living that Reiki promotes, you will see the changes that these values can cause in your life.

CHAPTER 1. Universal Energy In Human Body

What is Reiki Energy?

It is probably best if we start with energy and what that is. Energy itself is defined in many different ways by many different disciplines. Everything from spiritual and religious practices, all the way to the scientific properties of physics, energy seems to be everywhere.

Energy equals mass squared times the speed of light. That is Einstein defining the universe with physics. Starting by defining energy of course. We can define energy and energies in a spiritual way as well. The breath of God, or the life of a plant, can all be traced back to basic energies.

Energy defined leans to strength and vitality. This is the stuff of work to sustain activity. Vigor and liveliness lead to this vitality. It is the fire and passion of what makes us do what we do.

When dealing with perspective and different ways of thought, it is reasonable to say that Eastern society looks at the spirit of life differently than the West, we have to take into account that Reiki comes from this Eastern way of thinking.

It may seem strange at first to look at the Eastern philosophy as this his blend of color and life and energy resides in all things. The Universe resides in all things. Energy is the Universe. The Universe is energy. Back and forth the energies flow.

If you have ever sat in a field of flowers and grass, with the sun making you all warm, you begin to feel this energy. It is the buzzing and sound of the insects around you. It is the flittering of a small butterfly as it floats by.

The energies of us as we live is also a way of measuring this energy. Imagine your life as a shell with no energy. Our lives are powered up by our own energies. Without energy we are just a husk. Yes, there is something to be said for not believing. It is only in the moments that we see ourselves for what we are with and without.

Energy is

With this in mind we can begin to extrapolate as to what the energies of life are. Once we leave the debate of the mystical spiritual conflict versus cold, demanding, clinical science behind, we can begin to see life for what it is. A series of energy movements.

This philosophy is a corner stone in describing what Reiki energy is and what it does.

Consider the fact that energy can be either flowing or not, then we can begin to see that those who have a skill set can manipulate this energy. This manipulation is not a negative practice. Reiki tends to teach flow over stagnation, or non-flow.

This is what the Reiki energies are. Just as there are so many different life energies, there are so many ways to control your own, as well as that of others.

There is a pattern to life, and to the energies of all forms. Rei, in its spirit and energies, lead us into a pattern of wisdom. This symbol of Rei is an intelligence. A non-physical energy that leads us to a pattern of life. It is an instructor as well as inspiration. It is the higher knowing of what happens and why it happens.

The beginning of Reiki is the why life happens the way it does. This is the energy pattern of why life happens the way it does. Rei is our starting point. Energy and passion combined with intelligence giving us the result of wisdom.

Reiki energy literally starts with wisdom.

And now the power part. Ki. With the understanding of Ki, we begin to see spirit as power. Ever met someone who is so full of spirit, and they seem like they are lit up like a lightbulb? It is when we stop to look around us, that we begin to see that every one of us, every*thing* around us, has this power.

This spirit of Ki is connected to almost everything. Consider the lifeless form of your cellphone. It is just plastic, glass, battery and circuits. There is really no life there. Even when we power it up with energy there is still a lifeless quality to it.

It is when we breathe our Ki into our devices that they become something so much more than a box of plastic. They interact with us in return. Energy is exchanged back and forth. This is the power of the Ki in a more physical form.

We are attached to almost everything. Some expert theologians say we are connected to everything. There is the possibility that Ki does indeed connect us to it all.

This power comes with examination. Once we find the energy of Reiki, we can see if we are flowing with it or not. It is more than acceptable to remain in a state of non-flow with Ki energy and live a full life.

The energy of Reiki is a bit more than just getting by. The energy is about connection and ability to self-heal, and to ultimately heal others. It is about the universe and that flower growing in that pot over there. It is about why our hands move and why we are the way we do.

Ki is power. Power is energy. Life is energy. Life is Ki, for the lack of a better way of defining it. The energy of Reiki is this pattern that comes from wisdom and can be manipulated within others. Imagine an entire society that is constantly flowing with this energy. What would it accomplish? How would everyone get along?

There is a way to constantly sustain this energy flow. This is the technique of the Reiki, to get us to flow energy. We are not here to remove tumors or cure cancer, although within the realm of Reiki healing, this is possible. We are here to use this energy to get the person who is need of healing to flow with their life force again; to get ourselves flowing again.

This is totally possible. Energy is real. Reiki energy is real. The world around us flows with energy, and we only need to learn how to tap into it, connect, listen, and find our way to move with the flow of the energy for the highest and greatest good of ourselves and others.

CHAPTER 2. Origin of Reiki

Reiki is a traditional Japanese style of energy work that was primarily passed down orally for centuries. Knowing the exact origins are difficult since the tradition was based on word of mouth for so long. However, Mikao Usui is credited as the founder of Reiki, as he rediscovered the art in the 1800s.

During a cholera epidemic in Tokyo, Usui fell ill, and while he was struggling to live and recover, he had a spiritual awakening. Once he was recovered, he was led to join a Zen monastery where he learned a healing method that had been used for centuries. This healing method includes laying static hand positions on the body. Usui did not dive directly into studying Reiki at this point, however, he wanted to increase his spiritual awareness of healing before continuing.

According to legend, he went on a spiritual quest which led him to a mountain top where he meditated and fasted for 21 days in order to better understand Reiki. He had a pile of pebbles with him while he meditated, and after each day, he threw one pebble away.

After the 21 days of meditation and study, Usui set a firm intention that he wanted to see things clearly. It is said that he received an energy flash the beamed straight through his forehead and supplied him with the Reiki Symbols that are used in Reiki treatments.

These were symbols that he had previously discovered in the Sutras he had been studying. It is believed that he reached enlightenment at this point in his studies.

As he traveled back down the mountain, he tripped and hurt his foot. The legend says he was bleeding and when he placed his hand over his foot, the cut stopped bleeding and the pain subsided. Then he stopped in a village and ate an entire meal without experiencing negative feelings or discomfort even though he had been fasting for 21 days.

When he returned to the Zen monastery, he used his new gift to heal the arthritis of his superior. Usui then decided to start using Reiki to try and help the poor and homeless communities in Kyoto. Unfortunately, he found that most of them would quickly return to their lifestyle of begging.

He was reminded that healing has to be holistic and includes the body, mind, and spirit. Usui returned to meditation and discovered the 5 principles of Reiki. Then he devoted the rest of his life to teaching and practicing Reiki.

Another important contributor to the discovery and spread of Reiki was Chujiro Hayashi. A physician and retired Marine commander, Hayashi learned Reiki from Usui. Together, the two opened a Reiki clinic that combined Reiki with Hayashi's physician knowledge.

Hayashi kept detailed records at his clinic of what Reiki was used to treat and how different hand positions treated different conditions more effectively. With his notes and observations, he wrote the guide, *Reiki Ryoho Shinshin* which he included as a manual for students in his classes.

In his clinic, Hayashi expanded on how Reiki sessions could be given by developing the Group Session method. He would have a client lie on a table and multiple practitioners treat the client all at once. This created a much stronger energetic session. He also developed a new method for giving Reiki Attunements to his students.

Hayashi also changed the way that Reiki was taught. He would combine the Shoden and Okuden teachings and Attunements into one course, especially when he traveled. He traveled to Japan and was asked by his government to report on military information around Pearl Harbor.

Hayashi refused to provide such information and was dishonored by his government, being branded a traitor. To restore his family's honor, he performed seppuku or ritual suicide.

Howayo Takata is the woman who is most notably credited with bringing Reiki to America and the Western world in 1937. Takata was married to a bookkeeper at a plantation they both worked at in Hawaii.

After her husband died, it was her responsibility to support her family. However, after several years of hard labor and long work hours, she started to experience severe abdominal pain and problems with her lungs.

When her sister died, she was the one who had to travel to Japan and inform her parents, as they had resettled in Japan. While in Japan, she was admitted to a hospital and diagnosed with a tumor as well as gallstones. She was also diagnosed with asthma and appendicitis.

Rather than receiving surgery, Takata made her way to Hayashi's clinic for treatment. She had never heard of Reiki before, but the diagnosis she received at the clinic was very similar to what she got from the hospital, and this impressed Takata. She wanted to learn Reiki to keep healing herself and to bring it back to Hawaii with her.

For one year, Takata worked at the clinic and was taught by Hayashi. She was one of thirteen Reiki Masters trained by Hayashi. When she returned to Hawaii, she opened several clinics and started teaching Reiki. She would give sessions and treatments and taught students up to Level II Reiki. Throughout the country and world, she was known as a healer.

In 1970, Takata began to offer the Master Level training for a cost of $10,000. Neither Usui nor Hayashi required a high fee for their teachings, however, Takata may have used the fee as a way to establish respect and legitimacy for Reiki practitioners. She believed that treatments and teachings should not be given for free.

During her courses, she did not provide written material or allow her students to take notes. Another deviation from Usui and Hayashi's teachings. The Reiki symbols were forbidden from being written down. She based her teaching methods off the ideology that Reiki was an oral tradition. She also insisted that a student must only work with one teacher during the studies.

Since these were deviations from the way Usui and Hayashi taught Reiki, it is not entirely clear why Takata had such restrictions for her students or charged such high fees.

By the time she passed away in 1980, Takata had taught and Attuned 22 Masters. These Masters began teaching their own students. Takata made them promise to teach the same way that she taught her students. However, after a time, Masters started relaxing their strict teaching methods and began allowing for notetaking and manuals. Students are now encouraged to seek out additional teachers to learn new methods and get different experiences.

Despite the exclusiveness of her teachings, Takata is still credited with how far and wide Reiki spread in the US and Western World.

Today, it is estimated that there are over 1 million Reiki Masters in the world and as many as 4 million practitioners. The more the scientific and medical fields find in regards to the human body and energy, the more interest there is in alternative methods such as Reiki. It has been used for centuries, even if not on a huge scale, so clearly it works!

As you progress through your own Reiki teachings, you will find many different avenues to study and receive Attunements. Some Masters will only teach in classes that might be a single weekend per Reiki Level. Other Masters might have developed online courses with all the information you need, and once you work through the course material, they will provide you with distance attunements.

Reiki has also expanded into several branches that have varying levels of learning and ways to practice. Usui Reiki is considered Traditional Reiki and that is going to be the basis of the information in this book.

Each Master has different course material and probably varies in the tasks and learning activities that you will be required to perform. The best you can do is find a Master that resonates with you and a learning style that you enjoy.

CHAPTER 3. The Basics of Reiki

Reiki Basics

The basics of Reiki will be taught in your first-degree training and as you get higher in degrees and levels of Reiju (attunement) you will learn more about the gifts of Reiki and how to practice it well. The elements of Reiki come together to promote a way of life and a belief that will help you stay grounded in the right energy and platform of healing to help you on your path of healing yourself and other people.

The pillars and principles of Reiki are from Dr. Usui's original format for teaching Reiki and will demonstrate the basic mentality of what Reiki embodies and helps to connect you to in your practice. You will also learn about what are called the Five Reiki Elements, although these were not originally taught by Usui and are from an adapted form of Reiki. You will learn about it here as many Reiki Masters have started to teach these elemental concepts and so you may find a Master who would like to train you with these kinds of techniques.

All of the basics of Reiki, together with what you have already learned about energy and how Reiki works, will help you find the attitude, respect, focus and admiration you need for the Reiki healing process. As you read, ask yourself what part of these principles you are already working with in your life and how you can improve upon them.

The Five Reiki Principles

Reiki is meant to be thought of as a healing practice. It may have been born out of a world religion, but it is not a religious practice. There are basic principles of Reiki that are meant to help you receive Reiki through an open consciousness and purity of intention and spirit.

The five principles were created by Usui and are seen here in these pages. They have gone through many alterations and additions, but this is as close to the original concept as you can get. These principles are useful to memorize so that you can implement them into your practice sessions as you prepare to work with a client.

They serve as helpful reminders to keep you focused and in an attitude of healing and working as a channel of light and love.

These principles are simple and effective and are mantra for healing and growth. These five principles are what set you on the right path of healing and having an open heart to allowing Reiki to flow through you effectively for healing purposes. These affirmations, or mantras, are part of the basics of how your entire energy and life-force is able to accept Reiki and allow it to become a part of your every day life. It is a good practice to state these principles to yourself every day.

In Usui's clinic, he trained his students to meditate every morning and night on these principles. Your Reiki Master will likely not ask you to do this, but you may find that you will want to keep them handy in your mind for your healing practice and therapeutic work.

The Three Pillars of Reiki

The Reiki pillars give form to the principles and you could say that the principles are the foundation of the structure, and the pillars are what hold it up well.

The pillars are actually just simple prayer poses, or meditations that help you maintain the principles within your practice. They are simple and effective and will give you the balance and energetic opening you need to ask for Reiki to help promote healing in the self and others.

The First Pillar: Gassho (gash-show)

Meaning: Two Hands Coming Together

This is a prayer position. It is the palms touching together and held out in front of the body at heart level, or if you are performing this hand position in a less formal way, the hands are up against the heart pointed toward the chin. A more formal gesture is seen with the palms together and the fingertips pointing out at a 45-degree angle, as a sign of reverence for what is in front of you or outside of you.

Either one of these positions is considered a Gassho and is used for prayer, meditation, a sign of respect, and so forth. The term "Namaste" is actually part of a Gassho and is used in a similar fashion, stating the word along with the hand sign means "I respect you."

A Gassho is often performed in a Reiki session as part of your greeting with a client and can be used throughout the session, or as you open and close your healing work with yourself, your client, and the Reiki energy flowing through you.

The Second Pillar: Reiji-Ho (ray-zhjee-ho)

Meaning: (Reiji) Indication of Reiki Power / (Ho) Methods

This is a three-step meditation, or prayer, to connect you to Reiki to allow you to be guided by the energy rather than just using hand positions. Additionally, this pillar is useful in distance healing practices.

First, you close your eyes and place your hands in Gassho and ask Reiki to flow through you, repeating the request 3 times (you can ask in your mind). Allow the Reiki to surge through you.

Second, you bring your hands in Gassho up to your third eye and ask for the health and recovery of your client on any and all levels, if it is needed. Here, you invite Reiki to go where it needs to go for healing. Ask Reiki to guide you and show you the way.

Third, Let Reiki pull you where you need to go and let go of the attachments you might have to controlling it. If you are not feeling like you are able to let the Reiki flow and guide you, you can repeat Reiji-Ho again, or simply use the hand positions over the chakras to help you direct Reiki into your client. When you are being guided, allow Reiki to do the work until you feel like you are no longer needing to work in any areas and then stop, as you are guided to do so.

Finally, perform another Gassho of gratitude and respect for the experience.

The Third Pillar: Chiryo (chee-rye-o)

Meaning: *Treatment*

According to the rituals of this pillar, the practitioner will place the dominant head on, or above the crown chakra of the client being worked on (note: you don't have to physically touch a person in order to heal them with Reiki). From this position of rest over the crown chakra, the practitioner will wait for the inspiration, or impulse, to move in a direction.

Similar to Reiji-Ho, you are allowing the Reiki to guide you on your healing path with the person you are treating and when you perform this action, you are giving heed to the energetic "knowing" of the client (crown chakra) of where to go to treat them. Give free reigns to your hands and they will find the source of the pain, block, discomfort and place of treatment. You will remain in the places you are pulled to until you are released, as this will be when the pain is also released. Your hands will then move to the next place of treatment.

This pillar comes with more practice and experience in most cases but is accessible to anyone who is open to working with Reiki. It tends to be a more direct healing treatment method, as opposed to the Reiji-Ho, which will have more flow overall. Chiryo will be more focused and slow moving.

The Five Reiki Elements

The Five Elements are part of Chinese healing practices and are promoted in the Traditional Chinese Medicine techniques and Taoist philosophies. Wu Xing is another name for these elements together and they are earth, fire, water, wood and metal.

The reality of utilizing any element to understand the basics of Reiki is that it can show you another level of healing properties and practices in a fundamental and Universal way.

In other cultural beliefs, there are the five elements described as being earth, air, fire, water and ether, or spirit. You can look at either of these platforms to help you study a deeper level of Universal truth to help you in your healing practices.

The elements are a practical approach to learning the lessons of what causes malnourishment, or health and healing, to the aspects of our whole selves. Every level of our being (mind, emotion, spirit, body) requires connection to these elements and with certain realities, too much or too little of one element can cause an excess or deficiency in another. It is similar to the chakra system and how an imbalance in one creates a need in another.

Interestingly enough, the chakras are each represented by an element, according to the traditions of their origin. (root=earth, sacral=water, solar plexus=fire, heart=air, throat=sound, third eye=light, crown=ether). Obviously, that adds up to more than five elements, but the perspective is that the basic elements are the basis of all life and all matter and so to understand the way the body, mind and spirit work, it is helpful to go over what the elements can be representative of in the healing process.

Since not all Reiki practices using these elements, you and the Master you study under, may have a certain approach to understanding and utilizing these elements. There are even entire books devoted to learning healing with this kind of approach and you can find more information through Traditional Chinese Medicine practices (Wu Xing) as well as in other off-shoots of the original Reiki practice laid out by Dr. Usui.

It is not a requirement of Reiki that you learn these elements, but it can be a very useful tool in your practice.

Other Practical Basics

Meditation and Techniques

Reiki is akin to a meditation. When you are working with a client to promote healing, you are in a deep trance of Reiki flow. It is like leaving your earthly self, long enough to transmit the direct flow of ULF into the energy centers of another. You can get better and better with time, and one way to help you remain focused in your treatment sessions is to practice meditation in general, before, and after your treatments. This can also help you relieve any of your own energetic issues or blockages so that you can stay grounded and open to assisting others in your work.

The pillars and principles you have learned are essentially meditations to practice Reiki and so if you are incorporating these principles into your work, then you are on the right path to staying grounded, centered and focused as a channel of light.

The techniques you use in Reiki are also simple meditations that come with some practice and allowance of Reiki flow, so when you are practicing the pillars and the principles, you are effectively channeling Reiki. Other basic techniques that require a meditative mindset are the aura combing and energy assessment and other forms of assessment that utilize the third eye for "seeing" the problems and issues.

The technique of "energy sight" is highly common amongst Reiki practitioners and will begin to open up to you (if it isn't already) in your first-degree attunement when you begin to practice energy healing on yourself. You will often be able to see the auras, chakras, and what lies within them in a variety of ways. There really aren't any limitations to how these "issues" will present themselves when you are using the sight technique. You might see entire landscapes inside someone's energy field, or strange objects, creatures, or elements that need to be removed. It really just depends on each individual experience.

Practicing Reiki involves a lot of intuitive work and not just technique. You could say that opening yourself to channeling Reiki and using intuitive method is the main technique you will use to help you promote the healing process in another person. There are no practices that will help you better than following the flow of what Reiki shows you to do, and this is the powerful meditation of working with Reiki as a healing treatment.

Hands on Healing

The hand positions are incredibly simple tools assigned to certain placements and postures along the chakra system to show you where to work and where to let Reiki flow through. This process is not complicated and once learned will feel like a regular step-by-step approach to using Reiki healing techniques if you are not yet confident with letting Reiki chose where to go, as it asks you to follow along.

Mantras and Symbols

Mantras are a part of the principles and pillars of Reiki and these can come up during any session. Also, as part of the symbol drawing technique, you will chant the name of the symbol, like a mantra, three times as you are drawing it. The mantra is stated in the mind and not allowed, in most cases.

Mantras and symbols are a powerful and effective tool, but are not always necessary. They provide more focused intention and as you get better acquainted with the general flow of a Reiki session, you may find that you only need one or two symbols every so often, while in other healing treatments you may need to use symbols and mantras often to promote a bigger energy shift and transformation in your client.

All of these Reiki basics are intended to help you see the overall platform of Reiki and how it is structured to help others and the self. All of these basics are part of the doctrine of Reiki and as Reiki transforms and is spread, new ways of approaching Reiki are permitted and accepted, as you have read with application of the five elements from another healing practice.

CHAPTER 4. Benefits and Limitations

Reiki is a tool to use to improve your overall health. It can aid you in your spiritual, mental, physical, and energy recovery. It has been proven time and time again to aid in restoring one's body to peak physical condition, particularly when used in conjunction with other therapies and medical treatments. Reiki sessions will reinvigorate you and invite your body to a new level of relaxation. The benefits of Reiki sessions truly are incredible, but the art itself it is not without its limitations. Physical healing and mental healing are a part of the Reiki process, but it must be used in conjunction with other medicines and be practiced by a learned student of the art.

Benefits

One of the greatest strengths of Reiki comes from its ability to focus both the mind and the body inward. If you have ever tried meditation, the feeling of unity between you and the surrounding is similar to the feeling you have during a Reiki session. Your anxieties and stress melt away as you blend in with your chair; the limits of your body and your surroundings becoming blurred. It is this increasing unity with the world that helps alleviate the stress brought on from the drudge of everyday life. While in sessions your anxiety is completely eradicated, out of sessions this feeling lasts for several days, with anxiety and stress returning over time. There is added benefit in that a patient can expect to see better sleep for some days following a session. The relaxing nature and connectedness of Reiki lead one to find more comforting and more rejuvenating sleep. This sleep works as a cycle to improve the body's overall health as rest and relaxation are essential elements in persevering the mind, body, and spirit.

Many patients turn to Reiki as a form of spiritual enlightenment. The goal of expanding one's spiritual mind is as ancient as time, and Reiki serves this adventure admirably. The meditative qualities are largely what helps in this goal; however, the connectedness one feels between mind and body is the real secret that gives Reiki an edge over other spiritual pursuits.

There is an explosive realization in linking the body to the mind, enabling the soul to find spirituality more easily. Transparency into the self allows making meaningful connections between earthly events and the spiritual agent that surrounds us all.

Maintaining and improving mental health is another key aspect of Reiki treatment. The relaxation that comes through sessions is a place where the mind can focus on past events and put history into the context of one's life and the world around them. The feeling of connectedness helps put problems into context and reshape the way one sees their own life. Larger, more difficult mental experiences, such as loss, is also appropriately treated through Reiki. The grieving process is enhanced through the essential links between the body and the physical world around it, allowing cleaner clearer perspectives on one's emotions and their involvement with those they may have lost. Regarding other mental ailments, such as long-term depression and social anxiety, Reiki is an aid rather than a complete solution, but it has been widely reported that Reiki sessions do lessen the burden from severe depression and strong social anxiety.

On the physical level, Reiki can by itself alleviate the pain from minor body ailments, such as headaches, arthritis, and sciatica. These purely physical problems are soothed through Reiki sessions and meditation. Very often the stress of a condition like arthritis will lead to a worsening of the condition itself. Reiki helps rebalance the tension in your physical muscles by alleviating the mental strain the condition is causing. Other physical ailments that have had a positive effect from Reiki include menopausal symptoms, fatigue, and asthma.

In conjunction with other medicines, Reiki can have a large effect on speeding up the recovery from long-term illnesses. It can be used effectively to balance the damaging effects of chemotherapy. Chemotherapy attacks the cancer afflicting the body, but it cannot differentiate between the cancer cells and the cells the body needs to survive. As a result, the sickness associated with chemotherapy can be agonizing and attack all aspects of daily life.

Reiki helps remove some of this burden by refocusing the body on itself, helping delivery the precious life energy to spots of the body that have been harmed through chemotherapy. It was actually through my readings on how chemotherapy patients responded to Reiki that I truly went from being a skeptic to a believer. The results speak for themselves with patients reporting far better health than their counterparts that started on chemotherapy without having any Reiki sessions.

Limitations

Reiki has incredible uses, but it is not the singular cure that some practitioners have made it out to be. There are many limitations to the practice, but first and foremost comes time and dedication. Reiki requires regular sessions to be effective. It's also not guaranteed to have results during your first session. While you should experience connectedness to the world around you, a general feeling of greater well-being too, as you come out of your first session, you will realize that this feeling will be fleeting. As you have more sessions, you will notice the benefits of Reiki lasting for a longer period. For some, this essential limitation is enough to deter interest in Reiki at all, but I want to remind you, the practice is an extension of the body. As with anything that improves oneself, it must be done with a level of consistency to ensure positive effects. It is not a one-time cure, but anything that works on the body in the long-term is something that needs to be repeated, whether that is exercise, eating well, or Reiki sessions.

The reason that a steady flow of Reiki sessions is required comes down to the physical practicality of how Reiki works. Reiki is designed to open the channels of positive energy that exist within the body. It is meant to clear blockages and reroute flows that have been distorted over time. It often requires multiple sessions, and certain blockages can be very difficult to clear. It is possible to have a remarkable breakthrough on your fifth or sixth session if that is when the block is finally cleared.

There will be a sudden change in your health, but this sudden change will have come from the sessions that came before it. It is also possible that the channel for your positive energy is simply weak—this could be from inactivity of years of energy moving toward the wrong flow point. In these cases, too, multiple sessions will be required with the hope of improving the channel and increasing its capacity.

Effective in ailments such as asthma, Reiki should not be used as a replacement for an inhaler or be used to seek immediate effect in potentially life-threatening medical emergencies. While Reiki will be effective on asthma over time, an asthma attack is best treated with a prescription inhaler. Asthma is simply an example—there are other conditions such as a rapid onset migraine or minor physical symptoms like a pulled muscle. Both of these can be improved with Reiki, but it cannot be understated that these effects should not be expected to have an immediate effect. Some patients do respond better than others, but always be prepared for a backup plan, and remember the core principle that Reiki is used as a supplement, never as a sole solution, and never as a sole solution to a problem that needs to be fixed immediately.

Reiki has shown many uses in helping cancer patients with chemotherapy. It has shown to help AIDS patients as they toil through the pain caused by their medications. It has not been shown to be a singularly effective method of treating any life-threatening illness. No IARP-registered practitioners would claim that Reiki has these effects, but there are less honest practitioners that I have heard of. These practitioners give the art a bad name and generally taint all metaphysical sciences. As much as it saddens me to say, I have seen these types of practitioners before. They claim to be able to pull cancer out of one's gut using merely their hands—they are capitalizing on the hopes and dreams and backing it up using a proven method of improving the human condition. The technique such practitioners use gives false security to patients, and even though they may feel better in the short term, it in no way will be the sole solution to a larger problem like cancer.

Be aware of the limitations of Reiki—know what it can solve and what it can't. Know that it has incredible benefits but that these do come with their limits. If you go in with the right expectations and find the right practitioner, you will have no problems. You will be conducting your sessions in the right mindset with the right attitude for the problems that you are trying to solve.

People begin the practice of Reiki for various reasons; some use it to relieve stress while others use it to achieve balance during a transitionary time in their lives. The reasons may vary, but nearly everyone who begins decides to continue practicing for the long-term. Reiki helps every single person in different ways. Even if someone comes for one reason, they soon realize that there are a wide range of matters that can be dealt with using Reiki. The healing effect has an impact on every aspect of their lives. Let us take a look at some of these benefits of Reiki.

Reiki Promotes Balance and Harmony

It is an effective energy healing system that is noninvasive, and which enhances the natural healing ability of the body. Reiki can be energizing and helps to promote the overall well-being of a person. It restores balance and looks into any issue in-depth. Reiki does not provide superficial solutions but deals with any issue from its root. Practicing Reiki will help to restore any person's mental and emotional balance.

Reiki for Stress Release and Relaxation

Reiki induces deep relaxation and releases stress and tension from the body. When a person is receiving Reiki, they don't have to consciously do anything but just be. This helps them relax and take a break from their hectic lives. They feel at peace and lighter from within. Reiki gives you a space where awareness of the inner state of your mind and body increases. You get to learn how you can be more attuned to your body and make better decisions for your own well-being. It helps you in accessing the inner wisdom and knowledge that exist within every single person.

Reiki for Balance and Energy

Reiki can dissolve any energy blocks and promote balance between the body, mind, and spirit. Getting regular Reiki healing will help you become calmer and more at peace. This helps in dealing with stress healthily. The process of learning and retaining is also improved. Any emotional or mental wounds can be healed with Reiki. If you suffer from frequent mood swings, Reiki can alleviate them as well. Relationships can be strengthened and healed too. Your capability to love will be enhanced, and you will be more open to others. This will help all your relationships grow stronger and better.

Reiki for Detox

Reiki will help your body detoxify itself and improve the efficiency of the immune system. The modern-day lifestyle has made most of us live in a constant state of fight or flight. This, in turn, has made your body forget how it can regain balance. Reiki will help to remind your body how it can shift from the fight or flight mode to a "rest and digest" state again. This state of being does not mean that you will be unproductive or inactive. It will just help you in improving your sleep cycle and the digestive system. This is essential for good health and vitality. The more you induce this state, the healthier you will be without having to deal with stress or exhaustion.

Reiki for Mind and Improved Focus

Reiki clears your mind and helps improve your focus. It helps you feel centered and more grounded. Reiki also helps you stay centered and focus on this moment rather than living in the past. This will improve your capacity to accept everything that comes your way and to work your way out of any difficulties. Instead of acting out of habit, you will react to situations in a better way.

Reiki for Sleep

Reiki aids in better sleep. The first and most obvious outcome that you will experience from Reiki is relaxation. When you can relax, your body can sleep better. It also helps you think with more clarity and relate to other people more.

Reiki for Self-Healing

Reiki will accelerate the self-healing ability of your body as you restore its natural state. Reiki healing will help to restore the natural state of your body and will shift it in the right way. Everything from your blood pressure to your heart rate will see improvement. As you practice Reiki, you will see that you can breathe more easily and deeply. Science supports the fact that breathing better supports the state of mind. It is mainly because the oxygen flow to your brain is improved and this improves brain health. With deeper breaths, the body will moves into the rest and digest state induced by the parasympathetic nervous system. This is the state that your body is naturally supposed to be in and not the fight or flight state that is induced constantly by your current lifestyle.

Reiki for Pain Relief

Reiki helps to relieve pain and improve physical health. Even though the healing system is noninvasive, Reiki aids in good health at the deepest level. It improves the functioning of all vital systems in the body and assists it in performing optimally. You will see that it helps you gain relief from migraines, arthritis, and other ailments on a more physical level.

Reiki also relieves the symptoms of insomnia, asthma, menopause, and various other illnesses.

Reiki for Emotional Cleansing

Reiki aids in spiritual growth and emotional cleansing. It is not necessary to be a very spiritual person to benefit from Reiki; however, Reiki will help those who want support in their journey of spiritual or personal growth. Reiki is not a healing system that only targets a particular symptom; it addresses everything in the mind and body of that person. This is why it can induce subtle shifts from deep within. You will make better decisions in difficult situations and your attitude towards certain things will also see a shift. Reiki will help you gain a clear perspective, so you deal with issues more positively.

Reiki and Alternate Treatments

Reiki complements other treatments, whether medical or alternative. Reiki is a very effective and complementary healing system. It can be used even when a person is undergoing treatment from conventional medical methods. Reiki helps patients to relax both physically and mentally. This helps the patient to heal faster and more effectively under whatever treatment they are undergoing. Their sleep cycle improves, and their mind remains calmer. Since the system is noninvasive, it can be administered without even touching the patient. This is especially beneficial for patients who have significant physical injuries or have suffered burns. There are a lot of alternative medicines that have side effects when used on patients suffering from conditions like epilepsy, but Reiki is nothing but beneficial for them as well. Even a person undergoing chemotherapy can benefit from Reiki healing alongside their cancer treatment. Reiki aids and supports women throughout their pregnancy and even after they give birth; therefore, just about everyone can benefit from Reiki.

You Can Learn Reiki Yourself

You don't have to join classes or take courses to learn Reiki; to learn Reiki and practice it, a book like this is more than enough. The rest is just up to you and your openness towards the healing energy of Reiki. You can learn and practice Reiki by yourself to see some personal development or just to help yourself heal in any way.

On a physical level, Reiki supports the body's natural healing ability. It helps to release any toxins and blockage and also provides relief from pain. You will make better choices regarding food and also become more in tune with your needs.

On a mental level, Reiki helps you become aware of any negative thoughts and patterns. You will become conscious of your thoughts, and this will give you the power to control and change them. Your awareness will help you learn more about your thought process and help you consciously make better decisions even when the thoughts are negative.

On an emotional level, Reiki helps you accept who you are and love yourself. It is very important to practice self-love, and this is not the same as selfishness. Reiki will teach you to have compassion for yourself and others. You will connect better with the higher power, and it will give you a sense of belonging in a greater sense so you feel more present and connected and loved.

In general, there are many positive benefits of Reiki. It involves the universal force of light that is accessible to every single person. It is empowering and involves a healing and safe touch. Reiki complements western medicine and heals the body faster even after surgery. It helps to reduce pain and works like a sleeping aid. Reiki can reduce anxiety and brings peace and serenity. It will bring clarity of thought and also improves your capability to accommodate others. Reiki also helps in chakra healing and balancing. It is a tool for self-development and growth. Reiki also helps in aura healing and helps you access parts that lie deep within yourself. To put it simply, Reiki is limitless.

Reiki can be an incredible journey for every single person. You will see that it helps you become a better and stronger person just like it helped me. Reiki can be of extreme help when you are going through any tough situation in your life, and it will help you better deal with such things. As you embark on the journey of Reiki, keep reminding yourself of your daily progress and continue to reap the maximum benefits.

CHAPTER 5. Step-By-Step Reiki Learning Process

Level 1: First Degree

The first degree usually looks like a beginner process, where you will have an awareness of your energies. The process is as follows:

- What is Reiki?

- How it works

- A complete history of Reiki

- The principles of doing Reiki

- What are chakras?

- What is energy?

- How to place hands and heal yourself and other people

- Meditation that is guided

- Attunements

- How to do Reiki on animals, food, and plants

- How to practice daily

- Reiki ethics

Level 2: Second Degree

The second degree of Reiki is the continuation of the first degree. After getting awareness of your energy vibrations, you can learn the practical version of Reiki. The second degree contains the following teachings:

- Reiki symbols—mental, power, distant, and emotional

- How to effectively draw symbols on someone and how they work

- Attunement to the second degree

- Practicing the use of symbols

- How to heal someone from a distance

- How to prepare a room through symbols

- How to work with chakras and crystals

- How to heal someone on a deeper level

- Practicing healing on a regular basis

- How to set up your own Reiki practice

- How to keep a record

- Learning Reiki ethics at a professional level

Level 3: Third Degree

The third level of the Reiki practice is also called the master level. After completing this level, one can become a Reiki master. This master can be a practitioner that heals other people or a Reiki teacher. The process of becoming a Reiki master is explained below:

Usui Reiki master: You can become Usui Reiki master after getting first and second Reiki degrees. This degree requires a lot of experience in the field. You can become a Reiki master after giving one year of healing others. There are master symbols to open your energy canals.

Karuna Reiki master: This word is directly related to India and Buddhism. To become a Karuna Reiki master, you must first have to get attuned to the Usui Reiki. The Karuna and Usui Reiki symbols work together to heal anyone.

Reiki Healing Techniques

Gassho: Usually, the centering Reiki technique is performed for self-healing, but this is also a great tool to centralize your body before giving Reiki to anyone else. The name of this technique is Gassho. To perform this technique, you have to join your hands in a prayer position and keep your thumbs at your chest bone. Make sure your chin rests on your middle finger. While you are sitting in this position, concentrate on the chakras of your palms. Slowly exhale your breath and feel it on your hands. This amazing position quickly and efficiently controls your thoughts. You can automatically realize that your focus has also improved. However, if you feel that you have disturbing thoughts coming to your mind while doing this Reiki, let them pass. This technique can be performed for fifteen to twenty minutes every day, and it is an excellent tool to clear your thoughts.

Reiji-Ho: While sitting in the Gassho position, move your hands to the third-eye chakra. After doing this, place your thumb on the center of the third-eye chakra. This technique is really helpful to improve your intuition. Keep yourself in this position for some minutes and feel the Reiki energy moving in your body.

After performing both these centering techniques, move your hands and place them on your navel. This particular position is also called Hara or Tanden. This is the center of your body. If you focus on this part of your body, your focus will be improved. Doing this technique can improvise your Reiki. Whether you are doing it on yourself or on a friend of yours, this process can create a sense of balance. It can also be a practical position after the Reiki session, as it tends to grab the energy in the belly.

Clearing

Yes, you heard it right! You can also clear your space with Reiki. This process works to clear the negative energy in your room or any other place. It is really beneficial if you perform Reiki at a place where the energy level is good and is spread in a positive manner. You can clear a space to live there comfortably. You might have experienced something odd whenever you enter into a room. This strange feeling or sensation can be anything like imbalance. That is when you need to clear that space through Reiki.

The first step toward clearing a space through Reiki is to set up an intuition. Take deep breaths. The next part is to visualize as if you are grounded on the core of the earth. After this, visualize yourself being lifted up to the center of the galaxy. When you are meditating at this stage, imagine yourself at a balance in between both these positions. This alignment is really important. Visualization will lead to the calmness of your mind. Then imagine this room as a client and gently introduce your energy vibrations to the room. Behave as if this is your own room (in case it is not), then offer your intention to the room. Do Reiki to that room with your hands touching each wall, door, and furniture. After doing Reiki, visualize as if that room is filled with your positive energy.Finish your session by cutting cords and flicking away the vibrations you just created. You can also play a positive sound, like a bell or anything that attracts positivity to that room. Just remember that you can only clear an area when you are clear. You induce your energy to that room, so make sure you are positive before doing this.

Beaming

Beaming Reiki has nothing to do with touch. You can create energy and start sending to the person or thing you want to heal. In this type of Reiki, the energy is sent from the hands to the various parts of the body of that person. He or she may or may not feel energy moving inside the body. It does not matter. Reiki heals at a greater level.

Extracting Harmful Energy

The process of extracting harmful energy from the body is called shamanic energy extractions. This thing works to remove the bad energy, not the good one, out of the body.

Usually, bad energy is the vibrations that do not belong to the body. This condition can occur to anyone who is exposed to negative thoughts. It can even happen when a person does not open up to other people or stuffs his or her emotions. When this situation occurs, it creates a choking kind of situation. To be more specific, it creates blocked emotions or energy. The spiritual intrusion extraction is the removal of any such energy from your aura and chakras. Anything that is bad can cause it—for example, anger, jealousy, and even a curse. The symptoms of this energy block can be constant pain, suicidal tendency, depression, and more.

The process usually involves water cleansing or through crystals. If personal healing is not possible, distance healing can also be performed on a person.

Infusing

Reiki can also work on objects or nonliving things. Why stay limited when you can heal and lift up so many things through energy? Reiki can work upon anything and enhance the energy or aura of that particular thing. Performing Reiki on a number of things can enhance harmony, create peace, and soothe your place. You can use Reiki to balance anything that you tend to use every day. By doing so, that thing resonates with your energy and makes it easy for you to live peacefully.

Take your car as an example. Try balancing its energy through Reiki, and you may notice you are not feeling angry in the next traffic jam. Another thing can be your furniture. By performing Reiki on your furniture, you will feel more comfortable. If you have arrogant family members, Reiki can remove bad energy from the furniture that they use. You can also try doing Reiki to your bed so that you can sleep peacefully on your comfy mattress. You can even perform Reiki on your clothes, jewelry, or shoes to make you feel special and calm the entire day. Do you feel stressed every time your computer slows down? Then you can also try Reiki on your digital devices to keep you sane when they are not running properly. You can also do Reiki on your medications to heal you properly and create a positive vibe.

Smoothing and Raking the Aura

The aura is important when you are dealing with Reiki. You can smooth out or rake the aura through Reiki. And trust me, doing so can improve the Reiki procedure to 100 percent. It is like lifting up the aura of the person who is going to get healed. The aura smoothing can be done before and after the Reiki session.

Before giving Reiki to a person, build up your intuition and get ready to smooth out the aura. Just before you start doing Reiki, move your hands in the sweeping action. By doing this, you can connect to the energy field of that person. Take about a minute or two, and then start your Reiki procedure as you normally do.

When you are done with Reiki session or just after you remove your hand from the person's body, repeat the smoothing process again. This process acts like bathing because it clears any negative thought or energy out of the body of your client.

This entire process of smoothing removes any bad energy from the body of the Reiki receiver, and it stops that energy from bothering that person again. By doing this aura smoothing before Reiki makes it easier for you to do effective healing. Another benefit of doing this is that you can have a brief of the energy of that person just before doing Reiki to them.

CHAPTER 6. Importance of Reiki as Alternative Medicine

Space, or rather the entire Universe, is composed of energy. Science explains time and time again that energy is what makes up all living and non-living things. Essentially, energy is a reality. This includes your body. There is a host of electrical and energetic impulses coursing through your body all the time. It is this energy that reacts to the energy around you, as well as reacting to the Universal energy. The chakras are conduits for being able to align well with the Universe and the world around you.

Those that have reached Samadhi, or the highest level of enlightenment, are the few that have found the balanced joy of having completely balanced chakras at all times. Most people will not know this feeling. Instead, you will struggle like the rest of us, finding ease in some situations when the chakras are clearer, while other times, those same situations seem like a chore. The good news is that when you notice a chakra or two is imbalanced or not aligned, you can do some things about it. The hard thing is that your misaligned chakras will not be jumping for joy as you work to find balance. Healing yourself and fixing your chakras can be a mental challenge, if not physically challenging as well. Listed below are some of the great benefits of having aligned chakras, and more reasons why you should look to heal and balance your energy centers.

1.   Your physical health and well-being

Your life force, or prana, or energy, is moved through your body through the nadis. This energy courses through your body, passing through certain centers or "stations," known as your chakras. Similar to how you want to exercise and eat a good diet to help keep your arteries clear for proper blood flow, you want to do certain things to keep your chakra centers clear for proper energy flow. Imbalances or blockages occur during your normal, everyday life. For example, when you experience fear or negative emotions, you block energy flow. Also, if you have unhealthy lifestyle habits, you block your life force. Finding a balance in your chakras means you are able to better balance your spiritual, emotional, mental, and physical health.

2.   Your spiritual well-being

Just like your physical health, your spiritual well-being is important for ideal functioning in the world today. Being connected spiritually helps ensure you are calm and stable in your thoughts and actions. You receive energy from the spiritual realm first. It travels down into your body resulting in your mental and emotional experiences and, finally, your physical experience. This is why it is so important to address your spiritual health by balancing your chakras. This connection impacts all areas of your life. Your physical body and the spiritual realm are connected through your chakras. Making sure this relationship is balanced ensures your body is balanced. Typically, while balancing your chakras, you begin at the bottom and move to the top. This is like walking up a ladder from the bottom to the top, instead of trying to jump to the top of the ladder and ignore all the missing steps below. When you are successful at unblocking your chakras, your energy can flow freely in from the spiritual realm, balancing all aspects of your life. Only those that master their crown chakra can attain enlightenment or Samadhi. This is according to the Ashtanga yoga philosophy, as outlined by Maharishi Patanjali, a well-known Indian sage.

3.   Throwing out bad energy stored up in your body

Finding balance in your chakras means also finding balance in your mind and heart, as well. You live a healthier life, not because you are physically fit, but because you support your emotional and mental well-being. Clearing out negative energy blocked in these energy centers allows you to open up to healthier relationships, handle financial matters more effectively, and more. The waste that needs to be "recycled" from your everyday life needs to be removed. The more often you clear out this "bad" energy from your body, the clearer and more relaxed you will feel.

4.   Bring in more joy and love into your life

It may sound obvious that the Heart chakra is related to your ability to receive and give love; however, in order for you to feel joy and deep acceptance of yourself, you also need a clear second chakra or the sacral chakra. This is the place of true purpose and identity. Your heart is necessary for love, but your sacral chakra is necessary for fulfillment and vitality in your life. Sometimes, when this second chakra is blocked, you feel disconnected from your purpose, unsure about what you should do, lack creativity, and get overwhelmed emotionally. Those with a balance in this area often appreciate beauty and art and are typically more spontaneous. When you are searching for your purpose and happiness in life, it is wise to focus on clearing this center.

5.   Connecting to your inner self

This acceptance and clarity bring about joy and love. But you also need to heal and clear your first chakra to get a full appreciation of your true self. Your human body, or "mortal coil," is a tool for your soul's experience. The more you are connected to your inner self, or your soul, the better you understand this existence. This human body you reside in is a small piece of the Divine. Your aim in this world is to connect with the divine consciousness. When you understand this, you are able to detach from material objects and remove negative feelings like jealousy, greed, and anger. All of those negative attributes depress who you really are. Clearing them out of the way, freeing up your first and second chakra to disseminate energy properly, allows you to know your potential and tap into the consciousness of the Universe to live your destined life.

6.   Turn the weakness into strength

A chakra shuts down or blocks out negative experiences and feelings. Depending on the situation, it may shut down completely and need a "jumpstart." Sometimes, when you get stuck in a negative pattern, you keep this chakra closed off, not allowing you to grow and develop. Instead, when you unblock those affected chakras, you encourage the energy to flow in and out once more.

When your system works properly, you have the ability to turn your negative experiences into positive ones, learn from situations and turn bad habits or patterns into positive results. This is true and sustainable growth, but is only achievable when you are open, clear, and flowing.

7.   Improve your finances

One of the amazing benefits of clearing and balancing your chakras is your ability to manifest good things into your life. It is changing the negative and pessimistic views and comments into positive affirmations and requests. When you shift your focus on bringing to you what you need and releasing the things that no longer serve you, you are able to increase your access to the Universal intelligence and bring things to you that you need. This can be in the form of financial assistance. For example, repeating a daily, positive affirmation calling for money to manifest in your life through different revenue streams, you will see it come to fruition when you need it. Money is a common block for your chakras. It is a stress and a negative influence. Your financial matters sit in your first and second chakras, so clearing this block from there is necessary to a properly balanced system. To help you manifest positive financial matters into your life, make sure your first and second chakras are clear and choose a daily affirmation to call forward your financial needs.

8.   Turn your desires and wishes into your reality

When you are balanced and healed, you have access to your true purpose and potential. It is only then that you are able to bring your physical body in line with your mental body. This alignment creates a pathway for you to transform your life. It is this connection that allows you to accomplish your goals in life. You change your weaknesses or challenges into strengths and opportunities. You can bring to life all that you desire because it is what you are supposed to do.

9.   Improves your intuition

You have a little voice inside of you guiding you along this journey. This voice is your intuition and knows what your purpose is and what you need to do. The problem is that many people learn over time to ignore or suppress this voice. As you tap into understanding your true self, you give space for this voice to be heard.

And the more you clear and connect with your Crown and Heart chakra, the better you are at calling forth this intuition when you need it. This is different than waiting for the voice to speak, but rather encouraging the voice to start sharing. To help you tap into this intuition or internal guidance system, make sure you have your body and mind connected. Allow yourself to calm down and be still. Turn your thoughts to positive affirmations and intentions. Give yourself permission to release from your body and soul anything that no longer serves you. Anything that ruins your peace and suppresses your true self is not useful now and should be let go. When you are in this place, allow the positive energy to enter and circulate through your body and all the negative blocks leave your body.

10.   Learn how to express your emotions in a good way

Some people are great at revealing how they are feeling, but do so in a way that is overwhelming, or others struggle with showing their emotions and end up with either intense outbursts or complete shutdown. Sharing emotions is good and necessary, but it needs to be done in a calm and balanced manner. As you balance your chakras, you encourage positive energy to enter your body and negative energy to leave. As you do this, you allow negative emotions to be released. This helps remove the blocks in your energy centers. Sometimes, these emotions that you release are hard to express, but when you can release them, you can find a sense of completeness emotionally and physically. Once you let these emotions go, and feel through them, you are able to have a more balanced emotional state. You are more easily able to let go of anxiety, worry, sadness, anger, etc. Even stress is easier managed when your body is balanced mentally and physically. Stress is one of the leading causes of disease, so learning how to let this go is also vital to your physical health.

The Seven Major Chakras and Their Benefits

The seven chakras, as introduced earlier, are the Root, Sacral, Solar Plexus, Heart, Throat, Third Eye, and Crown. When one or more is blocked, you will receive messages from your body about it. If you are aware of these messages, you can act quickly on it to bring your body back into balance. Below is a breakdown of some of the benefits of the individual chakras on the body. More details for each chakra and finding balance will be shared later in this book as well. Keep in mind that some of the imbalances are either caused by an underactive or overactive chakra. This is why you will see something like not emotional and overly emotional on the list for what you would feel for an unbalanced chakra.

Your Root Chakra
If you are unbalanced, you feel:

- Insecure

- Unstable

- Insensible

- Unbalanced

- Afraid

- Nervous

- Attached to material items

- greedy

If you are balanced, you feel:

- Trusting

- Connected to community

- Connected to the physical body

- Secure

- Provided for

Your Sacral Chakra
If you are unbalanced, you feel:

- Insensitive

- Unemotional

- Not able to open up to others

- Overly emotional

- Promiscuous

If you are balanced, you feel:

- Sexual
- Accepted
- Confident
- Joyful
- Able to express emotions in a healthy and proper manner

Your Solar Plexus Chakra
If you are unbalanced, you feel:

- Indecisive
- Passive
- Aggressive
- Embarrassed about yourself

If you are balanced, you feel:

- Confident about yourself
- Certain in your thoughts and actions

Your Heart Chakra
If you are unbalanced, you feel:

- Cold
- Not kind or friendly towards others
- Heart palpitations or heart attack
- Jealousy
- Hatred
- Anger
- Grief and excessive sadness
- Fear

If you are balanced, you feel:

- A healthy state of appropriate sadness
- Forgiveness
- Awareness

- Caring

- Empathy

- Compassion

- Healthy relationships

- Peace

- Love for others and for yourself

Your Throat Chakra
If you are unbalanced, you feel:

- Lying

- Unable to talk or clearly communicate

- Shy

- Low self-esteem or self-confidence

- Bad listener

- Talks to much

If you are balanced, you feel:

- Confident in your self

- Able to share your thoughts and feelings clearly

- Creative

- Communicative

- Good at listening

- Honest to others and to their self

Your Third Eye Chakra
If you are unbalanced, you feel:

- Confused

- No imagination

- Overactive imagination

- Living in a fantasy world all the time

- Unaware of others' emotions and mental states

- Not smart or intellectual

If you are balanced, you feel:

- Intuitive

- Clear-headed

- Intellectual

- Wise

- Spiritual

Your Crown Chakra
If you are unbalanced, you feel:

- Rigid

- Thoughts are inflexible

- Depressed

- Bored

- Greedy

- Frustrated

If you are balanced, you feel:

- Connected to something larger than your self

- Engaged

- Content

- Awake

- Energetic

- Wise

- Satisfied

CHAPTER 7: Beginning the Session

Before you even begin your session, set somewhere between ten and twenty minutes to sit with your client and perform an intake. The intake is vital to a session as it is when you will be gathering the majority of your information. Clients should let you know of any health conditions or issues that they are or have experienced in the past. This includes illness, injuries, and surgeries.

An intake should cover some personal information about stress and emotional levels, as these can be indicative of energy blockages within the body, the same as physical ailments.

If it is the first time you are seeing a new client, the intake also serves as a time to get to know one another and to start building a trust bond. Trust bonds are the most important part of the client, practitioner relationship. A true trust bond is one of the best ways to retain clients, but it also ensures the highest vibration of work. Trust bonds can take some time to build but keeping the client comfortable and responding to their needs is part of that trust bond.

Once you have gathered the information in your intake, set the expectation for your client to get on the table. If this is their first session, giving them a quick rundown of what to expect, and a general overview of the hand positions is another way to ensure comfort.

Your client should begin to face up on your table, lying down, fully clothed, with their arms at their sides. Their legs should be uncrossed and flat on the table, or with the knees slightly propped up with a pillow or bolster.

Crossing of the limbs can impede the energetic flow in the body.

In the very beginning, you should perform and energetic scan of the body. This can alert the practitioner to areas of energetic blockages, areas that need a little focus, or potentially problematic areas in the body and energetic anatomy. This scan should be done before the practitioner begins using hand positions on the body.

The session can be performed with your hands directly on the client or hovering over their body. Some clients prefer not to be physically touched. Some of the hand positions should be performed over the body as they correspond to the pubic bone or the coccyx. This goes for other sensitive areas or injured areas. Make sure to move carefully, gently, and slowly. Lift your hands to move them from one position or another as sliding them along the body might be unsettling for your client.

The hand positions are static, and you shouldn't apply pressure. Your hands should rest gently on your client if you are physically touching them. If not physically touching them, hold your hands about four to five inches above the body. During the intake, you should ask if they prefer physical contact or hovering hand positions.

Each position should be held for three to five minutes. Intuitively feel out how long the position should be held. A full session is usually between 45 to 60 minutes, but it can be longer. During a session, pay attention to your client's body and how it is reacting. Changes in breathing, deep sighs, and even twitches or movement in the limbs and extremities often indicate positive energy changes.

Even though Reiki is intuitive and goes where they body needs it, following the hand positions can be important so you don't accidentally miss any areas of the body due to your own energetic influence. Intention for the session is important, and our own energetic frequencies can impact our intention. From the client's perspective, they often like to feel that their entire body is being touched and worked on.

It isn't necessary to have the client flip over midway through the session and work hand positions on their back, but some practitioners do like to work both sides of the body. If a client is asleep during a session, flipping them over can interrupt their energetic flow. To perform back positions on the front of the body, place your hands above the front and intend that the position is for the client's back.

Full Body Hand Positions

The following hand positions are a generalized guide. You can use your own hand positions, or adapt the ones in the picture as you like. This picture only shows hand positions for the front of the body, however, similar positions can be used down the back with the client lying face down as well.

Ending the Session

Some additional methods include placing the first and second finger of one hand over the third eyes chakra and the first and second finger of the other hand over the sacral chakra and then lift the hands off the body and into the air.

These final hand positions serve to balance internal energy but also close the client off to the flow of universal energy.

Sessions can be ended with a verbal affirmation to affirm that the client receives the healing and balance that they require from a Reiki session. You can also fluff the aura of your client at the beginning and end of a session to promote healthier energy in the aura.

After a session, give your client a few minutes to come back to their bodies and get up. Depending on their health or the intensity of their session, you may need to help them into a sitting position, slowly. Offer your client a glass of cool water. Anytime someone receives energy work, they should rehydrate, especially with the shifts in energy.

Make sure to drink water yourself and wash your hands with cool water to ground yourself. This serves to ground yourself again after you have opened yourself to energetic flow and frequencies.

After a session, leave another ten to twenty minutes to go through an outtake with your client. Ask them to share what they feel, or anything they experienced during the session. Everyone experiences Reiki differently. This is also a time to share any insights, visions, or feelings you received during the session in regard to your client.

Discuss what they might experience in the aftermath of a session and then talk about rescheduling a session or developing a treatment plan for regular sessions. Always remind them to stay hydrated the next few days after a session as well.

While you can't really overdose on Reiki energy, it is recommended that clients wait about a week between sessions. This will give the body and energetic anatomy time to adjust to the energetic shifts and changes the body experiences. Of course, for injuries or more serious illnesses, more frequent sessions may be necessary.

Considerations when Working on Clients

Anytime you perform any kind of energy work or bodywork on a client, there are some considerations to account for. This is true for Reiki as well.

While Reiki itself doesn't have any contraindications (specific situations in which Reiki shouldn't be performed because it may cause negative repercussions) these considerations are important.

Pacemakers give off electrical impulses in the body. There isn't any scientific validation for this, however, electronic devices can be impacted by energy such as Reiki. Avoiding performing Reiki near a pacemaker is a good practice to adhere to. This will ensure that the pacemaker keeps functioning properly during a session.

If working with a client who has a pacemaker, keep the hands and intention away from the heart center as a safety precaution.

Any clients who are on prescribed medications should carefully monitor any changes in their body, especially clients being treated for high or low blood pressure and using insulin for diabetes. Reiki can lower blood pressure and blood sugar. Advise your clients who are on medication to consult a doctor if any changes occur that may require adjustments in their medication. These risks are low in comparison to other bodywork methods, however, keeping your client informed about the potential risks will allow them to tread carefully and know to go to a doctor with any concerns.

During the intake process, you can have your client fill out a medical history form that includes any medications or current treatments they are undergoing. This form can also include a generalized waiver that informs your client of potential risks, but it is also important to verbalize this information for the client's benefit.

Keeping your clients aware and informed is another important aspect of that trust bond.

Prescribing and Diagnosing

A diagnosis is when a label is given to a specific symptom or set of symptoms that afflict someone. When a diagnosis is made in the medical field, it is often accompanied by a prescribed medication or treatment plan to fix the problem. Often times, prescriptions for a specific diagnosis are similar or universal.

Unfortunately, sometimes the conventional medical field forgets to take into account that every human body and experienced symptom is different and can react differently. This is the main reason that some people seek alternative treatments. Be aware that some clients might be coming to you frustrated that conventional medicine and diagnoses haven't helped them in the past.

Reiki is a powerfully intuitive tool. In many cases, you may experience a sensation or even a vision in regards to a specific area of the body, or a specifically known ailment. While giving your client this information is important, it is equally important to remember that as a Reiki practitioner you are not a doctor (unless that is a secondary profession).

Reiki Practitioners cannot legally diagnose or prescribe medications or treatments. This is a fine line because sometimes the information received in a session is very specific. For example, if you are working on a client who has chronic neck pain, and you get an intense energy vibration from the C4 and C5 vertebrae, then you may want to recommend that your client have a doctor or health care professional take a closer look at those two vertebrae. Recommendations are not diagnoses or prescriptions.

That being said, recommending treatment options, such as additional Reiki sessions, or recommending herbal tinctures, or supplements that you have knowledge on can instill a deeper trust bond between you and your clients. However, these can only be recommendations and suggestions.

Some suggestion or recommendation phrasing can sound like:

"I've had success with using this supplement to ease back pain."

Or *"There are some well renowned herbal tinctures that can be taken internally to reduce inflammation. I can provide you with a list if you'd like."*

Be sure to phrase any noted physical discoveries in a gentle and considerate way. If you discover a dark spot in your client that could potentially be a physical ailment, such as cancer or a cyst or abscess, stating that outright can be very alarming to a client.

Some phrasing options could be along the lines of:

"During our session, I noticed and energy block in this area of the body. It could be contributing to your pain and may deserve a closer look from a doctor or medical professional."

Or *"While I was working on you, I got a strong energy vibration from this part of the body. It might be a good idea to follow up with a doctor or health care professional."*

Keeping the conversation light and neutral gives the client important information about their session and options. It gives them the choice to pursue additional options outside of their Reiki treatments and may lead to a more definitive diagnosis or treatment without you crossing that professional boundary.

Each client and Reiki session is going to be different. These are the basic guidelines to follow when performing sessions on clients. There are also precautionary measures to consider whenever working with other people. Additionally, Reiki practitioners are not legally allowed to cross certain professional boundaries, knowing where those boundaries lie and how to still maintain a professional relationship with your client is key.

CHAPTER 8. Reiki Symbols

More practiced Reiki healers who have attained the second or Master level of Reiki are able to use the symbols sacred to Reiki. When using Reiki symbols the healer brings the person to be healed into the same zone of Ki, so the healer and the recipient are attuned to each other. This enables the healing energy of the practitioner to interact with that of their subject so the healer can be guided by intuition rather than simply carrying out a step by step generalized Reiki massage. When used during healing sessions they provide both protection and healing to the subject. The Reiki healer will use the symbols in order to focus their attention to connect with different levels of Ki using the appropriate symbol in order to activate and boost their Reiki energy. Reiki symbols have been passed down from Master to Master. When performing a Reiki healing the symbols have to be activated. This can be done in various different ways. The vital part of the successful use of Reiki symbols comes from the Reiki healer and the belief that the symbol can be used within healing and the intention. The symbols should then be applied initially on the healer's hands and then drawn or visualized on the crown chakra, the hands of the subject, and on any particular area that needs to be treated.

When initially introducing Reiki symbols into your healing sessions you can bring them into the healing realm of Ki by spelling out the name of the symbol three times, tracing the shape with your finger, using the palm of your hand to draw the symbol light on or above the person you are healing, drawing them through visualization through your third eye, or by simply visualizing and concentrating on the shape of the symbol. The most important aspect of using the symbols is that you intend for the symbol to assist you and draw on the associated energy during your Reiki healing. Masters of Reiki healing are so practiced in the use of the symbols that the physical aspect of the symbol becomes unnecessary and the intention and focus of the energies associated with each symbol becomes the center of their energy balancing. There are five traditional symbols of Reiki. Each has a different purpose and can be used in different manners to accentuate and focus the healing powers of Reiki. They were originally introduced by the Japanese monk Usui in order to assist students of Reiki in focusing their intent and to attune their Ki with their subjects.

The most powerful of all the Reiki symbols is the Master Symbol: Dai Ko Myo. Dai Ko Myo is used to bring healing to the soul and when utilized correctly can bring about life changes for the Reiki healer and the subject. It deals with the root causes of disease and illness by providing peace and enlightenment and aligning the soul and the spiritual self. The effect of Dai Ko Myo is to enable the subject to become more psychically attuned and intuitive to their own needs. The Power Symbol: Cho Ku Ray is primarily used in order to raise the level of Reiki power. It means I have the key. It enables the healer to draw energy from the environment and focus it where the healer intends. Again it is the intention of the healer to draw that power and focus it that gives Cho Ku Ray its power. When using Cho Ku Ray the words can be silently thought three times or the symbol can be traced over the healer or the subject.

Cho Ku Ray is a versatile symbol and can be used to manifest healing energies, to cleanse the spiritual body from negative energy – this can be both within the Ki of the subject, or in an area such as a hospital or an area where an accident or injury has occurred. Cho Ku Ray can also be used to cleanse herbal poultices, medical drugs, food, and water.

This symbol is often used in order to increase the healing power of other Reiki symbols and to ensure that energies that have been raised during healing treatments are protected and maintained. Cho Ku Ray is also excellent when focusing healing powers on specific areas of the body. If you want to use the Cho Ku Ray symbol on yourself then you should focus on the mirror image, reversing it, and that will channel the increased energies inward rather than outward. The symbol used primarily in order to deal with emotional healing and providing a sense of calm to the recipient of healing is the Mental / Emotional symbol Sei Hei Ki. Sei Hei Ki means the key of the universe. This symbol provides emotional cleansing and psychic protection. When dealing with afflictions that are governed by the mind as well as the body such as addiction, post-traumatic stress, and anxiety the symbol Sei Hei Ki is brought into play. A Reiki healer will use Sei Hei Ki when performing meditations prior to a healing session in order to cleanse their own Ki and make them more receptive and intuitive in their healing of another. The Mental / Emotional symbol provides balance and harmony by clearing emotional blockages, removing bad vibrations, and eliminating negative energies.

Reiki healing can be carried out both within close proximity where the healer will place their hands either above or lightly on their subject, or, remotely across distance. Healing can be carried out by focusing the life energies and sending Reiki across time and distance. Reiki healing can be transported to anyone and anything at any time utilizing the Distance Symbol: Hon Sha Ze Sho Nen. Due to the shape of the symbol this can also be referred to as the pagoda symbol. One of the main purposes of Reiki healing is to balance the life energies in the healer and in the subject. It is the unblocking and balancing of Ki that provides an access to the other aspects of Reiki. The freedom of energy flow within the spirit allows Reiki to benefit the whole body. The symbol used for balancing and grounding Ki and unblocking energy chakras to allow the flow of healing spiritual energy through the body is Tam-A-Ra-Sha or the Balancing Factor. If Tam-A-Ra-Sha is focused on a point of pain it can be used by a healer to reduce or remove that pain.

Whichever of the Reiki symbols you are using in your healing of another or of yourself the most important aspect is that the symbols are activated and that the focus is in the intention of performing the action of the symbol itself. Reiki symbols provide access to specific healing energies, used in combination they are a powerful tool to the healer and a source of positive healing for the recipient. When first working with Reiki symbols it might be difficult to remember the Reiki names for each of the symbols, using the alternative name for the symbol will not have any detriment to the symbol's use providing the intention is as strong, for example, if you're unable to remember Cho Ku Ray during a healing session it is possible to substitute the Reiki name with its alias: The Power Symbol.

More often than not, traditional Reiki masters avoid showing the Reiki symbols to people who are not yet attuned, specifically to the second level of the Reiki training. It is believed that the symbols were made public in a book that was published in Australia. Still, it is up to the Reiki master whether or not he/she will reveal the symbols to his/her students.

The Cho Ku Rei is the first symbol. It is regarded as the symbol of "power." Literally, it means "place the power here." It is a declaration to be awakened or to remember through letting go of things that hinder one from realizing his/her true nature.

The Sei He Ki is the second symbol. It is regarded as the "mental and emotional" symbol. It is also considered as the symbol for "harmony." This symbol emphasizes that one's focus should be in the present state and that each individual is believed to be a new creation at the present moment. The Sei He Ki is said to heal the mind, body, and spirit. It cleans and heals through eliminating the attachments that an individual has, which result in his/her illness or suffering.

The Hon Sha Ze Sho Nen is the third symbol. It is regarded as the "distant" symbol as well as the "connection" symbol. It is believed to come from a Buddhist chant, which means "a righteous man may correct all thought" or "right consciousness is the root of everything." Being in the right consciousness means being fully in the present state or in the present moment. Instead of "reacting," this symbol emphasizes "acting." Reacting depends upon one's ego or conditioning. More often than not, an individual's conditioning is the cause of his/her illness or suffering. Thus, by eliminating one's conditioning, he/she will be free to be in the present state to heal and respond.

These symbols are viewed as tools or a road map and not a destination or journey. In general, these symbols are activated by drawing each of them with one's finger/hand or one's mind. The symbol's name is either spoken out loud or just in one's mind, then visualizing to tap it three times. The pattern of activating the symbols is draw-name-tap-tap-tap.

CHAPTER 9. The Power Symbol

The Cho Ku Rei, pronounced as "sho-koo-ray," is referred to as the power symbol, or sometimes, the "light switch." This is because this symbol connects an individual to the energy similar to a switch when being turned on. The power symbol is said to make the energy come to surface while opening an individual to the Reiki energy channels.

The power symbol can aid in starting the flow of the Reiki. More often than not, practitioners use this symbol to begin their sessions by drawing it on their palms and hovering their hands to the air. Doing so is said to defeat negative patterns of resistance. Using this symbol in a particular area can lessen pain and clear spaces. The power symbol is also used for cleansing objects in an environment so that they can function for one's highest good. This symbol is drawn in an object to empower it with the Reiki energy.

Uses of the Power Symbol

The Cho Ku Rei is used for a number of purposes. Apart from starting a session to feel the connection between the Reiki source and energy, it is also used to center the power at each hand position as well as problem areas, if any. This symbol is also used by drawing it over an individual by the end of a session so that the healing energies would be sealed in.

Another use of the power symbol is to clear an area that is full of negative energies. For instance, the symbol is drawn to all the corners of a room, which is intended to be clear or filled with light.

The power symbol is also used for protection. This is done by drawing it on a paper and placing it under or on the things that are intended to be filled with the Reiki energy.

This symbol is also used during meditation by drawing it over on one's self. For instance, one can draw the Cho Ku Rei on a shower head before taking a bath. This allows the water to be filled with the Reiki energy while cleansing the individual.

Other Uses of the Power Symbol

Cho Ku Rei is also used to alter or enhance the taste and nutrients of food and drinks. This is done by putting the food or drink on top of the symbol for ten minutes. Many can attest that there is a discernible difference in the taste of food or drink, which was placed above the power symbol. For instance, a cheap bottle of wine can taste better when it is placed on top of the power symbol before consumption.

Another use of the Cho Ku Rei is enhancing the function of objects. For example, when a battery runs low, drawing the symbol over it can increase its charge level. Some people do this on their cell phone batteries. They draw the power symbol over their phones or their hands, and the batteries increase their charge levels.

Cho Ku Rei is also used to make cut flowers last longer than simply putting in a vase with water. This is done by placing cut flowers in a vase. The individual should then hold the vase around its base to channel the Reiki energy. Drawing the power symbol on a paper and placing the vase on top can also make the cut flowers last longer.

The Mental and Emotional Symbol—Sei He Ki

The Sei He Ki, pronounced as "say-hay-key," is referred to as the mental and emotional symbol. It is also regarded as the symbol for harmony. This symbol is used for healing mental and emotional customs and habits that are no longer working for an individual. It is also used for fighting off mental and emotional distress.

Sei He Ki is also used for acknowledging emotional issues and healing them as well. It also promotes positive behavioral changes. In addition, this symbol helps in releasing negative conditioning brought by past experiences through responding instead of reacting. According to Buddhists, ego is caused by conditioning. Consequently, eliminating the conditioning of life results in the freedom of an individual from suffering. Sei He Ki heals and releases the desires and conditioning to obtain oneness and harmony.

Using the Sei He Ki for healing is quite simple. One can simply use it while healing with the basic hand positions. It is also used during emotional meditation for releasing and heal patterns and forms of conditioning, which cause problems and sufferings.

Reiki Treatments and the Sei He Ki

The energy frequency that Sei He Ki produces is higher than Cho Ku Rei. The Sei He Ki is used for generating a balance between the emotional and mental planes. According to the surviving students of Usui, this energy of Cho Ku Rei creates a link with the spiritual, which is why it is regarded as celestial energy. Consequently, the energies from the mental and emotional planes are drawn together into harmony by the energy of the Sei He Ki.

When the Sei He Ki is drawn over one's body, there will be two effects. First, it enhances the energy flow through one's hands; and second, it directs the energy toward balancing the mental plane and releasing the emotional plane. Given that the Sei He Ki generates a high frequency, its effects are less discernible to the hands. In addition, although its energy is strong, it is finer and more delicate as compared to the energy of Cho Ku Rei.

The effects that Sei He Ki generates are diversified as the symbol can address tension, sleeplessness, traumas, stress, anxiety, and restlessness. It is also helpful in resolving emotional problems, including anger and sorrow. This symbol is also efficient in releasing emotional blocks, which may be caused by unresolved issues that were not dealt with properly. Furthermore, this symbol is also used for improving or altering personality traits and undesirable traits.

The Sei He Ki is usually applied in areas such as the heart, head, and solar plexus, which are considered the primary mental and emotional centers. According to the traditional Chinese medicine, there are different emotions held in various organs of the body. For instance, fear is often held in one's kidneys; joy is held in one's heart; anger is held in one's liver; grief is held in one's lungs; and sympathy is held in one's spleen.

As such, the energy of the Sei He Ki could be used specifically in those areas to address their imbalances and unwanted emotions. In Reiki, on the other hand, practitioners usually use their intuition to guide them to the areas that need healing.

Sei He Ki and Positive Affirmations

As one draws the Sei He Ki over the head, positive affirmations could also be used to help the subconscious mind accept one's intentions. Some of the most common affirmations include "You feel safe," "You are loved," and "You are calm, serene, and content," among others. There are a number of positive affirmations, which one can use as he/she works with the Sei He Ki on a specific area.

When using Sei He Ki with positive affirmations, practitioners start by sliding their hands underneath the head at the back of the client. The energy used comes from Sei He Ki through drawing it from above or visualizing the symbol over the client's head. Practitioners focus on the client's third eye as they pass along the positive affirmation or new thought pattern to the client. Others place one of their hands to the client's skull along the base while the other hand rests on the client's forehead.

Other Uses of the Mental and Emotional Symbol

Some other uses of the Sei He Ki include the following: (1) relationships—using the symbol as two related individuals lie in bed; (2) memory—using the symbol to remember such as when studying or preparing for a meeting; (3) goals—using the symbol to achieve one's plans, affirmations, ideas, and goals by writing them along with the symbol on a piece of paper; and (4) spirits—using the symbol to help lost souls or spirits travel "into the light."

The Distance Healing Symbol—Hon Sha Ze Sho Nen

Another aspect of the Reiki healing is the distance or absentee healing. Given that the Reiki system is a unique healing method, it can heal through the symbols, specifically the Hon Sha Ze Sho Nen, even without the physical presence of the healer.

The distance healing symbol allows one to send his/her healing energies to other people at a distance. It is used specifically when applying the hand positions is inappropriate such as when the client is sexually abused or with a burn patient. In cases where hand positions are irrelevant, the Reiki energy is sent from across a room or at a distance. This is referred to as "beaming," which is used specifically in Hon Sha Ze Sho Nen. This symbol is also used for karmic release. It is able to send the Reiki energy outside of space and time.

The distance healing symbols are composed of five elements, which translate to "no past, present, or future." The only precept of Hon Sha Ze Sho Nen is "now" or the present state.

Hon Sha Ze Sho Nen, unlike Cho Ku Rei and Sei He Ki, does not generate energy at a specific frequency. It sends the Reiki energy in such a way that one does not have to worry about distance or time. The surviving students of Usui claim that the energy of the Hon Sha Ze Sho Nen creates a state of mind that translates to oneness—that is, oneness with the universe, allowing a practitioner to transcend space and time.

The distance symbol is used to send the Reiki energy without putting one's hand to the client. It is able to send Reiki energy to someone in a different town, country, or continent.

Moreover, the surviving students of Usui claim that the distance symbol has various connotations. For instance, the associated kotodama is a "connection" kotodama, which allows one to send energy to another who seems to resist an emotional resist. For instance, one can visualize Hon Sha Ze Sho Nen over another's solar plexus to allow the emotions to connect and be released. If the other person is in need of improving how he/she expresses thoughts or emotions, a practitioner can visualize the distance symbol over the other's throat, heart, and solar plexus or throat to head to connect the emotional or mental areas with the center of communication. It may only take a few minutes given that the energy is not channeled as that with Cho Ku Rei and Sei He Ki.

When starting a treatment using Hon Sha Ze Sho Nen, a practitioner rests his/her hands on another's shoulders. The practitioner also visualizes the Hon Sha Ze Sho Nen in his/her head while saying its name for three times. This way, the Hon Sha Ze Sho Nen connects with the other person on a deep level or on all levels.

More often than not, using Hon Sha Ze Sho Nen for healing entails being guided by one's feelings instead of applying the symbol in an analytical or a calculated manner. It is important for the energy to flow and function when it deems appropriate.

Healing the Past

Just as the Reiki system of natural healing is effective in healing the present state, it can also be sent to the past for dealing with difficult situations that left a mark. For instance, Reiki can heal a situation involving a regretful argument with a loved one that still has an effect in the present state. An individual will be able to deal with such situation that transpired in the past and heal its effect simply by imagining the situation and sending the Reiki through distant healing. Sending the Reiki to heal the past does not mean that one sends the Reiki "back in time." It means that one is healing the effect that the bad or difficult situation caused, as well as how the individual interpreted the situation.

Sending the Reiki to the Future

One can send the Reiki to the future. For instance, if one will have a job interview, he/she can send the Reiki to the place of the interview ahead of schedule. This way, the individual will be filled with the Reiki once he/she is already in the interview proper.

Drawing the Reiki Symbols

The following steps can help in drawing the Reiki symbols:

First, draw the symbol in different ways. Simultaneously, one should imagine that the symbol is being drawn in the color violet, which is the color most associated with the Reiki. If it is difficult for an individual to visualize colors, he/she can intend the symbol to be violet.

Second, the name of the symbol should be spoken to one's self three times. This should serve as a mantra.

Third, the drawn symbol should be tapped using one hand or finger while saying its name. There should be a total of three taps. This way, the symbol is activated and generates its appropriate effect.

The symbols are usually drawn in various ways. One, an individual can draw the symbol with the palm of his/her hand, where the energy comes out. This is applicable when drawing the symbol over a room's wall.

Second, an individual can draw the symbol over the body, making sure that all fingers and thumb form a cone. The symbol should be drawn over the hand or a part of the body. It is important to take note that the Reiki energy can also come out of one's fingers.

If both hands are occupied, specifically when treating another person, a practitioner can trace the symbol, visualizing a Pinocchio-like nose. While imagining that the symbol is drawn through the "extremely long nose," the head movements used should be small.

Third, the symbol can be drawn using eye movements. A practitioner can trace the symbol over his/her hands or over a body part of a client or recipient.

When tapping the symbol, a practitioner can use his/her eyes or nose.

More often than not, an individual who mastered drawing the symbols can generate the desired effect simply through visualizing the symbols as a whole. Once the symbols become second nature to an individual, the latter can do away with drawing out the symbols.

CHAPTER 10. Ailments That Reiki Can Cure

Alternative treatment is a term that refers to various medical interventions that fall outside the scope of conventional medicine. Alternative treatment is increasingly becoming a common solution for people suffering from various ailments out there. The preference for alternative treatment can be attributed to the fact that there are various conditions that people might be suffering from, and the conventional is yet to come up with remedies for the same.

Furthermore, alternative treatment is considered less intrusive as compared to conventional; medicine with much fewer side effects. Ideally, alternative treatment is most effective when it comes to the treatment of non-life-threatening ailments and conditions such as stress. The treatment is also very effective as a compliment of mainstream medicine.

There are various forms of alternative treatment out there, and one such form is Reiki Treatment. Reiki Treatment is a unique treatment approach in which the energy from one person is transmitted to another through the arms. The Reiki practitioner places their arms on the affected body part of the sick person. The energy from the practitioner is then transmitted to the patient, and it is this energy that facilitates the healing process.

There has been a significant amount of skepticism when it comes to the effectiveness of Reiki treatment. This can be attributed to the fact that there is no clinical evidence that the treatment is indeed effective when it comes to addressing various conditions. However, perhaps the most reliable evidence that can underscore the need for Reiki comes from the people who have undergone this form of treatment at one point or the other in their lives. Many people have indeed come out and shared their stories on how this form of alternative treatment has had a positive impact on their lives.

Preparation for Reiki Treatment

Before you can use Reiki treatment on yourself and others, you must go through an initiation ceremony that will equip you with this unique healing ability. Most of the intricate details of the initiation process are considered high-level secrets and are revealed to the people attendees during the session. But generally, the process consists of four attunements that are administered over a four-day workshop. The attunements are meant to enhance the energy levels of the attendees to enable them to become Reiki practitioners.

Before attending the Reiki treatment workshop, there are various things that you should do. First and foremost, you should desist from taking alcohol or any other drug for that matter. Secondly, you should avoid eating meat, fish and processed foods. Ideally, you should maintain a diet comprising fresh vegetable products and fruits at least 48 hours prior to the workshop.

The initiation ceremony is headed by the Reiki master. The Reiki master guides the students through the attunement process. The master also uses various ancient symbols that are believed to convey universal energy to attendees, making it possible for them to be future Reiki healers.

Things to Do Before Commencing the Treatment Process

Once you have successfully gone through the initiation process, you can use Reiki to treat yourself and other people as well. There are several things that you must do in order to prepare for a Reiki treatment session. First and foremost, the setting and overall atmosphere of the room where the treatment is to be administered is very important. You should ensure that the room you are using for treatment is bright enough to facilitate energy flow. Bright colors such as white, yellow, or even sky blue can be used for the interior setting of the room.

It is also important to have a few plants in the room since plants can help the patient relax, and they also play a key role in the transmission of energy. Some good soothing music will also go a long way in enabling the Reiki practitioner to convey energy and the patient to receive the same. Reiki treatment is also most often than not an emotional affair, and patients might experience a flurry of emotions as the energy transmission process is initiated. To this end, it is important to have adequate tissues to be used by the clients during the treatment process.

Avoid alcohol and drugs

As a Reiki practitioner, it is important also to avoid alcohol and any other recreational drug at least forty-eight hours before attending to a client. This is because; alcohol is believed to inhibit energy transmission, thus undermining the overall treatment process. In addition to avoiding alcohol and drugs, enhanced personal hygiene is also important during the treatment session. Make sure you take a shower before attending to clients, brush your teeth, and avoid foodstuffs such as garlic that can undermine your breath.

Clothing and Jewellery

Your clothes can have a bearing on the effectiveness of the treatment process. Tight-fitting apparel can impede the flow of energy through your body, and consequently, you might not be able to adequately channel the right amount of positive energy to your clients. It is important to ensure that during the treatment process, clothing such as ties, tight pants, and shirts are not worn. Secondly, it is generally believed that jewelry attracts negative energy, which lacks the healing attribute that can help the client. For this reason, you should not put on any jewelry while attending to a client during a Reiki treatment session.

Invocation

This is a form of special declaration that you must make to yourself as a Reiki practitioner. Before the healing process, it is important to appreciate the fact that you are not a healer. As a practitioner, you are merely a vessel that can be used for channeling positive energy that can heal your clients. The invocation is very important since it reminds both the client and the practitioner that it is the universal energy that is available to everyone that performs the actual healing process. The invocation process might be in different wordings for different practitioners, but it must acknowledge the role of universal energy, otherwise referred to as Reiki in performing the healing process.

Undertaking the Actual Treatment Process

Before commencing the treatment process, there two things that are vital and you must remember. First and foremost, you should not subject anyone with a pacemaker to the treatment. This is because; the treatment might undermine the functioning of the pacemaker by changing its rhythm. Secondly, people suffering from diabetes should also be excluded from the treatment since it can interfere with their treatment for diabetes.

The General Position of the Client

The ideal position for the client is for them to lie flat on a table with both their arms and legs staying also resting on the table. The arms and legs should not cross since this position will prevent maximum energy flow. Once the patient is lying in the correct position, you should commence the treatment process by placing your hands firmly in the appropriate places. You should ensure that you are able to rest your arms at different parts of the body for at least five minutes.

Different Positions for Reiki Treatment

For a holistic Reiki treatment experience, the placement of the arm should cover the entire body. However, you can also offer localized treatment depending on the exact nature of the client's treatment requirements.

Head and Shoulder Positions (1, 2, 3, 4, 5, 6)

Position 1 entails the practitioner placing their arms over the central area of the client's face covering their eyes and check bones. Position 1 treatment is ideal for treating various conditions that might emanate from the nervous system, such as stress and cerebral nerves.

The position is also effective in treating addressing asthma, sinuses, and eye-related infections

In Position 2, the practitioner places their arms on top of the head. The position can be changed to ensure that the entire area on top of the head is covered. This position is used to facilitate the healing of heat-related ailments such as migraines and headaches. Position two can also be used to provide a remedy for digestive disorders, stress management, and even addressing eye-related ailments.

The third position is where the Reiki practitioner places their arms along the sides of the client's head. In this position, the practitioner covers the ears, and it is therefore considered very effective in providing a remedy for ear-related conditions such as hearing impairment. The eye also plays a key role in facilitating the balancing of the body, and thus, position three can also be used to correct balance issues. A range of other general diseases such as colds and flu can also be treated using this position.

Position 4 entails allowing universal energy to flow into the patient's body through the back of their heads. The practitioner thus places their arms at the back of the head and maintains this position for at least five minutes. This position can be used to treat mental disorders, including stress, depression, and phobias.

In the fifth position, the target area is the throat area. The rams are placed around this area and allowed to rest for the prescribed amount of time. Position 5 can be used to address breathing disorders; infections associated with throat are such as bronchitis, speech impairment and other such ailments that might significantly undermine the overall quality of life of the client. Finally, in the sixth position, the arms are placed on top of the shoulders. This treatment is good for shoulder pains and general body aches.

General Body Position (7, 8, 9, 10, 11 & 12)

Positions 7,8,9,10,11 and 12 are considered general body treatment positions.   These positions enable the practitioner to reach major body organs that are located at different positions. In the previous positions, the closest organ that the practitioner target is the brain.

However, in these other positions, the Reiki practitioner is able to facilitate the flow of positive energy to other areas, including the heart, kidneys, liver, lungs, pancreas, and stomach.

Precisely, in position 7, the arms of the practitioner are placed on the chest area, covering both the lungs and the heart. Positions 8 and 9 entail placing the arms over the lower areas of the frontal body, including the upper and lower stomach areas. Position 10 covers the genital area, while positions 11 and 12 cover the limb and feet areas respectively. However, it is important to note that while treating the genital area, there should be no contact with the client's body; instead, your hand should be placed above the genitals but close enough to allow transmission of universal energy.

Some of the diseases and ailments that can be treated by using positions 7, 8,9 10, 11 and 12 include digestive disorders, breathing disorders, ailments related to the reproductive system and joint pains, among others.

Back-Body Positions (13, 14, 15, 16, 17, 18, And 19)

After exhausting the head and frontal body positions, you should kindly ask the client to turn over so that they are able to lie on their stomachs. This will allow you to perform Reiki treatment in the back area starting from position 13, which is the back-shoulder area, positions 14 through to 17, which are the mid-back areas. Position 18 is the back-limb area, while position 19 is lower feet area. Reiki treatment administered at the back-body positions is important in the treatment of spinal cord infections, treatment of the reproductive system, varicose veins and even stress-related infections.

Balancing of Energy

A holistic Reiki treatment ends with a very important last step, which is facilitating the balance of energy flowing through the client's body. In order to do this, you will be required to place your arm at the top of their head and one at the bottom of the spine. By doing this, you will make it possible for energy to flow at all directions, ensuring that all body organs have the right amount of positive energy flowing through them. This will ensure that the client leaves your treatment room a much healthier, happier individual than they came in.

CHAPTER 11. How To Do Reiki on Yourself

For self-healing we are going to use the same hand positions at Level II that you already learned at Level I. However, at Level II these hand positions are merely a guideline. You are going to tune into your Reiki guides and follow their guidance. Using the symbols during your self-healing sessions will increase the power and effectiveness of your Reiki. Protection Don't forget to protect yourself, prepare your space, and call in your Reiki energy. Use the symbols to enhance your energy as you prepare.

State Your Intention

State your intention to your spirit guides of what you would like to accomplish. Here is an example but say what feels right to you in the moment.

Begin Self-Healing

Ask your guides to direct you and tell you what symbols would be beneficial to use at each stage. Before you start the hand positions you may be guided to draw a POWER SYMBOL over your Heart Chakra or visualize it over your entire body.

As you hold each self-healing hand position, ask your guides about the chakra in that area. Ask if you should use one, two, or all three of your Level II symbols by drawing them over the chakra. Follow your intuition as to how long you should hold each position and allow yourself to be guided to different positions as well.

When "drawing" the symbols, you can draw them on yourself as if someone else was drawing them over you. Alternatively, you can draw them out in front of you and direct them back toward you. Each time you draw a symbol over yourself, tap it into your body with your palm three times while saying the mantra of the symbol.

If you are unsure about which symbols to use, you may also simply draw all three symbols over each of your chakras. However, it is best to try to be guided by your intuition and your guides.

Specific Areas of Concern

If there is a particular area of concern, place your hands in that area and ask your guides if you should place one or more of the symbols there. (It doesn't matter if there is a chakra in the area or not.) For example, if you have trouble with insomnia, place your hands on your head (in whatever manner you are guided) and ask your guides if you should draw any of the symbols.

If you have an emotional issue but you are not sure what part of your body it is related to, ask your guides where you should place your hands. For instance, if you are asking about a relationship issue, you may be directed to place your hands over your Sacral Chakra. Alternatively, you may be directed to place your hands over your heart and to draw the MENTAL/EMOTIONAL SYMBOL over it. Perhaps you will be directed to place the DISTANCE SYMBOL over your Sacral Chakra to connect to a past life issue related to this emotional disturbance.

Concerns with Guidance

If you feel that you are not able to hear your guides or you are not sure whether you should do a particular symbol, it is always ok to go ahead and draw the symbol. You can also go ahead and do all three symbols over your entire body and then once again at each hand position, drawing them over the nearest chakra. End with the POWER SYMBOL, as this will enhance the other symbols.

Using a Pendulum

In a self-healing session, it is difficult to pendulum test your own chakras to see if they are open and properly rotating. If you feel that you really need the pendulum confirmation, ask Yes/No questions. Ask is my [*name of chakra*] open? A "no" answer, a very small or unclear "yes," or no movement at all may indicate that you need to send more Reiki to that chakra.

Sealing In the Reiki Energy

When you feel you have received enough Reiki at each of your hand positions and it is time to close, ask that the Reiki energy continue to flow to you after the session for as long as it is needed. Draw a POWER SYMBOL over your whole body again (if guided to). State that the Reiki session is completed in your highest of goodness.

Thank Your Guides

Ask again for the white light to cover you and protect you. Place your hands back in prayer position in front of your Heart Chakra and thank your Reiki guides and Masters, spirit guides, and all other healers that have helped you.

What Happens If I Fall Asleep?

If you do your self-healing sessions at night when you get into bed, it is quite common to fall asleep. This is fine. It is actually a good sign. It means you are relaxed and your Reiki energy is working on you, actually making you feel sleepy. Your Reiki guides will continue your session, giving you the symbols as needed, and will close your session when you have received all that you need.

SELF-HEALING HAND POSITIONS

To reiterate, do not be so concerned with doing the exact hand positions, but rather follow your guidance. However, I have included the hand positions as you may wish to use them as a guideline in your self-healing. These are the same hand positions you learned at Level I. However, at this level you are going to tune into your Reiki guides and use your psychic senses to direct the placement and duration of the hand positions. You may do these sitting up in a chair, lying down, or even standing.

1.   **Back of the head** – Place both of your hands on the back of your head in a slight V-shape around the back of your Third Eye. The base of your hands should be at the base of your skull and your fingertips should point in and up toward your crown. Imagine yourself as a channel, allowing the Reiki energy to flow from your hands to your head. This is soothing and relaxing. Visualize the back of your Third Eye as a cone of energy. It is a

deep, vibrant indigo (dark blue) light. Visualize it rotating at the proper speed and direction for you. Ask your Reiki guides for a stronger clairvoyant connection. If you have issues with over-thinking, insomnia, or other issues in this area, ask your guides why are you experiencing this. Ask for the Reiki energy to assist you in healing this and ask your Reiki guides if you should draw a symbol here. Perhaps use the Mental/Emotional symbol to calm your mind followed by the Power symbol to enhance the energy.

2. **Hands over your crown** – Place your hands over the top of your head with one hand on each side and your fingertips meeting at the top of your head (Crown Chakra). The Reiki energy is working on your mind, head, and crown. Visualize your Crown Chakra as a light that goes straight up to the sky. It is a deep, vibrant purple. Ask your Reiki guides for a stronger connection to Source. Ask your Reiki guides if you should draw a symbol here.

Perhaps use the Distance symbol to connect you to Source followed by the Power symbol to enhance the energy.

3. **Hands over your eyes** – Cup your hands over your eyes with your fingertips at the top of your forehead. The Reiki energy is working on your eyes and your Third Eye, helping you to see more clearly physically and spiritually. Visualize your Third Eye as a cone of energy in the middle of your forehead. It is a deep, vibrant indigo (dark blue). Visualize it rotating at the proper speed and direction for you. Ask your Reiki guides for a stronger clairvoyant connection. If you need clarity in an area of your life, ask your Reiki guides for help. Ask your Reiki guides if you should draw a symbol here. Perhaps use the Distance symbol to enhance your clairvoyance followed by the Power symbol to enhance the energy.

4. **Hands across the back of your head and neck** – Place your hands side by side on the back of your head. One hand should be at the base of your skull (top of your neck) and the other above (covering the back of your Third Eye). The Reiki energy is working on your mind, head, and Third Eye. Visualize the back of your Third Eye as a cone of energy. It is a deep, vibrant indigo (dark blue). Visualize it rotating at the proper speed and direction for you. Ask your Reiki guides for a stronger clairvoyant connection.

5. **Hands cupped over your throat** – Cup your hands in a V-shape around your throat. You are working on your Throat Chakra, which will enable you to speak up more confidently and clearly. Visualize your Throat Chakra as a vibrant turquoise light. Visualize it rotating at the proper speed and direction for you. Ask your Reiki guides for a stronger clairaudient connection. If you have issues with not being able to speak to someone about a matter, now or in your past, ask your guides for assistance. Try to release any hurt feelings or resentment you are storing and forgive those involved.

You may want to do this if you have, for example, a throat issue such as a sore throat. You may also ask for assistance for an upcoming meeting. Ask your Reiki guides if you should draw a symbol here. Perhaps use the Distance symbol to connect to another person and forgive them.

6. **Hands on your shoulders** – Place your hands, one on each shoulder. You may cross your arms if this is more comfortable. (Either way is fine.) This is soothing and releases the stress carried in the shoulders. Visualize any stress and tension being released.

Ask your guides for assistance with any issues in your life that you feel may be causing this tension.

7.   **Hands over your heart** – Place your hands with your fingertips touching over your Heart Chakra (a little above the center of your chest). The Reiki energy is working on your Heart Chakra. Visualize your Heart Chakra as a deep, vibrant emerald light. Visualize it rotating at the proper speed and direction for you. If you have any heartache or past issues stored in this area, talk to your guides about it and ask for assistance in healing. You may also visualize the color pink (which represents love) being given to your heart. Try to release any hurt feelings and resentment you are storing and forgive those involved. Ask your Reiki guides if you should draw a symbol here. Perhaps use the Mental/Emotional symbol to calm your heart followed by the Power symbol to enhance the energy.

8.   **Hands over your Solar Plexus** – Place your hands with your fingertips touching over your Solar Plexus Chakra just below the center of your chest.   This is your confidence center, your advertising center, how others see you in the world. If you or your business is not receiving the attention that you would like, ask your guides for assistance. Ask your Reiki guides if you should draw a symbol here. Perhaps use the Power symbol to enhance the energy.

9.   **Hands over your navel** – Move your hands slightly lower so that your fingertips touch over your navel. You are directing Reiki to your internal organs. Visualize your internal organs working efficiently and effectively. If you have any issues such as indigestion, ask your guides why you are experiencing this. Ask your Reiki guides if you should draw a symbol here. Ask if there are any specific organs that need strengthening. If so, perhaps you will be guided to draw the Power symbol.

10.   **Hands over your Sacral Chakra** – Place your hands on either side of your groin area. The base of your hands should be on or near the hipbones and your fingertips should be over the pubic bone. You are directing Reiki to your Sacral Chakra. Visualize your Sacral Chakra as a deep, vibrant orange light. Visualize it rotating at the proper speed and direction for you. If you have any relationship issues, past or present, they will be stored here. Talk to your guides and ask for assistance in healing. Try to release any hurt feelings and resentment you are storing and forgive those involved. Ask your Reiki guides if you should draw a symbol here. Perhaps use the Distance symbol to connect you to a past relationship that you need to forgive and release.

11.   **Hands over your lower back** – Slide your hands behind you to rest at your lower back (just above your hips). Your fingers should be pointing downward and touching the upper buttocks. You are directing Reiki to the back of your Sacral Chakra. This area represents finances. A lower backache is an indication that you are disconnected from Source and do not trust that you are in the flow of abundance. It often comes from feeling that we have to support others. Visualize the back of your Sacral Chakra as a deep, vibrant orange light. Visualize it rotating at the proper speed and direction for you. Talk to your guides and ask for assistance in healing.

Trust that there is abundance for all. Ask your Reiki guides if you should draw a symbol here. Perhaps use the Power symbol to enhance the energy.

12.   Hands over your Base Chakra – Slide your hands underneath each buttock cupping the fold where it meets the top of your leg. If you are lying down it may be easier to draw your knees toward your chest. You are directing Reiki to your Base Chakra. This area represents your early childhood, where you are going in life, your soul purpose, and how balanced you feel. Visualize this chakra as a deep, vibrant red light. Visualize it as a light going from your tailbone down to the ground. If you know you harbor ill feelings for things that happened in your childhood, talk to your guides and ask for assistance in healing. Try to release any hurt feelings and resentment you are storing and forgive those involved. Ask your Reiki guides if you should draw a symbol here. Perhaps use the Distance symbol to connect you to a family member who you need to forgive.

13.   **Hands over your knees** – Place one hand over each of your knees. If you are lying down it may be easier to either draw your knees up toward your chest or to lean forward, covering your knees from a seated position. If you prefer you may just envision that you are touching your knees without actually doing so. We have small secondary chakras in our knees. If you have issues with your knees, ask yourself what you are not being flexible about. What are you afraid of moving to or from? The right knee is indicative of issues having to do with emotional relationships or spiritual matters. The left knee is indicative of issues having to do with practical or physical matters. Ask your Reiki guides if you should draw a symbol here.

14.   **Cup the soles of the feet** – As you cup the soles of your feet visualize tree roots of white light going from your feet into Mother Earth to ground you. This completes the circuit of energy and is very balancing. Ask your Reiki guides if there are any symbols needed anywhere else or if there is another area that you should send Reiki energy to.

15.   **Close the session and thank your guides** – Ask your guides to continue sending you Reiki for as long as it is needed. Disconnect your energy and thank your Reiki guides and Masters, spirit guides, and all other healers that helped you.

CHAPTER 12: How to Do Reiki on Yourself

Most people begin their journey of Reiki healing by practicing on themselves. It is necessary to start with yourself before healing others, as you must be physically and emotionally healed to be able to accept the healing energy of Reiki and channel it through your body. Though many people choose to take courses to ensure they are connecting to Reiki energy and using it to its full potential, it is possible to learn Reiki for beginners on your own. If you find yourself struggling, don't be afraid to look up tutorials or signup for a class nearby. This can help you take your Reiki connection and education to the next level.

Step 1: Connecting with Reiki Energy

Creating with Reiki energy is about connecting with a heightened state of consciousness. In this state, you are aware of your connection to the life energy that flows through all the Universe. It should flow through effortlessly. Though connecting with Reiki energy is only the first step of practicing Reiki, it can be the most challenging for beginners. Do not become discouraged if you struggle with connecting to this heightened state, especially if you have not practiced any type of meditation before.

There are two parts to connecting to the Universal energy. First, you must speak to the Universe, let go of your ego, and open the connection to the wisdom and energy of the Universe. Once you are an open conduit for energy, you may use a visualization technique to feel the energy flowing through you.

Reiki Invocation

When you enter the state of mind that allows you to connect to Reiki energy, you are connecting with the consciousness of Universal Energy. To do Reiki Invocation, it is as easy as speaking to this energy of the Universe and asking it for permission to conduct its energy as a healing channel. When you speak to the energy, you should have a calm and clear mind. Beginners sometimes start their session with a few minutes of meditation to get them in the right frame of mind.

Once you are relaxed, you will be able to speak to the Universal consciousness aloud or silently.

It does not necessarily matter how you ask to connect to this Universal Energy. You should choose to speak with the energy in a way that aligns with your own beliefs. However, the overall goal should be to pass on a pure form of healing and unconditional love. Once you have decided what to say and are ready to speak to the universe, place your palms together and position your hands in front of your heart chakra, as if in prayer. This is done using the heart chakra because healing must come from a place of love. The heart is the core of the emotions and the core of the soul. Once you are ready, you might say something like:

"I call upon the energy of the Universe and the energy of all the Reiki conduits of the past, present, and future to take part in this healing session. I call these energies near to me to create a stronger connection to the Universal energy.

I ask that these energies give me the infinite wisdom to channel this energy. I ask that the power of the Universal Energy flows through me and allows me to conduct unconditional love and pure healing, as well as grants me the knowledge to use and direct this energy where it is needed most.

I ask to be empowered through the blessings and divine love of the Universe."

It is important as you ask for this permission that you allow your shift to focus. You should not be focusing on yourself or your own ego being granted the ability to heal. Instead, you must raise your own consciousness and allow your questions to raise your vibrational energy. You must be in line with the Universal Energy so that the energy can flow through you as if you are a channel for its healing benefits.

Notice how as you speak to the universe, you are asking permission to be a conduit. You are not asking to be a healer or to make your own decisions in healing but are instead asking to be a conductor for the knowledge and wisdom of the universe. For this to be effective, you must allow your ego to float away and align your beliefs with the Universal consciousness, which is a higher state of knowledge and truth. As you settle into this greater power, you must let go of those beliefs that do not align with the laws of the Universe.

Visualizing Universal Energy Entering Your Palms

The Universal Energy is not something that you can physically see, as it exists beyond a physical level of reality. This is the reason you must allow your mind to enter an altered state of consciousness to connect to it. Visualization can help you 'see' this connection beyond the realm of reality. As you bring that into your mind, you will physically feel the powerful energy of the Universe coursing through you. Here is an example of a visualization you may use:

Begin by closing your eyes and breathing in deeply. As you let go of this deep breath, see bluish-white energy beams as they surround you. These energy beams stretch from the ground, like threads connecting the grounds of the earth to the sky and beyond, connecting all that exists in the Universe.

As you become aware of these connections, feel yourself bathing in this light. Take another deep breath. As you release it, focus your energy on your palms, speaking to the Universal Energy around you. Breathe in the infinite light and call it into your palms, visualizing the light entering your body. As it flows through your body and out your palms, they glow with an energy that has a cool, white color. Now, you should be able to feel the Universal Energy radiating through your palms.

As you do the visualization technique, keep in mind that it does not matter what the energy looks like. While visualizing it can help, you should sense or feel how the energy appears. Not everyone can physically see this energy, but that does not matter.

It is your willpower and your willingness to connect to the Universal energy. It is your thoughts and willpower, as well as your willingness to be used as a conduit for the energy of the Universe, which creates the reality of your ability to heal.

Step 2: Performing an Aura Scan

The way that people perceive the existence of auras is often incorrect. Your body does not create an aura or give off a type of visible energy. Rather, the aura describes a Universal energy. This energy surrounds all living things, but it is not really around it. A person's aura is not projected, as it exists within the body, too. The body is overlaid on the spiritual energy that is an aura.

Your aura is part of your energy system. It absorbs and puts off information, working much like the brain in the way that it is able to transmit and receive signals from the world. Everything that is inherently you exists within the aura, affecting its overall health. It is a collection of your vibration, as well as your memories, experiences, thoughts, and emotions. When you are experiencing a negative emotion, it can distort your aura and affect its health. For example, some negative thoughts may show up on your aura as a muddy, dark blob. Once it takes hold, this may present as a physical symptom.

Many people are aware that auras have different colors that transmit information about the mind and body. In addition to different colors, auras have properties including size, pattern, shape, and texture. The color also does not have to be solid, such as the case of certain textures or discolorations.

Doing an Aura Scan on Yourself

Once you have connected with the Universal energy, you should feel the energy around you. Close your eyes to help with your visualization of this energy. Then, position your hands so they are just above your head, with your palms facing your body. You should either use your dominant hand or both of your hands for this exercise. Hold your hand(s) out in front of you, anywhere from 2-10" away from your body.

The first time that you move your hands down your body do a quick overall pass from your head to your hips. The base of the spine holds the root chakra, which is the lowest. Notice how you feel overall to gauge your energy. Then, do a second pass and be aware of the differences you might feel in different areas. Some areas may feel as if the energy is thicker or thinner, either speeding your hand along or slowing it down as you pass through. You may also sense subtle vibrations or temperature differences. If an area feels cooler, it means that the energy is flowing out. If it feels hotter, more energy is being drawn inward.

When you do notices differences, it is because your energy may need assistance or because it is in a state of change. This is when you move onto the next step using a targeted approach. You will have more success with aura scanning the more you practice. As you have more Reiki sessions, you will also find that you are more in tune with your body and what it needs for your energy to flow freely.

Step 3: Setting Your Intention

Setting your intention is as simple as stating what you want. By knowing what blockages or disruptions you are experiencing, you can trace this back to the root problem. By using a targeted approach and directing Reiki energy, you can heal specific ailments. Some examples of problems commonly healed during a Reiki session include:

- Achieving Spiritual Balance
- Reduction of Pain
- Reduced Stress
- Promote Healing of Trauma
- Promote Healing of Obesity
- Restoration of Relationships
- Improved Sleep
- Connect to a Higher Purpose
- Ability to Overcome Addiction

- Increased Positivity in Emotional State

You can think of your intention as a message. You are communicating to the aura, whether your own or another person's. This communication states your desired outcome and by directing your energy to that outcome, it strengthens the results. For your message to be heard, it must be clear and strong. As the Universe grants this request, the aura reflects that intention and heals the body and/or mind.

Setting your intention can be greatly improved by using Reiki techniques in combination with visualization. As you are focusing on your intention, visualize the outcome. Visualize how the outcome will change your life. Feel yourself becoming happier and focusing on more positive things, like going out dancing with your friends or having more time to spend with your significant other. Focus on the pain going away or on resolving whatever is holding you back.

For visualization to work, it must be incredibly vivid. Imagine how you would feel if your intention were to come true. Feel the relief of pain, whether emotional or physical. Imagine how you would look and feel if you were able to overcome your weight loss struggles or how refreshed and invigorated you would feel if you were able to get a full night of sleep. If you are healing someone else, visualize the changes that may come about and how they would feel if you were able to heal them. Combining visualization with setting your intention can have profound benefits and increase your Reiki healing power.

Step 4: Activating Reiki Symbols

Reiki symbols are symbols that you create with your hands that improve your ability to heal, transmit energy, and more. There are several symbols commonly used during Reiki, depending on your intended purpose and whether you are practicing on yourself or someone else.

To learn how to tap into Reiki power on a deeper level, it can be helpful to learn these symbols. While they will be described here, it would be impossible to describe how to do them in writing. You can find tutorials, charts, and other guides online that will help you with activating Reiki symbols the proper way. You could also take a class or speak with a Reiki teacher about learning these symbols.

The most commonly used Reiki symbols include:

- Cho Ku Rei (Power Symbol)- The power symbol can amplify many things. It is commonly used at the beginning of a Reiki session to help amplify healing energy, as well as provide spiritual protection that people need when they are connecting to the aura of others to heal them. It may also be used to empower other symbols or infuse food with energy.

- Hon Sha Ze Sho Nen (Distance Symbol) - This symbol is about enlightenment, peace, and unification. As it unifies, healers typically use it when they are healing someone across a distance. It can also be used to send attunements across distances, allowing people to open their chakras and be receptive to the wholesome, healing energy of the Universe.

- Sei He Ki (Mental & Emotional Reiki Symbol) - This symbol is ideal when you are trying to heal yourself (or someone else) mentally or emotionally. It is attuned to the energies of love and wellbeing in the universe. Not only does it create a calmer mental state, but it may also be used to help someone release negative energies or remove addictions.

- Dai KO Myo (Master Symbol) - As the name suggests, the Master Symbol is the most powerful in Reiki. Often, it is only Reiki Masters that can connect with this symbol. It is used to create wondrous life changes, to heal the soul, and to relieve the body of disease and illness in the aura.

Step 5: Guiding the Energy

One of the biggest mistakes that beginners in the world of Reiki healing make is believing that hand positions take priority over the other parts of the Reiki healing process. Things like being able to connect to the higher consciousness that allows you to access the energy of the Universe and setting your intention are much more important. However, it is possible to guide Reiki energy, especially when you are targeting a specific area of the body.

To direct Reiki energy, simply place your hands over the area you want to heal. Visualize and feel the energy flowing as you state your intention. If you are doing a full body Reiki session, then simply moving your hands over the body will be enough. As you guide the healing energy to the areas of your body that need it most, it is important to state your intention for each individual area you are trying to heal. Repeat steps 3-5 as many times as you need to before closing the connection. You will be finished when you can do an aura scan without feeling blockages or disruptions in energy.

Step 6: Closing the Connection

Another mistake that Reiki beginners often make is failing to close the connection between themselves and the Universe, or themselves and whoever they are trying to heal. When you fail to close the connection, you may absorb any negative energy that was released from your aura or the aura of the person you are trying to heal. If you do not close the connection, you can carry these emotions around and it may make you feel ill or exhausted.

The key to closing the connection is releasing any of the negative energies that have accumulated in your system. You can do this easily by visualizing all the negative energy flowing out of your body through your palms, releasing any negative energy that is stored in your system and leaving you in a rejuvenated state. As you connect with your typical energy, you will find yourself returning to your normal state of consciousness.

Many people also wash their hands with cool water following a session to help them remove residual energies that may linger behind on the hands.

CHAPTER 13: Energy-Shielding, Cleansing and Protection With Reiki

Many of the healers I know are natural psychics and empaths. This means that they are particularly susceptible to absorbing the energies of others and being influenced and overshadowed by the general, pervading energetic vibration of the environment in which they live. This environmental vibration might include the toxic thoughts of less compassionate souls, the pain and suffering of others, the worries and fears of others - particularly in these fretful times – as well as chords and attachments from energy vampires. I know it all sounds a bit extreme, dramatic and not particularly pleasant, but please bear with me.

Practitioners who are new to working with energy will sometimes be frightened by all these things, but there's no need to be frightened as long as you know how to clear your energy, keep it clear for as long as possible and shield it from further intrusions.

As we mature in our spiritual development, we discover that learning how to keep our energy clean is often as simple as learning how to keep our bodies and our homes clean. As long as you have the tools, you can use them effectively and live in a nice, clean, energetic environment where everything and everyone thrives and grows.

Many Reiki masters and practitioners believe that none of this cleansing and clearing is necessary, as Reiki can take care of all the energy clearing and protecting we could possible need. There is some validity in this, for example, using the Power Symbol can be extremely effective for both clearing and protection. However, different methods serve us at different times and in different situations, and its fine to have a range of tools and resources to uplift the energy within and around you.

Below are some of the tips I have found effective for energy-clearing, mostly using Reiki:

Personal Energy-Clearing Tips

Visually draw the Power Symbol on the palms of both hands and carefully run them over your head, face, torso, arms and legs in a soft stroking motion

Draw the Power Symbol in front of you, behind you, to your left and to your right, and feel yourself held within its energy. Feel any negativity being draw out of your energy field and cleansed and neutralised harmlessly. Stop when you feel lighter and clearer.

With your hands in the gassho position, call in the presence of Reiki. Build the energy by drawing or visualising the Power Symbol in your hands, and once you feel the energy flowing powerfully, hold your hands a few inches above your head and imagine a vibrant Reiki shower raining down on you, washing through your energy system and removing from it all forms of negative energy.

Energise some small crystals with Reiki, for example, clear quartz, black tourmaline or labradorite and set the intention that they will keep your energy clear. Start by sitting quietly with your eyes closed, holding the crystals between your hands in the gassho position. Call the Reiki energy into your hands and humbly ask that the stones be cleansed and energised to carry and amplify the power of Cho ku Rei. Repeat the mantra in your mind several times until you feel the energy flowing into the crystals. (If it's more convenient time-wise, you can combine this with your gassho meditation). Hold the position and the intention for 20 minutes and then carry or wear the stones on your body for the rest of the day.

Fill a large glass bottle with filtered water and hold it in your hands. Ask the Reiki energy to flow into the water and repeat the Cho Ku Rei mantra in your mind several times until you feel the energy flowing into the water. Hold the water and the intention for 10-20 minutes and then sip the water throughout the day.

Add several drops of lavender essential oil to a small spray bottle filled with distilled water. Hold the bottle between your hands in the gassho position and ask the Reiki energy to flow into the water and the oil. Repeat the Cho Ku Rei mantra in your mind several times, visualise it in the space around you and draw it on the bottle with your finger. Continue to draw the symbol and repeat the mantra for 20 minutes and then use the spray to cleanse your aura whenever you feel the need to refresh your energy or uplift yourself emotionally.

Treat yourself to regular self-healing, using the Power Symbol until your energy field grows stronger and more resilient. Draw the Power Symbol into each of your chakras and visualise it clearing and unblocking any stagnant energies held in each one.

Space-Clearing

Draw the power in each upper and lower corner of the room you're working in. Draw a Power Symbol over the door and on all the walls, depending on how intense the need for protection and the size of the room. Use your intuition

Call in the Reiki energy to run through you, and direct it out into the space around you

Use intuitive hand positions to fill the walls of your room with Reiki energy, then draw the Power Symbol on each wall and on the ceiling, and energise them all with energy from your hands

Use the Reiki-energised energy clearing spray (above) as a room spray.

Energy-shielding and protection

Wear Reiki-energised crystals, not only for energy-clearing but also for added protection – You can now even buy palm stones, which are engraved with the Power Symbol. Do some research into Reiki jewellery and see what you find and which pieces you feel drawn to

Draw or visualise a giant Power Symbol in front of you and carefully step into it

Draw the Power Symbol in front of you, behind you, to your left and to your right, and feel yourself held within their energy. Visualise each symbol turning into a solid gold structure and see golden threads joining the symbols together until they form a protective circle around you

Visualise a golden cloak made up of little Power Symbols and see yourself putting it on, over all of your energy bodies. Take your time building up the picture and see it going over your shoulders, and covering your head and third eye chakra. See yourself zipping it all the way up to your chin. Sit quietly for a few minutes, giving yourself time to notice any vibrational shifts or changes in your energy

CHAPTER 14: Basic Bioenergetics

Reiki is included in what is being called energy therapies. I prefer to use the word "bioenergetic" because I consider that in many cases these therapies handle terms that are difficult to identify with what is commonly understood by energy (electric, magnetic, light, heat, etc.). Within the concept of "bioenergy", we will understand "non-material influences" of different types that exert their effects on humans in very different ways. These influences in the West have been called energy. Probably trying to make use of the concept of "energy" as opposed to that of "matter". In this way, all those who do not use a material vehicle directly to exert their effect are considered as energy therapies. In other cases, the concept of the "spiritual" is used as opposed to the "material". Thus, it is common to mix or not differentiate energy and spiritual therapies. In this manual, we will use the term "bioenergetic" to refer to both one and the other and we will see that Reiki can fit into both classifications.

The "non-material influences" I referred to have been contemplated by different cultures since ancient times. Some of these influences have been understood and explained, more or less completely, by science. Some examples may be solar radiation or natural radiation of different types, which influence the state of health in different ways. In other cases, these influences turned out to be "non-tangible" rather than "non-material". The clearest example may be that of microorganisms or germs present in certain diseases. Science has studied many of these "energies" by giving them names and explaining them to a greater or lesser extent, but there are others, of which ancient cultures speak to us, but to which science has not given a definitive explanation or cataloging.

Each culture has given these influences different names and has given them an explanation from their cosmology. In this sense it is interesting to note that in the West there has been a separation between cosmology (study of the physical universe) and metaphysics (study of the spirit), but in other cultures the spirit is inherent in the physical world, so that the one does not It can be understood without the other.

Today many people are interested in studying the knowledge that comes to us from these ancient cultures, assimilating or understanding them from our own mentality, thus creating "Western bioenergetics".

This knowledge comes to us impregnated in the language and spirituality of these countries, and their understanding and adaptation to our way of life, our religious concept, and our science are complicated on many occasions.

In the effort to access the information contained in this knowledge it happens that sometimes we distort and confuse their meaning. Other times we find that the approaches made to us from these traditions seem to directly contradict what our science and culture teaches us, making reconciliation impossible. In other cases, more than it may seem, we can observe how the human being has understood since ancient times things that only recently science dares to raise, being the old permits perfectly identifiable with current scientific approaches.

If we ignore possible frauds, purely personal opinions, and intentionally falsified information, all the Cosmo-logical approaches that we find in other ancient cultures are compatible, in one way or another, with current scientific knowledge. It is only necessary to be able to see the pyramid from all angles and understand that there is the last vertex that unites all the ways of seeing the Universe: the need to understand the outer and inner world, the ultimate reality and thus be able to approach the state of balance longed for by the human being.

Of the cosmological systems that come to us from other cultures, some of them attract attention because of their apparent globality, universality and practical immediacy. Among them, we can highlight two that have been mostly chosen: the Tantric and Taoist culture. The one and the others have reached the West by the hand of Yoga and Traditional Chinese Medicine, two practices that we have adopted in our culture as an alternative means of enhancing our health.

Originally the ultimate goal of one and another system is not limited to seeking the improvement of the health of the individual. What we find in his teachings and practices is a description of the manifestation of the spirit in this world and tools to achieve its total integration into our lives. For what purpose? Reach the state of harmony in each and every aspect of our life and come to live with a special connection with the universe. This total harmony will be, from now on, what we will consider as integral health.

Probably, of these two knowledge sectors, the closest to Reiki is Taoist. Its founder, the Japanese Mikao Usui, was a student of esoteric Buddhism arrived in Japan from China. One of the disciplines he studied during his youth was the Kiko, a variant of the Chinese Qi Gong. The Qi Gong is one of the disciplines encompassed in Traditional Chinese Medicine, deeply influenced by the Taoist view of nature. One of the practices of Kiko is the accumulation of Ki (a concept that we will discuss later) in the body in order to use it to strengthen one's health or transmit it to other people for healing. Possibly in this practice is the root of what would later be the Usui Reiki Ryoho. Studying the Taoist conception of nature and health, we are probably studying the basis on which Usui supported his natural healing system, so this will be one of the driving pillars of this manual.

On the other hand, since Yoga is a practice known to the public for a longer time in the West, certain parts of the Tantric tradition are already well known and are used extensively to try to explain bioenergetic therapies. I refer specifically to the bioenergetic anatomy of the Chakras and the way in which they relate to our environment. Considering that this is a system already known to many people interested in one way or another in "bioenergetics", we will also refer to its bases in this manual.

Unfortunately, many people, from their ignorance, trust the solution of all their problems to the practice of a technique (of Reiki or another type), without understanding that there is no real healing if there is no personal commitment to our health. It is not enough to know how to cook to eat properly. Similarly, it is not enough to start in Reiki to regain health.

With the concepts of basic bioenergetics and other knowledge added in the different parts that make up the manual, we intend to provide sufficient tools that allow the person who begins to practice the first level of Reiki to assume the task of enhancing their own health and that of those who are in charge.

Below are the basic foundations of the philosophies to which we have referred, as well as its relationship with Reiki, with special emphasis on the vision that health and disease offer each of these cultures.

CHAPTER 15: Attunements

Group or Individual

I personally prefer to perform individual attunements. I take each student into a separate area where I give them their attunement. Some Masters attune their students in groups where the students are lined up in rows or in a small circle. If attunements are given in a group and some are attuned before the others are finished, all must remain in quiet meditation until the whole group is finished.

Distant Attunements

Experiences during an attunement

What a student experiences during an attunement is similar to that of a recipient during a Reiki session but stronger. Although some students will feel nothing, the majority of students will feel or experience their attunement.

- Physical Sensations – You may feel heat, cold, or tingling sensations. For example, you may feel a muscle twitch, or you may sweat.

- Dizziness – Occasionally students feel slightly dizzy. If this happens, just relax and your Reiki Master may instruct you to visualize tree roots of white light going down into Mother Earth to ground you.

- Emotionally Overwhelmed – the Reiki energy may bring up and resolve issues within you as it clears your chakras. You may even see a glimpse of a past life or your soul purpose. It may also be a very happy emotion that makes you want to cry. Emotions are good. Allow yourself to release.

- Laughing or Crying – You may experience uncontrollable giggling, laughter, or may even want to cry. Just accept and allow yourself to feel what ever you are experiencing.

- Seeing Colors – Some sense bright lights or balls of light. This is simply the Reiki energy coming into you and your clairvoyant sense powering up. You may even see visions or receive messages.

- Seeing Spirits – Some may see their guides or Reiki Masters in spirit. Students may even see Dr. Usui during an attunement.

After an Attunement

Immediately following any Reiki attunement there is a period where the cleansing can be intense. This often coincides with the 21 days of self-healing. Your guides continue to clear your chakras and align your energy during this period. If you had blockages (physical or spiritual), your Reiki guides will remove these blockages first. As your chakras are cleansed and aligned, anything that you didn't deal with may surface. This is a good thing as you are finally resolving and releasing negative energies that may have been causing you issues for years. Cleansing takes place on all levels – physical, mental, emotional, and spiritual. The more the Reiki energy is allowed to flow, the more beneficial this will be. During this time, go easy on yourself and allow the process. Drink lots of water as this will help you to release toxins and flush out any negative energy that has surfaced. Your self-healing sessions will help you to release and cleanse more quickly. Take time to meditate daily. Allow yourself lots of sleep and rest. Taking walks in nature is very healing and may help you through this process. Most students report some moments of emotion during this time. They usually report feeling wonderful, more energetic, healthy, and alive.

Preparation Before an Attunement

Some preparation the week before will help you to get the strongest connection out of your attunement. However, even if you don't do any preparation, you will still receive the energies, become a Reiki channel, and receive your Reiki Level One certificate. Your Reiki powers will also continue to enhance long after the class.

These suggestions are not something to stress over, but if you have the time they may help strengthen your initial experience and minimize any negative feelings afterwards

Preparation for an Attunement

1.   Limit or cut out animal protein for the 3 days prior. Fish is fine. This is to clear any negative energies from food.

2.   If you have ever fasted and enjoy this process, fasting on juice or water beforehand is good. (1-2 days or just a few hours). If you are not used to this then just try to eat healthy.

3.   Limit or stop any caffeinated drinks for 3 days.

4.   Limit or no alcohol for 3 days.

5.   Limit or no sugar or junk food for 3 days.

6.   Limit or stop smoking cigarettes for 3 days.

7.   Quiet negative outside distractions, news, horror movies, etc. for 3 days.

8.   Try to spend some time appreciating nature each day.

9.   Start as soon as possible and meditate daily, an hour if possible. If you are not able to meditate, just sit quietly and contemplate. Ask to release anger, fear, worry, and other negative feelings. Then spend some time contemplating or meditating on why you want to receive a Reiki attunement and what you wish to receive from your Reiki attunement. (e.g.

to increase your psychic ability or to be able to heal yourself and others, mentally and physically, etc.)

10.   If you use other rituals or methods to get your psychic powers stimulated, go ahead and start to prepare yourself. (e.g. crystals)

Again, many people do nothing beforehand, so don't stress about this, but a quiet contemplating period before would be good and at least avoid a heavy party weekend!

CHAPTER 16: Meditation and Reiki

Meditation can be termed as the process of channelizing your thoughts or turning your attention to a specific part of body, mind or spirit inside or outside yourself. It plays an important role in self-healing and enables you to understand yourself and the Divine guidance. It is just a mechanism that allows you to build full concentration on a particular task and eliminate all distractions.

Once you are attuned to Reiki, you can begin practicing certain meditations that will ensure that your chakras are well balanced. These meditations also make your aware of the relationship that exists between your mind and body and therefore, helps in bringing them together. Meditation ensures that all blockages and imbalances are corrected via the flow of life force energy. It helps you experience ultimate peace and harmony – something like you have never experienced before!

Each chakra has a particular type of energy that is unique to that particular chakra. By performing meditation along with certain visualization and affirmation techniques, you can cleanse your chakras and open them up to receive life force energy.

In order to practice this chakra balancing meditation, you would need to find a quiet and secluded place. You must try and make enough time for meditation. The recommended time is half an hour a day. Put out the dog, switch off your phone and do everything else required to make sure that you do not get disturbed. Create your sacred space before you begin your meditation practice. Here is one of the simplest, yet impactful Reiki meditation techniques:

Sit upright in a chair or in Sukhasana and close your eyes. Hold your hands in front of your chest in a 'Namaste' position and let the soles of your feet join together.

Use the power of your intent to heal and unconditional love in order to connect to the Reiki energy within yourself.

Visualize white light originating from your fingers.

Now visualize your third eye chakra, experience unconditional love in the third eye chakra and meditate on it.

Next, enable the unconditional love of Reiki move up as a bright light above your crown chakra. Bring your awareness back to the third eye chakra.

Relax and release your thoughts on completing this meditation.

Let warmth and peace move through your body. Experience the magical healing energy travel into ad through your body.

After you have completed this meditation, imagine yourself being encircled by white light from head to toe. This white light acts as an energy shield that is going to protect you from any negative energy that may be trying to block the flow of energy through your body.

Take a few deep breaths and move your toes, fingers, hands, legs and then slowly turn your attention towards your eyes. Open your eyes slowly and come out of the meditative state knowing that Reiki energy is flowing through all your chakras and will keep you healthy on all levels.

Let us look at some of the benefits that meditation has to offer:

INCREASED FOCUS: Irrespective of whether you are practicing a few minutes of meditation per day or indulging in a full day of meditative practice, your focus is bound to improve. This is primarily a result of regression of stress hormones in the body which when present force your brain to move in all possible directions. Meditation empowers you to understand when your mind is wandering and provide you the opportunity to correct it.

DECREASED ANXIETY: Well, meditation equals reduction in stress hormones and hence decreased anxiety. That's no rocket science!

Wait! There's more to it!
As you meditate, you loosen the connections of neural pathways that lead to your medial prefrontal cortex. The medial prefrontal cortex is the part of the brain that is responsible for processing information that impacts you directly such as an upsetting or a frightening moment.

Loosening this link via meditation enables you to look at the situation in a more rational manner.

ENHANCED CREATIVITY: Ample research has been conducted to prove that people who meditate are more creative and also open to new ideas.

ELEVATED MEMORY: When you meditate, you will be able to filter out all the distractions. This means you will be able to recall the stuff that you want to remember and filter out the stuff that does not need to be remembered.

INCREASED COMPASSION: People who practice meditation are more compassionate and empathetic towards others.

DECREASED STRESS: Studies suggest that mindfulness meditation leads to a substantial decrease in stress levels and as a result, lesser visits to the doctor.

CURE INSOMNIA TOO: That's correct! Meditation has the potential to cure chronic insomnia too. All you need is thirty minutes of dedicated practice each day.

MEDITATION CAN CHANGE YOUR BRAIN! Yes – meditation can change your brain, and this is in fact, one of the greatest benefits of meditation. It decreases mind wandering, preserves an aging brain, elevates concentration levels and improves self-control.

SPECIFIC BENEFITS OF REIKI MEDITATION:

- Here are some specific benefits of Reiki meditation:
- It brings about a deep sense of relaxation.
- It dissolves all energy blocks.
- It accelerates the natural healing process of wounds, etc.
- It changes negative training and behavior.

- It releases emotional wounds.

- It demolishes all disease.

CHAPTER 17. Carrying the Energy

You can carry the energy of the crystals with you wherever you go. This way, you can keep your connection to the crystals. However, do note that you might have to cleanse the crystals regularly.

There are many ways you can carry your crystals with you. Here are the most popular methods.

The Bag

You can place your crystals inside a small bag or pouch that you can carry around with you. You can place this bag in your pockets or wherever you find convenient so that you have them close to you.

Do note that when you pick a bag or pouch for carrying your crystals, you should not use the bag for any other purpose. The bag will hold all the positive energy of the crystals and should not be tainted by any dirt, impurities, or objects.

You can even take the crystals with you as you head to work, go about your day, or perform your daily tasks. Keep them as close to you as possible. You can carry all seven crystal with you or choose the crystal that you would like to focus on. I personally recommend carrying all the crystals and letting their energy empower you, even if some of your Chakras are not blocked.

You could also carry the Chakras to power your energy throughout the day or to help you in a particular scenario. Let us assume that you have to make a big presentation and you are feeling nervous; then you could carry as Aquamarine (for the throat Chakra) in the bag so that you may be able to convey your messages and ideas clearly.

You do not have to remove the stones from the bag. As long as the stones are close to you, they will spread their effect to you.

The Ring

You can even place an individual crystal or stone into a ring and wear them everywhere you go. not only can you draw on the power of the stone, but a ring is a stylish addition to your clothing as well.

You can even choose to wear the ring at all times of the day or for a specific time. If you are able to, you can create rings for seven crystals for each of your Chakras. This way, you will have the ability to change your crystals depending on what Chakra you want to focus on and have different colored crystals to match your attire.

Before you decide to wear your ring, place it on a bed of salt so that you can remove any contaminants or negative energy.

You should also power up the ring before using it. Take the ring in your hand and think of all the positive energy and emotions that you would like to imbue the ring with.

The Necklace

The necklace works in the same way as the ring. The one advantage of the necklace is that you can use different designs for the chain to fit your requirements.

Additionally, you do not have to reveal your chain all the time. You can simply place it inside your shirt and keep it hidden away, unlike a ring that is always visible on your hand.

You should remove contaminants and negative energy from the chain as well by following the same steps that you did with the ring; simply place the chain on a bed of salt.

Power up your chain by focusing on it and sending your positive energy and thoughts into it.

The Bracelet

Make sure that you place the bracelet on a bed of salt in order to remove any previous contaminants. Next, focus on the bracelet and add your positive energy and thoughts into it. However, do note that as there are many crystals in one bracelet, you might not be able to power it up completely by simply focusing on it.

Ways to Use Your Crystals

- You can place the crystal directly on the area of the ailment. Let us assume that you have an intense migraine. When you think of migraines, then you are associating them with the crown Chakra. One of the crystals used for the Crown Chakra is the Clear Quartz. Your next step will be to meditate using the Clear Quartz. You can do this in two ways.
- In the first method, you use it when you are lying down and working with all the crystals. You place the Clear Quartz above your head in the way that we had seen in the chakra powering technique we had seen earlier.
- In the second method, you assume the easy pose and focus only on your crown Chakra. Here, as you are not using all the crystal stones, you can place the Clear Quartz on top of your head. However, be mindful of the balance of the crystal as dropping it means interrupting the meditation process.
- You can purchase multiple crystals and place them in various places that you frequent. You could keep them at work. You could place them in your car. You could even have a few of them sprinkled around different parts of your home to create a positive energy field. Speaking of energy fields, there is one way you can enhance your home.
- Add them as decorations in different parts of your home. Not only do they create a positive vibe, but they also add a beautiful aesthetic to your home.
- You can also create water infused with crystals. Just make sure that the crystals you are using do not dissolve in water (which typically they don't if you have referred to the guide in this book). You can use this water in two ways.
- Take a bowl of water. Place your crystal or crystals inside it. You can use the water from the bowl to wash your face in the morning or whenever you feel like it.
- Take a glass of water. Place your crystals in them. You can drink from the water to rejuvenate your body and your Chakras.

CHAPTER 18. Using Reiki with Others

After working with yourself for a while, you will find that Reiki comes incredibly natural to you. Once you have reached the stage where you feel completely confident in this practice, you will be able to start using Reiki with others. The major benefit is that the life force will be felt in the giver and the receiver during practice. You can help your family and friends, while simultaneously reaping the benefits of Reiki yourself.

Why You Should Practice with Others

The relationship formed between two entities practicing Reiki is often referred to as a healing alliance. The most common experience of the giver is harmony. As you form alliances with others, you will find more peace and harmony in your own life. You may also experience feelings of oneness with others or nature or the world as a whole.

What To Do

You will find that there are a number of similarities between the way you would practice Reiki on yourself and the way that you would practice it on someone else.

Step #1: Discovering Their Intent

In order for Reiki practice to be effective for the other person, you must be very clear about what they are expecting from the session. The best way to do this is to have a long conversation beforehand about the other person's intentions. Ask questions like:

- How would you like to benefit from Reiki treatment?

- Do you have any specific ailments or illnesses?

- What if Reiki brings a sense of positivity to your life?

- Do you have a sense of purpose in life?

- Are there any pressing issues on your mind?

- How is your life at home? At work?

- Do you feel stressed?

Asking open-ended questions like these gives you and the receiver the chance to explore their deepest desires without much restriction. As you uncover what they desire most, ask follow-up questions until you have a clear picture of their intent before you begin Reiki practice. In order to establish a sense of trust, it is important to make it clear that you will not repeat anything said in a Reiki session to anyone else. This may make your partner more comfortable.

Step #2: Active Practice

Once you have finished this, you will do something known as spiraling. Take your left hand and place it on the right shoulder. Take your right hand and point your middle and index finger outward. Use these to draw counterclockwise spirals, starting at the left shoulder and moving toward the tip of the left hand. Then, start at the shoulder again and move toward the left foot. You will repeat this on the right side. This is intended to balance the energy before flipping the patient to heal the back chakras. Once you have asked your healing partner to turn so they are laying on their stomach, hold your hands above the body and perform a Byosen scan again, paying close attention to the chakras located above the back brow and the lower back. Now, stand with your hands about six inches above either of these chakras. Feel the flow of energy between each until they feel balanced. Next, take the middle and index fingers of your right hand and make a "V" shape. Keeping your hand on the left shoulder, draw a line that spans between the throat and root chakras. Pause for a moment at the back chakra and repeat this process twice more. Then, awaken your partner.

Step #3: How to Know if It is Working

Sometimes, you will not receive confirmation that the Reiki session is doing what it is intended to do until a day or even a week after the session. This is especially true of earlier practices, which will not be as strong in nature. In other cases, you will feel sensations through the course of the situation, which may include tingling, vibration, or temperature changes. Sometimes the sensations of Reiki will be felt together and other times the giver and receiver will experience this as opposites, such as one feeling hot and the other feeling cold. Whether you do or do not experience something, do not lose faith that the Reiki session is working. It will work, but sometimes the results take time.

A Few Tips to Keep in Mind When Practicing Reiki with Others

#1: It Is Never Okay to Make Promises

There are a number of factors that affect how effective a Reiki practice is for the people involved. As the giver, you must not make promises for how the session will end. You cannot guarantee that the receiver will find confidence or be healed in some way. All that you can do is help them set the intent for the session and then provide the practice in the best way you can. Other than that, the results are going to be up to them.

#2: Start with Willing Friends and Family Members

The receiver does not have to be sick or anxious in order to reap benefits from a Reiki session. This means that you can practice with anyone, as long as they have an open mind. Remind your willing participant that their results are going to rely heavily on their state of mind and intent during practice. Finally, be sure that they know that the results are always unique to the person and their situation, so you cannot guarantee anything.

#3: Practice with Plants and Animals

The spiritual life force of Reiki flows through every living being, including plants and animals. If the person that you practice with is unavailable, try with a pet or even a plant.

While the technique will not be exactly the same, try to use the same visualization of the chakras as an internal tube of light.

#4: Remember That You Cannot Control the Entire Session

As the healer in the Reiki practice, you do not have much control over the results. Imagine for a moment that you are a boat taking spices to India. If the sailors hit something and the boat drowns, is it the fault of the boat? No, it is not. In this situation, you are the boat. You can transport the Reiki energy to the receiver, but you cannot make it improve their life. If they are holding on to past grudges or do not honestly feel that Reiki will work, it is not going to benefit them as much as they would like it to. Additionally, it may take more than one Reiki session for the benefits to be felt as fully as they would like.

CONCLUSION

You can say – this all sounds nice, but you'll probably also be wondering "HOW THE HECK DO I ACHIEVE ALL OF THIS?"

And to your question, I'll now provide you with a simple, yet definitive, answer - arm yourself with patience, a positive intention, and the desire for self-improvement.

Do not let fear hinder you, and don't let the chance of 'failure' haunt you or stifle your progress.

Every worthwhile goal in life always looks like an insurmountable mountain. But the truth is that, just like any mountain, your goals can also be conquered.

The key is to not focus on the goal, but the journey. You must understand that the real prize resides within who you become along the way to your desires, as opposed to fulfilling your goals.

Life is a continuous, endless journey of the human soul. Yet growth is not automatic, nor is it a gift bestowed upon us by default.

No, growth and personal development are not accolades and rare gifts, they are prizes that awarded by the Universe to those that are willing to escape from their comfort zones and reach for things that look outside of their grasp.

And in conclusion, I would like to quote the words of a teacher living in India, Vatara Sathya Sai Baba. He said something like this: "The difference between you and me is that I know that I am Gods, and you do not know that you are also Gods." Each of us is a part of the Supreme Cosmic Creator, and therefore a Co-Creator within the framework of our competence. Our most important task and competence is ourselves and our life. This is what we must create for ourselves. Reiki is a great tool to help us remember that we are Gods too, and begin to build ourselves and our lives!

BOOK 3

Introduction

Kundalini is an ancient Sanskrit word from India that relates to the arising of specific energy and force of consciousness that is lying dormant or coiled at the base of our spine from the moment we are born. This energy is believed to be the primary source of life (our bioenergy or, traditionally, panic energy). Ancient yogic studies suggest that Kundalini energy stimulates the formation of life in the womb, following which it coils at the spinal base of the child. When we perish, it uncoils and gets back to its source.

This energy may arise and manifest from the spinal base (or at times even our feet) when we engage in regular and disciplined spiritual practices, or even in response to specific life events. When the Kundalini arises, it is typically believed to uncoil slowly like a snake, but it can rapidly and explosively move into the heart, head, and gut. This phenomenon can be confusing, scary, or blissful, and is generally followed by long periods of new sensations, feelings, and transformations in the person who has successfully awakened it. You may feel like the body's wiring is ramped up from 1oo to 200. Also, it takes time for the practitioner to adapt to the changes as a result of Kundalini awakening. In Eastern traditions, this energy is synonymous with spiritual awakening or realization. However, in other societies, it is viewed differently.

The spiritual concept of Kundalini energy has found references in several religious philosophies and traditions (though it may not have been directly referred to as Kundalini), including Taoism, Native American philosophy, Tantric Buddhism, Gnostic tradition, and many indigenous societies. The compelling visual of a snake rising within the human body can represented in esoteric or symbolic art and is an aggregation of many cultures and philosophies that has evolved over a period of time. Our body's ability to raise and intensify energy from within has been studied for several thousand years. It is known to be a natural process.

Kundalini awakening can lead to a string of consequences, both good and bad. It can trigger considerable positive changes and transformations in a person's emotional, mental, sensate, spiritual, physical, and psychic abilities. It can lead to stress in the body's vulnerable regions and bring about a significant shift in mental perspective. Awakening Kundalini can also cause several strange and unusual sensations such as vibrations, violent shakes, spontaneous movements, and several other similarly unexplained phenomena.

When Kundalini energy activates, it moves along our spine through a central path known as "Sushumna Nadi." Sushumna is the pathway housed along the spine through which the energy travels from one chakra to another, all the way to the crown chakra right above the head. There are many parallels between our physical functions and the functioning of Kundalini energy. For instance, the Sushumna pathway is comparable with our central nervous system. The purpose of this channel is to link the circulation of energy from the initial to the final chakra. Likewise, the purpose of our central nervous system, nestled in the larger part along the spinal path, is to create an exchange of signals between our brain and the other body parts.

Kundalini awakening offers practitioners an opportunity to embark on a spiritual path. It allows us to slowly release several delusions, patterns, perspectives, and conditions of our distinct self. Without training, the practitioner's consciousness may venture into the realm of the unknown and unfamiliar which can be disorienting. It can make individuals who go into these unknown and empty states scared, sick, or lose their mental balance.

Therefore, it is essential to understand the potential of Kundalini correctly to apply its awakened energy toward positive physical, mental, and spiritual goals.

What Are Chakras?

Chakras are our body's energy centers, which are known to facilitate the flow of Cosmic energy into our body. There are several ways to activate these energy centers and enjoy a multitude of physical, mental, and spiritual benefits. Some of these ways are yoga and meditations. The human body is known to have seven primary chakras (translated as 'wheels' in ancient Sanskrit).

Long before the emergence of modern technology and scientific studies, ancient traditions believed that all living beings held a life force within them. This life force, or energy centers, keep rotating inside the body to facilitate our physiological, mental, psychological, and spiritual activities. In a balanced individual, all seven chakras release equal amounts of energy to each part of our body, mind, and spirit. However, if a chakra is rotating too slowly or rapidly or is too open or closed, the person's health suffers.

A greater knowledge of our body's energy centers allows us to be more in sync with the inherent physical cycles and circulation of energy that can be used to direct physical, emotional, mental, and spiritual well-being. You can learn how to balance these chakras which will lead to a healthy, positive, and harmonious life.

Chapter 1. What Is Kundalini and Its Story

Kundalini is a word that is flying around the spiritual Cycles like wildfire. Most people simply accept the word without actually understanding what the word simply means. So, in this section, we are going to talk about what the word kundalini means. Now to be able to comprehend kundalini, you have to be able to imagine who God is or who the source of the universe is. You have to be able to imagine the universe as it is made up of multiple continents, you have to be able to understand the whole universe as a unified portion and infinite ocean.

The universe is very fragmented in the same way that of a zygote, and also, a fungus is fragmented. This helps to give rise to polarity within the universe. Keep polarity include polarity between male and female conscious and unconscious between life and death. The polarity of life and death is what actually gives birth to the rise of kundalini because kundalini literary is life, and it is life force energy. Kundalini is the opposite of death, which is an empty dead nothing else. So, it is very important to understand this.

In the human race, you can use the word death to mean different things. The death that human physical experience is simply the transition of perspective; it is not death in the way that we think. Kundalini is simply the animating fault of the universe. It is the opposite of the prefix of any life form, regardless of the dimension of life. It is present even in the beans like demons and spirits. Now life has a lot of characteristics with death. One of the characteristics of kundalini is simply animation. Stillness and movement are animations.

Therefore, Kundalini can either be still, and it can also be moved. In other words, something that is stiffed can still be very much alive. All the qualities that belong to kundalini involve growth, change, reaction, reproduction creation. Now, most of the problems that we have in the universe are that polarity exists within us; we don't have integration between life and death.

So, you can imagine yourself as a fragment of this unified consciousness which simply means you are a fragment in the polarity of life. Now another way to understand kundalini is to imagine an infinite ocean. Sometimes it looks like it is invisible from the internal energy. You are indivisible or inseparable from God or the universe. Now, your existence and your body are comprised of the same energy that is called God, which manifests itself in the physical form, which is called the life force energy.

Now when somebody imagines himself, he sees himself as a life force energy, which you can call the soul. When people talk about the soul, they just imagine the soul like a cup of energy in just the same way that they see the body as a column of energy, when in reality, they saw a stream of energy that is Simply Creating and expressing a physicality.

Some qualities of the soul include transcending life and death. For instance, perception needs to transform before death; if not, you will not be able to perceive death. This means that life is simply one aspect of the soul, now you should understand that you can't have the soul and life at the same time. You can lose life because you are life itself, which means you are kundalini.

To mention energetic levels which just raises above the physicality, the life force stream of energy, manifest in the physical body which will be for a man who was in the physical body arrange himself into radiance and into chakras which are the basic structure and

---

energy blueprint of the physical body. For the sake of understanding, some days, imagine the ancient Hindu philosophers.

Now the Hindus call the energy centers chakras because each of the chakras will be resolved to conduct a certain area of the human body, it was believed that we can feed life force energy into the different parts of the body through the chakras. The chakras were seen as something that could receive and give out energy in different ways.

Now kundalini is simply a Hindi word that originates from the yoga world of spirituality and can be translated as the coiled one. The reason is that the people of the Ancient World believe that the energy could be dormant, and if it was dormant and resting close to the base of the spine or the backside of the root chakra, then it means that the chakra is out of alignment.

Now, based on the way that the energy test is felt in the body when it moves, it's very easy to imagine the latent energy that these people will absorb as a coiled-up snake at the base of one spine.

Now, kundalini is restricted or limited to one chakra but even if it is capable of being dormant, and this is not the case. It is much easier to perceive the kundalini in the different areas of the body that are related to the chakra because those areas of the body are related to physicality and Sensation. Also, if you are allowing your kundalini energy and the stream of life force energy that is animating your body, it will begin to move like a Streamwood, which looks like a snake.

So, imagine if you could allow that Stream wood to be out of the way. Now when the kundalini is allowed on a lower energetic level, the energy will rush through. The radiant and physicality will be fair with the running of the spine to make the lower and the upper chakras to connect as a part of one current.

If you master your kundalini energy, then you'll be capable of allowing gushes of life force energy to flow through your body consciously. And it will give rise to the class if the sensation of shivering throughout your body it also tends to have a quality that is very similar to liquid fire. Now the second and biggest argument relating to kundalini is that it is simply latent energy.

Now the kundalini energy can't actually be asleep If you are dead. So, if you are dead, your kundalini energy will simply be still. Now kundalini is not latent energy that you need to activate, but it is simply awake and active even when it is still. The energy can be simply resisted. Now suppression is the kind of resistance that kundalini goes through. Kundalini tends to be still to the positive when it is creating room for other forms of consciousness that are prohibited or stopped by the observation of things.

Now when consciousness needs to be in a state of observation, kundalini will be still. Now kundalini needs to become still when it is resisted with the free will because that it is where it gets its consciousness from. Now, if somebody is in the state where they are deciding whether they want to be alive in the physical state, then their kundalini will be still. For instance, where someone is in a coma, their kundalini will be still.

The impression of kundalini, which forces it into the state of stillness through the true existence, is going to feel like absolute crap. The primary question that you need to begin to ask yourself about your kundalini is how you are resisting life. Resistance is simply nothing more than the opposition. You can see it as any oppositional Force that you are very aware of. Now you have to realize that there is a reason while your body is expressing itself in this reincarnation.

Kundalini contains a man's creative potential; therefore, you need to be bothered with how you are resisting your authenticity and your purpose for existing on Earth. Now the various forms of yoga breathing, self-surrender and meditation, and all other conscious exercises, doesn't actually awaken your kundalini, but it releases your resistance. And there is a reason while this conscious exercise works. Because if you have written in a specific way, it will release resistance every meditate in a specific way; it will release resistance.

If you are doing yoga in certain ways, it will release resistance. Now there is one major problem with this kundalini practice, and it's the way that it's being used in the modern world today. So many people are using kundalini practices to be able to make up; therefore, it cannot change. They don't try to solve the core resistance and make changes that they need to make so that they can fully live. But they try to use the kundalini practices just like a board that is actually sinking because there is a huge hole in the bottom of the boat. Now even if you take a bucket of water out of the deck of the boat every single minute, the boat is going to stay floating for a long time, because you're not attacking the root, while boat is sinking through the hole that is in the bottom of the boat.

Now that is the way most people treat their kundalini; they simply avoid the problem that is wrong with the kundalini and just try to do some yoga practices. If you speak and talk in your authenticity and allow your full Force to come through your body, then there'll be no reason while you will do those actions associated with kundalini practices.

So, try to correct that notion that kundalini is always awake, and it is always in a state of animation. Nothing is more important than your kundalini energy or life-force for being in alignment with your unique authenticity. Everybody comes into this life as a unique expression of self-consciousness. This means each person comes into this world with a unique essence and our unique purpose and unique thoughts and unique feelings around and unique desires and unique needs and unique role in the universe, all these are embedded in that essence. Our life experiences the process of unfolding of oneself authentic expression.

This is while Awakening is not different from stepping into full authenticity. Authenticity is part two Awakening regardless of what road you are taking to the content authenticity. You have to know who exactly you are, which is more than yourself physically on this earth.

You can only be authentic to the degree that you currently know yourself. This means that you can only be authentic to the degree that you are aware of yourself.

Most of us are freaking dejected and depressed that we don't even know who we are. We are not aware of ourselves. What we are in the world today is what will make us safe in our world and in the social groups that we have formed. As a result, we will become copies of other people who will become strategies.

All of this happens to build resistance for you and to make you deny yourself with your physicality and spirituality the reasons for being your desires, your unique needs, your instant truth so that your kundalini will be resisted. To resist your kundalini is to be without any energy and to be dead.

Nothing allows kundalini more than action that is backed by authentic inspiration; this is what living out your Life Processes all about. Some people experience what is called kundalini Awakening. Now kundalini Awakening means allowing d resistance in the being to be released, which allows them are the full embodiment and is to be filled with life force energy.

They are in alignment in 1 second with the essence. So, let's say that somebody attends a very intense kundalini meditation center and try to incorporate that into their life it will be very difficult because since they haven't made any change to their actual life, they get dumped back into the state of assistance.

In other words when they are trying to increase the process of allowing their kundalini, and the awareness that came with it, when the life doesn't mirror their authentic truth they get into problems and try to be back in that state of being and thinking of those thoughts and those actions and taking that life becomes absolutely unbearable.

This is what many people call "kundalini syndrome." Not if you awaken anyway, you are going to change the way you can and cannot interact with the world. This is why this heightened sense of sensitivity is a very important part of the Kundalini Awakening. It gives rise to the disparity between the two states of being. It is a wide gap, so most times, it feels part of as if you are trying to strangulate yourself.

It is a painful level of consonant dizziness. Now when you have this kundalini syndrome, it means that you are experiencing a resistance relatable to the area of life that you've had the most resistance before. So, if you have the kundalini syndrome, then it means that you are likely to experience those symptoms relating to whatever aspect of your life that you've had the most resistance in before. If it was on the mental level, then you're going to experience more mental symptoms.

If it wasn't on the physical level, then you are going to experience more physical symptoms. From a universal perspective, the sensitivity that is experienced as a result of a kundalini Awakening is an awesome thing. And it is not as a result of too much energy in the body. Kundalini is a recent occurrence with any awareness on how to adapt to change one's life by that sensitivity.

It is the same thing as having consciousness without any idea on how to integrate that consciousness with a world that is operating from a constant level of unconsciousness. Some of the things you've tolerated before you could only tolerate them now because you made yourself desensitized.

The thing is half of the things you thought you could do then, you could because you were in the state of resistance that you were used to. Half of the things that you were doing, you were doing them because you were not aware of how horrible they were. Haven't you noticed that sometimes the food you eat suddenly becomes horrible to your body and sometimes the things that you thought were normal suddenly seem barbaric?

So, you need to really adapt your life to that awareness. Most of the things that you were climatized to, you had to go into resistance to your own life force energy to acclimatize to them. The Kundalini Awakening makes this on bearable. It is no measure of health to be adjusted to a profound dysfunctional situation. All the mistakes that most people make it that the try to decrease the kundalini energy into the body instead of getting somebody to do what they want them to do, what is to make changes in their highlighting consciousness.

So, it isn't about the kundalini, but it is about the resistance to the life force energy. If you have been on the path of Awakening for a long time, and you are familiar with the discomfort of that shifting and integration. If you're matured where you are very used to holding state for this painful growth, then you are not going to get the kundalini syndrome.

And even if you have some symptoms of the shift in your consciousness, it is not going to stabilize you. On the contrary, if you haven't been on the path of Awakening for a very long time and you're not used to stretching yourself to integrate polarities, then it's going to destabilize you.

Now, if you are not used to making changes in accordance to the instability that is the inevitable nature of an uncertain universe or change in Motability, which is the foundation of who you are then chances are you are going to suffer from The Awakening process especially if it is a spontaneous and instantaneous shift in consciousness.

Do not think that if you are experiencing any kundalini syndrome, then something that matches with what is all about. But think of it as the more you practice this Awakening, which can be quite painful, then the easier it's easier for you to shift your consciousness. And the higher your frequency shifts, the more your consciousness moves, and the more consciousness get to where you are, the less likely that a shift in consciousness is going to take you to a whole new state.

This is why we are working in accordance to our awakening. In general, it is a pretty good idea to surround yourself with one person or multiple people who are Masters of energy and have been on the path for a long time. An example is a spiritual teacher or somebody who can guide you through the process itself or help you to integrate the process once they occur.

The Kundalini Awakening is not different from any form of spiritual Awakening. The very negative manifestation of the ego is the oppositional force of the kundalini. You can describe Awakening as an incarnated form, and kundalini practices are certain processes that enable that Awakening. It is one part of going to the top of Awakening. If you're on the part of consciousness, then you are a part of India raining. Kundalini is not a supernatural force in our lives; instead, it is life force energy. Therefore, it is left to you to resist or not.

Kundalini yoga is often called the yoga of awareness. It is both a physical and mental practice. Kundalini exercises are precise, repetitive, and prescriptive. Kundalini yoga, you are mostly chanting working with the breath to elevate your conscious awareness.

Chapter 2. How Kundalini Can Help Your Body and Soul

Surely, such a sacred practice has to have a positive effect on the body and the mind along with the spirit? The answer is that it definitely does, and they even outnumber the spiritual benefits!

There is a plethora of ways in which yoga benefits the body—too many to count, in fact. So, let's explore 15 different benefits of yoga in daily life.

1. Improves flexibility – This is one of the most fundamental benefits of yoga. You may not be able to touch your toes or bend all the way forward in your first class, but you will notice over time that your body begins to loosen up, and with that will come a decrease in muscle pain as well.

2. Builds strength – Yoga is the best way to build a healthy amount of strength while balancing it with flexibility. The strength of your muscles contributes greatly to your posture, how you walk, and how you power the daily physical tasks that you may have. Lifting weights builds muscle too, but that (more often than not) takes away from your flexibility.

3. Improves posture – People underestimate the weight of their heads! When you slouch, the amount of tension of your heavy had leaning beyond your spines center of gravity can have lasting effects. Yoga encourages and promotes healthy standing and sitting positions, so you will learn over time how to sit and stand properly which will increase the longevity of your back and neck especially.

4. Stops joint/cartilage breakdown – The body is more like a machine than anything else. Like most machines, it has to be well oiled and taken care of with great compassion. Your cartilage is a spongey substance that cushions the area between your bones within joints. Yoga takes you through full ranges of motion that will loosen those joints and promote proper maintenance of your cartilage. Without going through the motions, your cartilage will likely wear with age, and eventually will be scraped down until you're experiencing the trouble and pain of two bones rubbing together without any cartilage between them. Many elderly experience this, hence why they most so slowly. Yoga can solve this problem!

5. Spinal Protection – Spinal disks are the shock absorbers of your back and require a healthy amount of movement to stay limber and effective. In yoga, there are many motions that involve light twisting and turning to ensure that your spine stays strong and supple through the years. Back problems affect millions of people, so it only makes sense to find a solution that can remove you from that statistic!

6. Promotes bone health – This is important for women especially! You've seen the commercials about the prescription pills that are supposed to combat osteoporosis. Well, this is a natural, much less rigorous way to prevent it. The stances and poses that you take in yoga help to strength the bones of your arms and legs especially, which is where osteoporosis likes to start. In addition to that, yoga as a whole help to lower the amount of stress hormones produced in your body, which lowers the rate at which calcium is lost in your bones.

7. Blood flow goes up – Although yoga isn't the same as running or lifting weights, it actually is much more effective at evenly distributing oxygenated blood throughout your body. In fact, going through the motions in a session promote a higher blood flow to the areas of your body that may not always receive it as they should (hands and feet). A consistent practice will also lead to more oxygenated blood circulating healthily through your organs and tissues, and even can help with people who have had heart or kidney problems and don't get the appropriate amount of blood to certain areas of their bodies. In addition to that, this increased flow reduces your chances of unhealthy blood clots.

8. Assists immune/lymphatic system – Everything in yoga from the contraction and stretching of a muscle, to transitioning between poses allows a fluid within immune cells to break free and "drain", if you will. As it drains, your body will be able to fight off infection more readily. It also makes it so that cancerous cells are broken down faster, and also so that the toxic waste within these cells is disposed of more quickly.

9. Improves heart health – Regularly increasing your heart rate during exercise can lower your risk of heart disease as well as the chances of depression because of the endorphins released during exercise. Yoga isn't an aerobic exercise by default, but there are variations that can be done in order to simulate a situation where your cardiovascular fitness is challenged. And even for yoga that isn't ass vigorous, it still lowers your resting heart rate and improves your overall endurance.

10. Lowers blood pressure - If you have HBP (high blood pressure), you too can benefit from yoga. The constant movement combined with the cardiovascular challenge will regulate your blood pressure, and eventually will lead to an overall drop due to the consistent practice of raising and lowering it with different forms of exercise.

11. Regulates adrenal glands – Cortisol is a stress induced hormone that appears when in a time of crisis, embarrassment, etc. Yoga reduces the amount of that this hormone sticks around. Which it first becomes present, it's helpful and makes you more alert, and even boosts your immune system. The real trouble comes when the situation that caused the increase passes and the cortisol sticks around. An overabundance of cortisol has been related to depression, osteoporosis, HBP, and insulin resistance (which can lead to diabetes). It also has been said that a constantly uninhibited influx of cortisol can lead your body to a state of crisis, and in this state the body stores most things that you may eat or drink as fat for safety purposes. Nobody wants that!

12. Improves moods – It is no secret that any form of exercise improves your overall moods, and promotes a happier existence. The consist practice of yoga will promote an increase in those "happy" hormones like serotonin and the endorphins that fill you with joy, which can be a great combatant of depression.

13. Encourages a healthy lifestyle – There is a spiritual, mental, and physical aspect of yoga. When combined, these things will trickle into other areas of your life from how to eat to how to you think act around others. Yoga encourages a heightened self-awareness, and in gaining a great appreciation for yourself, you will be more likely to begin taking better care of your wellbeing.

14. Fights diabetes – Yoga lowers your bad while increasing your good cholesterol. It makes your body more sensitive to insulin, while managing your cortisol and adrenaline levels which usually contribute to weight gain and the urge to take in more sugary foods. With a lowered blood sugar comes a lessened chance of attaining a heart disease, kidney issues, blindness, and other sugar-related diseases.

15. Improves focus – In yoga, there is no moment but the present one. The only way to master a pose is truly to focus within yourself, and to maintain that focus throughout your sessions. As your mind becomes accustomed to going to that present moment space, it will begin to show in other areas of your life as well, which can greatly improve things as small as driving to things as large as your professional career!

As you can clearly see, implementing yoga into your life would bring nothing but goodness into it. Now, imagine these health benefits coupled with what Kundalini Yoga can do for you.

Benefits

This works. So, just to further prove how amazing of a practice yoga can be, I've added another 15 benefits to utilizing yoga as your physical activity for the day.

1. Relaxes your system – The relaxational aspect of yoga shifts the balance from engaging the sympathetic nervous system (fight or flight responses) to the parasympathetic nervous system (relaxation, lowered heart rates, calmness).

2. Improves balance - Proprioception refers to the ability of a person to stay aware of where their body is in space as well as how to counterbalance certain actions to keep from falling. Yoga greatly improves your proprioception, which leads to the ability to balance your body for great stents of time.

3. Maintains the nervous system – With the mastery of yoga comes a level of bodily control that many can't fathom. There are yogis in the world that can harness the usually involuntary power of their nervous system and make voluntary changes, like lowering one's heart rate at will, or forcing blood to accumulate at a specific location in order to heal or even to incubate something (for women who want to create a healthier environment for pregnancy).

4. Releases tension – Our daily cause a lot of tension, and we don't even notice it! Everything from how you drive, to how you sit, to how you hold your face, and other subconscious actions require your muscles to operate in a certain way. Yoga will essentially help you to see where you hold tension, and in practicing you will also see it relieved over time.

5. Improves sleep experience – Along with the stimulation that comes from improved focus is the byproduct of the meditation that occurs during yoga. This byproduct of increased relaxation and decreased stress can also lead to easier, deeper sleep.

6. Improves immune cell functionality – The meditative nature of yoga increases your body's ability to respond appropriately to foreign pathogens. As needed, your body will begin to produce more antibodies and other defensive structures within the body to properly maintain homeostasis.

7. Improves lung health – Those deep breaths aren't for nothing! A constant practice of total lung expansion during yoga decreases the average amount of breaths per minute, while also increasing the level of oxygen within your blood—resulting in improved respiratory health.

8. Combats digestive trouble – Many issues of the abdominal area can be stress induced, and if they are, they can be handled by regulating your cortisol levels. As we know by now, yoga has a phenomenal effect on stress hormones. Movement promotes faster processing of foods and other materials in the body, allowing for a more regulated digestive system which can prevent constipation, colon related issues, and trouble with your digestive tract.

9. Grants peace of mind – Because of the level of inner peace attained after consistently practicing yoga, your general levels of sadness, anger, and frustration will go down. You will learn to live more in the moment, without taking things as personally or as seriously because you will learn that most of what stands before you cannot be controlled, and that your original frustration comes from attempting to control it all.

10. Increases self-confidence – Many of us deal with the burden of thinking we aren't good enough. Yoga not only promotes the idea that you are good enough, but also that you don't need to be anything but who you are in this very moment. We live in a society of constant movement, and of chasing everything without being grateful for what you have. Yoga gives you a sense of gratitude for self, which will show in your future social interactions as confidence.

11. Assists in pain management – This can occur on a physical, mental, and spiritual level. On the physical level, yoga is great for those who experience joint pains, arthritis, and other muscle or bone related aches.

12. Grants mental fortitude – You will find that in staying dedicated to yoga, you will have gained a new level of discipline. Within this discipline lies a greater strength of mind, which most have said is the best benefit of yoga. This will translate to all other aspects of your life, and you will find that you can do more now on a social, professional, and sexual level than you ever thought you could.

13. Provides grounding – The trick to having a successful start with yoga is to find a good teacher. This teacher will essentially facilitate the beginning of your growth as a student of yoga, and will serve as a mental, physical, and spiritual guide for those who feel lost.

14. Replaces drugs with healthy habits – As you have read, you've seen now that yoga serves as a great, natural combatant to several diseases and ailments that can plague your life. Usually, each sickness comes with a list of pills that have to be taken in order to suppress or maintain them. But one thing that you must remember is that yoga is thousands of years older than modern medicine, and yet the people who lived thousands of years ago, still will able to overcome overwhelmingly more powerful illnesses! So, rather than jumping on the prescription pill train, try implementing some yoga into your daily life and see how differently you feel. The only side effect of yoga is a happier, longer life!

15. Creates greater sense of self – In gaining a greater understanding of yourself and the world that surrounds you, you will begin to be able to dissect and pinpoint where your own troubles and challenges exist within your life. It is said that rage and hostility can be just as contributory to heart problems as poor eating and physical stagnancy. So, even if you are currently experiencing something that you don't want to experience, your new level of understanding about yourself will help you to figure out what the cause of your problem is and to do everything within your power to remedy that situation within you.

If these benefits aren't enough to prove how awesome yoga is for you and your wellbeing, I don't what to tell you! All that can truly be said is that if you really desire a greater quality of life as well as an even more powerful sense of self, this is the path for you.

Chapter 3. Kundalini and Chakras, The Connection

Chakra Healing & Alignment

With the knowledge of what each chakra does and what chakra blockages mean in reference to your overall goal of awakening, you should now be able to take things a step further in reference to your own chakra healing. The following is a guided meditation for chakra alignment that you can read along to (or record yourself reading aloud and play back as you go) and try out. Essentially, we'll walk through one method for aligning your open chakras and inviting the serpent to rise.

Close your eyes and breathe deeply. Imagine that you're on a beach by a cool, clear lake. Picture the surroundings of this tranquil place, where you're alone with maybe a lake house behind you that feels like it's yours. Knowing that you're in a beautiful yet safe and secure space makes you feel utterly relaxed, strong, and at peace.

Suddenly, you realize that you're not on the beach – you're actually sitting in the lake and the water comes up to mid-chest level. You feel completely content with this decision, as the water feels somewhat warm and comforting in the summer breeze. You close your eyes in the meditation as well as in the real world.

If you cared to open your eyes, you'd see that the water is in fact so clear that it almost looks like there's nothing there. You'd see that it almost looks like you're just sitting on a ground of colorful gravel, but when you move your arms, you know better. When you move, you can see (and feel) the ripples.

In this clear and calm lake, you sit. As you find peace in being there and trust that nothing will harm you, you relax in a way that you haven't been able to do in a long time. You allow yourself to breathe deeply and roll your shoulders down to release any tension there. You roll your head from side to side to release strain in that area, too. Eventually, you bring your neck and chest to center, and you start to visualize your central channel.

In this inner column of energy, you visualize a free-flowing wave of white light. You have the sense that the white light is flowing so strongly and purely that it's turning the water around you white, too. You peep open an eye and confirm your intuition. The water you're sitting in is still the same temperature and texture, but it now looks like a bath of milk. You breathe in that purifying feeling and close your eyes once more.

Remembering that free-flowing column of white light, you take your visualization back to that space. Knowing that your chakras' blockages have all been cleared helps you feel confident moving forward, and you allow yourself to get all but mesmerized with the beauty of that inner white light. However, the light cannot last, and you know that this channel, this powerful column, can be used for something even more important than just centering you in this moment.

In this calming, milky lake in the middle of your safe, secure space, you begin to hum bravely. You don't really know the song you're humming, and it might just be one tone hummed with the sound "ohm." Whatever the song is, it's been with you always, and it's a supportive song that feels right for this moment. As you hum your song, it's like you're charming a snake, for kundalini seems to love the sound.

Sure enough, the small snake that lies coiled up at the base of your spine starts to move up, uncoiling and winding through your chakra energy wheels in search of the source of the sound. Normally, you might be afraid of the image of a snake within you but knowing that your body is rooted in this natural, imaginative space somehow protects you and shields you from any harm. You trust this fact and know it in your heart to be true.

Unafraid and excited, you hum more and more while kundalini rises and winds through the root chakra to the sacral, around the solar plexus, and then up to heart and throat. You notice that the serpent stays a while around throat chakra, and you assume that it's because kundalini enjoys the sound of your humming so much. Ultimately, kundalini knows it must continue, so in the peace of your body (resting in the peace of the lake, homed in the peace of this still, safe space), kundalini rises once more.

Kundalini comes up into your face to lick the third eye and crown chakras before turning and coming right back down through all the same chakras once more, down through third eye to throat, heart, solar plexus, sacral, and root. As the first cycle of serpent's winding is completed, you feel filled with potential, and you sigh with relief. You seem to feel that everything is right in the world and that your direction is being revealed to you as you draw this very breath.

In the cool, completely clear water, you open your eyes and see that the world has become so much brighter, sounds are clearer, smells are crisper, and the water feels lighter than air. You stand and reach out your arms to the world of this space and simply breathe in its beauty, knowing that you are full of the same exact potential, the same prana and shakti inspiring both you and nature. You breathe deeply and open your eyes to the world.

Reaching Higher Planes of Consciousness
If you have goals of accessing higher planes of consciousness, kundalini awakening is a great place to start. In fact, kundalini awakening itself instigates awareness of these higher planes, and some people even gain access to them, but it always helps to have a guide at your disposal. For those interested in reaching these states of consciousness with the help of eager kundalini. The following 8 steps will lead you to the access you seek, when performed for the right reasons.

First, clear your mind completely. Before you embark on the journey to other planes of consciousness, you'll need to make sure that you don't bring any unnecessary emotional baggage with you, so check it at the door! Close your eyes and breathe into a meditative focus. Try to eliminate as many thoughts as possible from your mind; let them dissolve like salt in water or like snow on hot pavement. Let them evaporate from your mind until a still and calm inner space is achieved. This still space is absolutely essential to attain moving forward, so you'll want to ensure it's a strong one. Hold this space in mind for as long as possible before even moving onto the second step.

Second, evoke the central channel. Meditatively shift your consciousness now to see this central channel illuminated within you as best as possible. If you're still working through any recent blockages, you might see those as darker spots in the channel, but hopefully, no spots exist whatsoever. Love is a vibration you'll want to carry with you as you journey into other realms, for it is part of what's so unique about being human. If you ever get lost, you can always follow that vibration back to where you came from, but that matters later. For now, just focus on breathing and boosting that central channel with as much love and light as possible.

Third, allow the serpent to rise. Once it's comfortable to do so and once it knows the channel is ready, kundalini will come out to play. At this point, you can meditatively visualize kundalini following its winding path through your chakras once more, up from the base to the crown and back down again. See how many slow and steady cycles you can withstand witnessing before you are pushed into action. Simply watch the serpent complete its inner course and trust in its energetic potential for you. Express love to kundalini and trust in the universe and then follow the next step.

Fourth, accept and express gratitude for your body, and don't let yourself forget about what your physical body does for you even on a daily basis! It's a source of great strength and support, and it will remain solid and secure on the earth plane while your consciousness and soul explore others. Breathe in that truth and breathe out your trust. Additionally, express a powerful wave of acceptance and love for your body. Feel grateful for all that it does for you and be proud of what you've accomplished with it! Whether your past life experiences come to mind or your conquering of chakra blockages to allow for kundalini awakening does instead, simply remember all your body has done for you and be proud! Know that future experiences with this earthen form will absolutely benefit your growth.

Fifth, check your goals against your higher self. You must have come to this experience in search of higher planes of consciousness for a reason, and that reason might not be backed by the purest of intentions. Try to be as honest with yourself as possible as you search to define the real reason why you want this type of access to other planes of consciousness. Once you've divined the answer, check it against your higher self. Some people ask this question in the form of, "WWJD? What would Jesus do?" You'll ask it in terms of, "What would my best self do?" Use that insight to inform your experience as you likely decide to move forward.

Sixth, state the goal you have in mind to kundalini. Once you've checked and altered those goals based on your interactions with your higher self, you should also check to make sure that your kundalini can handle such cosmic connectivity right now. Check in with kundalini again and make sure it's not overburdened, exhausted, or that it got accidentally rerouted from its path winding through the central channel. As long as kundalini is operating normally, then things should be good to go! Don't push things, however. It sure sounds fun to visit higher planes of consciousness, but if shakti isn't there with you somehow because you jumped the gun with kundalini's readiness, you'll surely regret it, for the experience will be nowhere near what you imagined.

Seventh, let kundalini take you there. As kundalini expresses its approval of your goals, let go of the reins and let kundalini take control. Trust that this vehicle of source energy will get you where you need to be, and feel the company of your angels and guardians, too, for they'll surely be able to make this trans-plane journey with you.

Eighth, make sure that you've developed a tactic to return. Accessing higher planes of consciousness (and other planes of existence) can be an experience similar to astral projection and travel at times, and you'll have to remember where you came from so you know where to return to. You won't want your consciousness floating out in the ether for anyone to imprint on or get interested in. In order to ensure that doesn't happen, make a return plan before you even "leave" for the higher plane. If you've seen the film Inception, take a note from their book and bring a "token" with you that will remind you which world is real. It might sound crazy, but the more awakened you and your kundalini become, the more immersive meditation experiences of this nature you'll have for yourself.

Astral Projection & Travel

Different from travelling to higher planes of consciousness with kundalini's help, you can also astrally project and travel with the same type of aid. When going to other planes of consciousness, the soul and mind go to another level of thought that impacts the body in ways standard words or knowledge would never be able to do. But when using astral travel, one can actually go to other dimensions, realities, worlds, and more. This section will serve as a guide for those who seek to develop abilities of astral projection and travel, for these gifts are more complicated than they may seem at first.

First, clear your mind completely in a meditative state. Let your mind become clear of thoughts and emotions. Let any urges, desires, needs, or calculations exit your mind as well. The goal is to have calm, serene silence within the mind. Before you travel to other energetic planes, you need to make sure that you're as pure of an energetic expression as possible. You don't want to end up going out into these other planes with energetic blockages that keep you from coming home just because of one thought that stuck out before you left! Try to eliminate that possibility from happening by maintaining this calm, composed mind before moving any further in the process.

Second, evoke the central channel and raise the kundalini. With your calm and collected mind, remember that central channel. Let it become illuminated with the same warm white light and then allow kundalini to feel invited to rise. Without any blockages in its way, the serpent cautiously yet comfortably winds and winds to your crown chakra and then back down again.

Third, allow yourself and the kundalini to meld together in a hypnotic state. With kundalini flowing through your chakras and activating the central channel, close your eyes and try to visualize what's happening in detail on the inside. Watch kundalini methodically rise and fall. Feel supported by those efforts but also allow those conscious thoughts and emotions to fade away once more. You want to get hypnotized by this motion; get lost in it! All that matters is that you and kundalini are one, and its motion within you begins to create a vibration that pronounces: I'm ready for travel.

Fourth, remember that your mind has so much more power than your body. Before you embark on the astral voyage, you'll want to partially ground yourself with this knowledge, and the best way to do so is to "ground" yourself (so to speak) in the astral body. With those eyes closed and your mind in this hypnotized state, begin to connect with the body that's not yours. What I mean is this: when you visualize squeezing your fist, it's not your actual body that moves, but you are imagining a body that's yours (that's not actually your physical body) doing the work. In this sense, I want you to connect with the version of your body that exists in the mental realm and that's affected when you visualize things. Try to move each finger and toe of that imagined body separately. Create several other exercises for yourself to root with this astral body, and your trans-plane journey will become all the easier. A few other things you can try are imagining doing jumping jacks, doing a cartwheel, counting on your fingers, juggling, and doing an intricate dance.

Fifth, connect to your subtle energy. You've worked to connect with your physical body, you've done the same and connected with kundalini, and you're connected with your astral body, but what about what's left? There's always an additional layer of subtle energy vibrating all around you due to the other carbon-based life-forms (and technological devices) in our world. Try to get in touch with that energy layer now. With your still-partially-hypnotized mind and your openness to the whole experience, allow yourself to feel a buzzing at the edge of your being as your astral body begins to separate from your physical body. This buzzing or vibrating is a good sign. It says that things are going exactly the way they should. Not everyone feels these vibrations before astral projection, however.

Sixth, let visualization take control. With your eyes closed, start to see your body as if you were floating above, it looking down. Let your soul, essentially, become elevated and weightless as it rises above your own body. Like the rising kundalini, your soul floats up to its highest potential and back down, just starting to explore the space around you. It wanders through your room and house but does not get outside your home to start. There's still a bit of safety-making and grounding work to do before that final step into the ether can be achieved.

Seventh (and maybe most important!), always keep your root in mind! There will be a silver cord that attaches your astral body to your physical body, and that will sometimes be the only thing that can help you get back home. Don't forget to mind this physical and energetic root cord. As you have been exploring your room or your home, did you notice that cord yet? If so, that's wonderful! If not, you may not be having a full, pure astrally projective experience quite yet, but keep running with the visualization to see where it takes you!

Eighth, allow yourself to explore the astral plane you've found, with baby steps first, of course. Now that you see your silver "grounding" or homing cord, go ahead and see what's around. Look around your neighborhood and maybe your city. Stay on the earth plane at first so that you don't get too overwhelmed. Eventually, you can try to explore completely different planes, realities, and dimensions, but your home density is always a safe and familiar place to start.

Chapter 4. Daily Kundalini Yoga Techniques

Kundalini yoga is a specific yoga practice designed to awaken, balance, and harmonize Kundalini energy. Individuals who embark on a Kundalini yoga journey often report that they begin experiencing the awakening symptoms after just one or two sessions. This awakening furthers as they move deeper into their Kundalini yoga journey. This form of yoga also helps support the Kundalini energy, keeping it awakened, full, and thriving in the individual practicing it.

Kundalini Yoga

Not all yoga practices are made equally. Some are designed to stretch out the physical body, some are designed to facilitate a mind-body-spirit connection, and others are designed for specific purposes, such as Kundalini yoga.

Kundalini yoga does not emphasize the physical as much as other practices, such as Hatha yoga, do. Instead, it incorporates meditation and mantras as a foundational part of the overall practice. The combined experience of the mind, body, and spirit being brought together through these three practices encourages Kundalini awakening and supports Kundalini flow. The body is supported and awakened by the yoga poses, the mind is supported and awakened by the mantras, and the spirit is supported and awakened through the meditation.

Introduced by Yogi Bhajan in the 1970s, Kundalini yoga is still relatively new to the Western regions. It is, however, rising in popularity as more individuals seek to incorporate the mind, body and spirit connection in their lives.

The 10 Bodies

There are ten bodies associated with Kundalini yoga. All ten bodies are awakened through Kundalini yoga, allowing individuals to begin to continue feeling full Kundalini flow. These bodies are as follows.

The Soul Body

The soul body is your flow of spirit. This is where you connect to your Soul and to infinity. The soul body is considered to be the foundational body and your true self. It provides you with the ability to live from your heart. This body responds to any form of heart work, as well as the raising of your Kundalini energy.

The Negative Mind

Your second body is your negative mind. This is one of our strongest bodies, as it consistently works toward assessing the environment and circumstances you are in, and if there is any danger present as a result. This body is responsible for your ability to stay alive and gifts us with what is often called "a longing for belonging" which is a phrase coined by Yogi Bhajan. Your negative mind can be balanced through integrity and discipline.

The Positive Mind

The third body you have is your positive mind. This works toward assessing what is positive, beneficial, and affirming in your environment and circumstances. This body allows you to see where opportunities lie and where you may be able to access resources.

The playful mind is responsible for bringing willpower and playfulness into your life. Everything you do with your navel point, or your core, contributes to your positive mind. You can also balance it through increasing your self-esteem.

The Neutral Mind

Your neutral mind is responsible for guiding you through assessing the information coming in from both your negative and positive minds. The neutral mind is compassionate, recognizes polarities, and works on intuition. The neutral mind can be balanced through meditation, which is a foundational part of Kundalini yoga.

The Physical Body

Your physical body is your temple. This is where all of the other nine bodies come together to exist in harmony. This body allows you to be able to balance yourself and your life. You can also sacrifice for your hopes, dreams, and the greater community through your physical body. The physical body possesses the energy of the teacher. It is balanced through regular exercise. The physical body also loves to share what has been learned with others.

The Arcline

Your arcline body is like a halo that wraps around your head around your earlobes, brow, and hairline. If you are a woman, you have a second arcline that exists across your breast line. Your acrline body allows you to intuit the world around you, as well as project yourself upon it. You can use this body to help you focus and meditate. Any practices associated with the pituitary gland or the third eye (pineal gland) support the awakening of the arcline body.

The Aura

Your aura body is your electromagnetic field of energy that extends around the physical body. It is responsible for holding your life force energy, as well as for shielding you and providing protection. Through your aura body, you can elevate yourself both energetically and consciously. Natural fibers worn on the body as well as meditation both contribute to awakening and balancing your aura. You can also incorporate the color white into your life and practice, which is believed to magnify and expand your aura.

The Pranic Body

Your pranic body is supported by your breath, which brings life force energy into your physical body. This allows you to experience accomplishment and energy in your life. You interact with this body every time you breathe in and out. The pranic body is awakened and supported by pranayama practices.

The Subtle Body

Your ninth body is your subtle body, and it is responsible for helping you see beyond the physical matter and into what else exists. This body is deeply connected to your soul body, as it carries your soul body after your physical body dies. There are many wonderful teachers and gurus who continue to teach us through their subtle body despite no longer being in the physical realization. Your ability to master anything exists within this body. If you want to experience mastery, do a Kundalini practice for 1,000 days in a row. Then, your subtle body will be balanced.

The Radiant Body

Your tenth and final body is your radiant body. This body is responsible for giving you radiance, courage, and nobility. When you meet someone who is naturally charismatic and magnetic, they have a balanced, radiant body. To balance and awaken your radiant body, you need to have commitment. Through the art of being committed to your practice, truth, kindness, and excellence, you balance and awaken your radiant body.

Embodiment

Though not technically a body itself, embodiment is an important element of awakening the 10 bodies. Embodiment suggests that all ten bodies are awakened and balanced. This is the ultimate goal with Kundalini. When you practice Kundalini yoga, you are awakening, balancing, and strengthening your ten bodies.

Yoga Poses to Awaken the 10 Bodies

The following yoga poses are written in the sequence in which they should be completed. There are 14 poses in total, all of which are designed to help you awaken your Kundalini and your 10 bodies. It is important that you remain mindful toward your breathing and use each of these as a pose to meditate in. You can also repeat a mantra to help you further integrate your mind, body, and spirit together.

Easy Pose

Easy pose, known as Sukhasana, is the first pose you are going to start with. This pose requires you to sit on the ground with your legs crossed and bringing your hands in front of your heart. Bringing the hands in front of the heart in this way is known as the prayer mudra. Rub your palms together a few times, warming them up. Then, relax your thumb joints into your sternum.

Stretch Pose

Gently move from easy pose down to your back, with your legs stretched straight below you and your arms straight down by your sides. When you are ready, bring your heels together and point your toes away from your body. Gently lift your head about 6 inches off of the ground and look down toward your toes. If this feels like it is too much or like it is bringing discomfort, you can slide your hands under your lower back and use them to support you. As you do this, practice the breath of fire (explained below.) Hold this sequence for about 1-3 minutes. If you are pregnant, do not practice this pose or the breath of fire.

The breath of fire is a pranayama. To do it, you want to inhale while pushing your navel away from your spine, then exhale pulling your navel back toward your spine. This allows you to completely fill your diaphragm, lungs, and throat with air and then exhale all of the air from your throat, lungs, and diaphragm.

Knees to Chest Tuck

While laying on your back, after you finish the stretch pose, you can move into a knees-to-chest tuck. Simply bring your knees up, wrap your hands around them, and then gently pull them toward your chest. If you are feeling confident, you can lift your head up. Your nose should be pointing between your knees. Use the breath of fire and hold this position for about 1-3 minutes. If you are pregnant or are experiencing a heavy menstrual cycle, you should substitute the breath of fire of long deep breathing. Breathe in for about six seconds, and out for about six seconds. Do not hold your breath at any point.

Ego Eradicator

When you are done your knees to chest tuck, you want to come back up to a seated position with your legs crossed in front of you. Begin creating the easy pose by bringing your hands back into the prayer mudra in front of your chest. Then, curl your fingers in and point your thumb up toward the air, as if you are giving someone two thumbs up. Your fingers should only be lightly curled, with the fingertips gently touching the palms and the majority of the palms remaining exposed. Then, put your hands up above your head and out to the sides. This opens and exposes your chest and core. Close your eyes and practice the breath of fire for about 1-3 minutes before moving into the next pose. Again, if you are pregnant, refrain from using the breath of fire and instead practice deep breathing.

Hold Your Toes

Now, you want to uncurl your legs and stretch them out to the sides in front of you. Your legs should be spread in a wide "V" shape in front of you. Keep your feet flexed with your toes pulled back toward your body. Do not push yourself to stretch further than is comfortable in this pose. Allow yourself to relax into it and trust that the more you practice, the more flexible you will become and the easier this pose will get. When you are ready, take a deep inhale and stretch your arms over your head. Then exhale and stretch your hands out to your feet, holding onto your toes and relaxing into the pose. Hold this for about 1-3 minutes.

Grasp Your Shins

Cross your legs once more, returning to easy pose. Hold each of your shins. Then, inhale and flex your spine forward, curling it over as if to expose your back. When you exhale, flex your spine backward, as if to expose your chest. You should be getting a good relaxed stretch out of this, so keep it calm and intentional. Do this pose for between 1-3 minutes before moving on to rock pose.

Rock Pose

To complete rock pose, you will need to tuck your feet under yourself and sit on your shins with your knees together in front of you. You should be sitting on your heels with your feet relaxed. Let your hands gently come to a resting position on your thighs before flexing the spine as you were in the previous pose. Your eyes should be closed and, if you feel comfortable doing this, gently rolled toward your third eye. Continue this stretching pose for about 1-3 minutes.

Grasp Your Shoulders

Remain in the same seated pose as you used for rock pose, with your heels underneath you. Keep your torso and head pointed forward, looking directly in front of you. When you are ready, lift your arms up and gently grasp your shoulders with your hands. Your left thumb should be behind your left shoulder with your fingers rested above your left collarbone. Likewise, your right thumb should be behind your right shoulder with your fingers rested above your right collarbone. Sit in this stretch pose for a few moments. Then, on each inhales twist toward the left, and on each exhale twist toward the right. Your arms should remain lifted, keeping your biceps parallel to the floor during this pose. Do this for 1-3 minutes.

To take this pose a step further, stay in this posture and return your torso and head to center, looking directly in front of you. Your hands should remain in the same position, with your elbows extended out toward the side. Each time you inhale, lift your elbows up, drawing a line toward the sky. When you exhale, draw your elbows down, returning to your original position with your biceps parallel to the floor. Do this stretching pose for about 1-3 minutes.

Shoulder Lifts

Take a few moments to return to a crossed leg position. Then, gently rest your hands on your knees and allow them to completely relax. Refrain from drawing your knees up in this position, as these shoulder lifts can sometimes result in tight hips causing your knees to draw up toward the sky. Allow them to relax toward the floor instead. When you are ready, inhale and lift the left shoulder toward the sky. As you exhale, lower the left shoulder and simultaneously lift the right shoulder. Continue this for 1 minute before reversing the process. As you reverse it, lift your right shoulder on the inhale, and drop it to lift your left shoulder on the exhale. Continue the stretch on this side for another 1 minute.

Double Shoulder Lifts

After completing your alternating shoulder lifts, you can begin lifting both shoulders at the same time. For this, you want to lift them and try to pull them toward each other on the inhale. Then, drop them and push them away from each other, allowing them to relax on the exhale. Continue doing this double shoulder lift practice for 1 minute.

Turn Your Head

As you continue to hold the easy pose with your legs crossed in front of you and your hands rested gently on your knees, you can begin turning your head. This will stretch out your neck, upper spine and upper back area, allowing you to experience a nice relaxing sensation. Each time you inhale, turn your head to the left. When you exhale, turn your head to the right. Your head should remain level, and your nose should draw a line around your head that is parallel to the floor. After you have done this for one minute, reverse the breath. On each inhalation turn your head to the right, and on the exhalation draw your nose across the front of you, turning your head toward the left. When you are done this reversed breathing part of the pose, bring your head to come back to a resting position in front of you, slowly exhale, and relax your body.

Frog Pose

This will be one of the more advanced poses of the yoga session. The frog pose requires you to come up into a squatting position, resting on your toes. Your heels should be drawn up toward the sky and touching each other beneath you. Your fingertips can be placed on the ground between your knees, with your fingers separated wide and each tip firmly planted into the ground. Evenly displace the weight between each of your fingers and toes to allow for a centered pose. Your head should be lifted with your chin pointing upward, allowing you to gaze toward the sky. Don't lift your head too hard, but rather allow for a nice relaxed upward focus. As you inhale, stretch your legs out slightly allowing your glutes to rise toward the sky. Remain on your toes for this pose. As you exhale, come down to the original position. Continue holding this rhythm with your breath for about 54 repetitions. However, if this is beyond your skill level, you can always aim for 13 to 26 repetitions. Continue adding more to your practice each time until you reach the 54 repetition mark.

Laya Yoga Meditation

With most of your poses now completed, you can enter the meditation part of the process. Here, you want to sit back into the easy pose. Left your wrists rest on your knees as you point your palms toward the sky. Then, bring the tip of your thumb to the tip of your index finger and create a circular shape. This is called the Gyan mudra. Now, chant the following mantra. As you are chanting take the time to visualize energy that spirals all the way from the base of your spine to the top of your head. This is the realized energy of Kundalini.

The chant is as follows:

"Ek Ong Karah,

Saa Taa Naa Maah

Siree Whaah, Hay Guroo."

You want to continue chanting and meditating for a total of 11 minutes to experience the full effect of this process. Carry the visualization from the base of your spine to the top of your head during the entire process, allowing it to unfold naturally in whatever way it manifests for you. Refrain from forcing the energy, but rather set the intention and allow it to show you how it wants to be realized, rather than the other way around. This is a great opportunity to explore the practice of releasing blocks by allowing the process to unfold.

Savasana

Lastly, you want to end your Kundalini yoga sequence with savasana pose. This pose requires you to gently lie down on your back, with your feet down and gently separated and your arms relaxed out to your sides. Breathe intentionally but with a natural rhythm here and relax as the energies flow through your body. Instead of trying to create or force anything, receive all that comes your way. This will allow you to integrate the entire yoga experience. From this pose, you can gently guide your awareness between the ten bodies, balance, and wholeness.

Chapter 5. Guided Kundalini Meditations

Kundalini Exercise 1

This is a sequence of exercises that ignites the fire within in hopes of waking kundalini. The mantras used is related to the name of truth and acts to stimulate our entire being with its vibration. The yoga poses and visualization act to engage your energetic body as well as your physical body to really get the energy moving.

Practice these exercises after your body is sufficiently warmed up after some light yoga or breathing exercises.

- Kneel onto your knees, sitting on the heels of your feet.
- Inhale and bend forward touching your brow to the ground
- Breathe deeply for ten breaths, relaxing into the position.
- Chant the following mantra, internally or out loud: Sat, Sat, Sat, Sat, Sat, Sat, Naam.

As you chant, each Sat should be vibrated into a chakra, starting with the root and rising through the other chakras until we reach the crown chakra and chant Naam. Continue this exercise for ten minutes, then move onto the next step for Kundalini exercise 1.

After you have completed, the Sat Naam exercise, you can begin the next sequence. This practice is simple and helps to relax after the Sat Naam practice.

- Raise your brow from the floor.
- Slowly stretch your legs outward, extending them in front of you.
- Straighten your back and raise your hands above your head.
- Bend at the hips and try to grab your toes, hold this position.
- Breathe deeply for seven breaths.

Each of the seven breaths should engage a chakra. Visualize the breath penetrating the root chakra, then upward through the other chakras until your seventh breath. After the seventh breath, immediately move onto the next sequence.

This part of the exercise is a winding down of sorts. You will feel the energy in your body shift dramatically. Take note of the changes you experience as you relax.

- Raise up from touching your toes then lay down on your back.
- Relax your body with your hands at your sides. Breathe deeply.
- Lay here motionless for seven minutes.

As you lay quietly, visualize kundalini lying dormant. Not unlike your motionless body, she lays asleep. Visualize her as a literal snake, just let the details come as they will.

Once you have reached seven minutes, rise up slowly, visualizing kundalini awakening. Sit quietly with your visualization and see what happens. Sit quietly and breathe normally.

This is the end of the first kundalini exercise, but after you relaxed, you can perform it again and again. It is best not to perform this exercise more than three times per day.

Kundalini Exercise 2

This sequence of exercises is designed for purification of the body and chakras. It acts as an overall clearing and opening, making way for the kundalini energy to rise. This purification is much needed in a world of synthetic drugs and foods. This exercise pairs well after long work weeks or before healing baths.

- Stand up straight, balancing your weight on our feet.
- Stretch your leg behind you with the top of your foot staying on the ground.
- Bend the other leg until you have a ninety-degree angle at your knee, your weight will be on the bent leg.
- Place your palms together, and hold at your chest, focus your vision on your brow.
- Deep breathe in this position.
- Stand up and switch legs performing the same exercise.

This practice is a physical work out that helps to get the body moving and engage the chakras in preparation for the next sequence.

- Sit down and cross your legs comfortably.
- Put your hands on your hips and raise your diaphragm.
- Breathe deeply in this position for three minutes.

The next sequence is more intensive, you can view the first sequences as a warm-up for the next ones.

- Stay seated and breathing consistently.
- Interlock your hands at your chest, forearms parallel to the floor.
- Inhale as deep as you can.
- Forcibly exhale all the breath as fast as you can.
- Inhale fully and hold breath.
- Exhale completely and forcibly.
- Continue this practice for three minutes.

We should be raising the energy up through the chakras as we practice this, the forced breaths engaging the solar plexus chakra and heart chakra. The next sequence contacts the throat and third eye chakras.

- Stay seated with your legs crossed.
- Extend the arms out at the sides like wings.
- Roll your eyes up gazing at your brow.
- Breathe deeply and hold this position for 3 minutes.
- Press your hands together and straighten your spine.
- Push firm on your hands and hold this position for three minutes.

This exercise is excellent for purification purposes but also works directly with kundalini energy. Visualizing kundalini being purified with this practice can add to the potency as well.

Exercise for Blockages

This exercise is great for clearing blockages in your chakras and nadis. It acts as a great precursor to kundalini works, while also engaging the kundalini. Practice this exercise on a weekly basis. It ensures your chakras do not become clogged.

- Sit with your legs crossed and raise your hands over your head. Practice a range of motion stretching your arms in circles.
- Stretch your arms straight up and bend at the waist, reaching for your toes. Rise back up and then bend back down again. Do this ten times.
- Now stand up and raise your hands above our head stretching from side to side.
- From the standing position, bend forward and touch the ground. Do this ten times.
- Raise your arms overhead, crisscross your arms, and stretch them thoroughly.
- Clinch your fists at your heart and roll your shoulders forward and backward.
- Lay down and pull your knees to your chest and roll back and forth on your spine.
- Stay lying down flat and pull your knees alternately to your chest. Pull one leg in as you stretch the other leg back out straight and parallel to the floor.
- Still lying on your back, bring your hands up as if to clap. Open the arms wide and repeat the motion.
- Lie flat with your arms by your sides and totally relax.

This exercise becomes quite fun as you move through the steps quickly. It can almost become a dance of sorts. This exercise can be performed before an intensive yoga or meditation session to get the energy flowing smoothly.

A Note on Ancestral Lineage

This exercise is great for breaking ancestral blockages as well. Consider all the people in your ancestral line, only a small fraction of them that you have actually met. These lines can get blocked just as energetic channels get blocked by day-to-day life. There may be criminals or other troublemakers in this lineage.

The advanced techniques of working to clear our energetic ancestral lineage are powerful and complex. Use the blockage exercises above to heal your ancestral lines visually. You can imagine the line of ancestors going all the way back to the source of consciousness, healing it along the way. You may even want to leave offerings or call upon your ancestors to assist you in this work.

Ancestral practices are very complex and would need a whole book to explore properly. For now, use the blockage techniques to clear your family line.

Chakra Balancing Exercise

Stimulating the chakra system at least once per day is good practice to ensure that your chakras will not become blocked or unbalanced in the future. Deep breathing exercises and a consistent yoga routine go a long way to achieve this balanced system, but we also must practice more intensive exercises as well, especially if we have yet to awaken the kundalini energy.

- In a standing position, place your feet shoulder-width apart.
- Squat down so the thighs are parallel to the floor.
- Reach towards your toes, placing the palms on top of the feet be sure to keep your back straight.
- Lift your head and look forward.
- Move to kneeling position, sit on the heels, and stretch the arms straight over your head.
- Interlock your fingers except for the index fingers, which should be pointing straight up.
- Chant the sound Sat from the solar plexus chakra, and pull the navel all the way in and up, toward the spine.
- On Naam relax the stomach.
- Continue for three minutes.

This exercise is great for stimulating the entire chakra system. If you wish to practice the above before moving on to the second sequence, then do so until you are fully prepared to perform the entire exercise. This is your practice, so make it what you want and go at your own pace.

- Kneel sitting on your heels, rest the hands on the thighs.
- Begin inhaling in short sips through your pursed lips until the lungs are full of air.
- With your breath held, raise up and rotate the hips around in a circle.
- Exhale and sit back down on your heels.
- Move to a lying position and bring the hands to the Navel Point. The left hand is closest to the body, and the right hand is over the left.
- There are about two inches between the body and also between the hands. Rotate the hands around each other in a clockwise direction, keeping your hands an inch or two form your body.

This is a great exercise for learning to feel the chakras as well. Step 16 is essentially asking you to use your hands in circular motions to feel and manipulate the chakras. Move on with the next steps after you have sufficiently felt and moved the chakras.

- Remain on your back and extend your arms straight above you.
- Make fists of your hands and pull your fists into your chest.
- Release your clenched fists and repeat three more times.
- Resting on your back, place the left hand on the heart and the right hand over the left.
- Breathe deeply and engage your heart chakra.
- Release your fists and place your hands at your sides
- Lay comfortably for five to ten minutes.

This exercise acts to clear away chakra blockages while also acting as a great warm-up exercise to start your day or begin your kundalini practices. These complex exercises have so many steps because this is the amount of effort needed to stimulate the kundalini energy.

The kundalini exercises above are the methods that will skyrocket your practice from a humble beginner's practice to a full-fledged advanced routine. When these exercises are practiced consistently and approached with respect and seriousness, you will surely open your chakras and awaken the kundalini energy. These practices should all be performed on an empty stomach to avoid cramps or indigestion. This is why we recommend performing them in the morning when you first awake. Your belly will be empty, and you will have a fresh canvas to work with as you start your day. Not to mention these exercises really get the blood moving, you may even be able to skip your coffee!

Neck Lock

The neck lock is an essential lock applied throughout many yoga exercises and traditions. This lock can be applied during yoga, meditation, and breathing exercises as you like. Do not apply a neck lock if you are required to move or rotate your head during your routine.

How to perform neck lock:

- Sit in your preferred practice space, keep your back and neck straight.
- Lift your chest upward as you deeply inhale, exhale but keep your chest in place.
- Pull your chin toward the back of your neck, lengthening the spine.
- Be sure your facial muscles and neck muscles are relaxed.
- Hold this position.

The neck lock is relatively simple. Simply adjusting your neck in this way helps to open the throat chakra and manipulate the energy there. Be sure not to force your head down or created tension when performing this lock; it should not cause pain.

When you perform the neck lock, you allow your neck to be opened and to be positioned in its natural way. This helps you maintain better posture in general and keeps the energy that is created in the upper areas of your body, offering a perfect posture for meditation, or simply sitting day to day.

Knot of Shiva

The knot of Shiva is located at your brow. This is fitting since Shiva's masculine energy is housed in the upper chakras. Untying this knot is the goal for this lock, it is thought that this knot blocks the gateway to the intuitive faculties. WE untie this knot by relaxing the muscles in our brow. This seems simple, but it is much more difficult than you think. We must completely relax the eyes and surrounding muscles, you will feel your eyelids lower, and your head will feel 'open.' Maintain this lock as long as possible and also implement it while meditating. This lock is great for work with the third eye chakra.

Diaphragm Lock

The diaphragm muscle forms a physical layer between our hearts and lower bodies. This area also houses an energetic layer between the upper and lower body. The diaphragm is almost like a barrier or gateway between the upper and lower chakras and working with this area is great or stimulating the heart or solar plexus chakras, helping energy flow between them.

How to perform diaphragm lock:

- Perform this lock on an empty stomach.
- You must also only perform this lock with no breath in your lungs, meaning while you've had fully exhaled.
- Sit comfortably with your back straight.
- Inhale completely and exhale fully through your nose. Hold this exhale, do not breathe in.
- Pull your entire abdominal region, especially the area above your belly button, back toward your spine.
- Maintain this position and keep your back straight.
- Press the middle of your spine forward gently.
- Hold this strongly tightened abdominal area for as long as you can without straining your muscles.
- Release and relax, inhaling slowly.

This is a fiery lock that gets the internal flame moving, this fire touches the upper and lower chakras, notably opening the heart chakra for compassion, and the solar plexus for motivation. Use this lock during deep breathing exercises.

Knot of Vishnu

Performing this lock correctly is similar to the knot of Shiva exercise. The knot of Vishnu is located at the chest, near the heart chakra. We need to untie this knot to open our hearts to joyful love. This knot is also thought to open our hearts to a less serious and playful side of life. To untie this knot, we can breathe deep into our chest, using visualizations of the heart chakra releasing to loosen the threads. We can also release this knot by pressing our fingertips just under the collar bone to the left or right of the sternum. Massaging this area takes a page from the acupressure approach to this practice.

Root Lock

This lock is a powerful contraction of muscles that stimulates lower chakra energy, allowing is to rise into creative energy. This redirection of energy is great for any yoga or meditation practice. Ending a yoga or meditation practice with root lock exercises is common throughout many traditions. This lock is helpful for any sexual issues that need to be resolved, even helping to redirect sexual energy to desired places.

How to do root lock:

- Contract the anal sphincter muscles and lift upward then inward.
- While keeping these muscles tightened, contract the muscles around the sexual organs. This will instantly send a tingling sensation up your spine.
- Flex your lower abdominal muscles near the navel area.
- Release and relax your muscles.

You can perform these steps simultaneously or in a flowing motion, tightening and releasing the lock. Combine with breathing exercises, holding the lock as you exhale, and releasing it as you inhale. This lock is a great exercise for your sexual organs, physically and energetically. It is a great way to get in touch with your body and bring your primal energy upward through the chakras.

The rook lock is great for stimulating the root chakra and sacral chakra, but it is also good for bringing this energy to the other chakras, in a sense, locking the energy from getting to the lower chakras. This is also a great lock for learning to feel the energy as it moves.

Knot of Brahm
The knot of Brahm is located at the root chakra near the base of the spine. This knot needs to be untied to keep energy moving smoothly for the lower chakras. This knot can be loosened by using the root lock exercise above, as well as a meditation on the root chakra. Untying this not allows us to be freed from our disruptive primal desires.

The Great Lock
This lock is named a great lock for a reason. It is a combination of all three of the lock exercises listed above. You typically start with the root lock then move upward performing all three locks simultaneously. This lock is incredibly powerful and should be performed only on an empty stomach, and after you have warmed your body up with some casual yoga and meditation.

This lock is the ultimate exercise to stimulate the entire seven chakra system. It is an excellent way to end a meditation session or to be implemented into the session itself. You can also switch in between the locks in an upward motion, root lock, diaphragm lock, neck lock and then back to root lock, to stimulate the entire chakra system.

The great lock is thought to balance our entire energetic and physical makeup, engaging the entire body. When practiced properly, it can achieve amazing results, getting the entire system moving and opening the chakras all at once. This practice is a great exercise to prepare you for the kundalini awakening, having all the chakras engaged at once prepares the energy centers for a more intensive flow of energy.

Introducing these locks into your practice is an advanced practice that needs to be handled with care. If you experience any pain, you should release the lock immediately. Gradually introduce these locks into your routine as you progress on your path to self-transformation. Once you have mastered the great lock and are able to transition from lock to lock smoothly, you will be able to take your practice in any direction.

Chapter 6. Meditation, Exercises and Poses

Pranayama

Breath is so important for balancing the energy channels and the whole chakra system. All of the benefits of pranayama listed above are just some of the physical and mental advantages. When you utilize Kundalini breathing for awakening, you engage that spiritual life force even more. Before you get started practicing, let's learn a little bit about what Kundalini breath looks like.

The main types of Kundalini yoga breathing are:

- Alternating Nostril Breaths: This basic Kundalini breath is a great place to start before advancing to more challenging techniques. It is relaxing and helps you achieve calm, connecting you to breathe awareness. Essentially, you close one nostril with a finger, or thumb, then breathe deeply through the other, open nostril. Then you switch sides. Repeat.
- Breath of Fire: This breath is as intense as it sounds. Rapid and forceful, this breath style engages your abdominal muscles to quickly pulse out air in exhalation after each very quick inhalation, like if you are jogging and your breathing becomes quicker and more intense. It is much more invigorating and purifying.
- Deep, Long Breath: As the name suggests, this breath takes a lot longer than a fiery one. If practiced, it can aid in opening the third eye and crown chakras. The practice involves pressing the tip of your tongue to the roof of your mouth and breathing in and out only through your nostrils. The fewer breaths per minute you take, the more likely you are to crack open the third eye.
- Mantra Breath (so-hum): The mantra style breath brings Kundalini upward gradually as a deeper focus breath meditation. You do not intone the words aloud, you think them. The 'so' is your inhale word to think as you breathe in and 'hum' is your exhale word to think as you release the breath through the nose.

On top of these styles of breath, there is the layer of where and how it travels through the body. This is a related, but different breathing context. You could say, the above-stated breathing styles are the vehicles, while the ideas listed below are the highways for them to travel on. These highways bare resemblance to the ancient Greek symbol known as a caduceus.

You are likely familiar with this symbol as it has been the universal symbol of medicine in the United States for some 200 years, however, it has actually been known as The Rod of Asclepius since around 2500 B.C.E. It is more likely that this symbol represents the concept of a "universal solvent." It is two snakes, intertwining around a tall, central, staff (Rod of Asclepius). You may have noticed, as you are reading this, some similarities to this symbol and the idea of Kundalini energy rising up the spine (staff) like a snake. This imagery directly correlates to the concepts of Ida, Pingala, and Sushumna. The channels called Ida and Pingala are like the two snakes, twirling around the spine's main energetic channel, Sushumna. Below are some distinctions about each energy highway.

- Ida - This is the feminine energy channel; cooling, passive, of the mind and associated with the lunar (moon) energies.
- Pingala - This is the masculine energy channel; heating, active, of the physical and associated with the solar (sun) energies.

- Sushumna - This is the main highway, running through the spine as the Ida and Pingala twist around. This channel is what activates and balances your chakras and when Ida and Pingala are flowing in synchronized harmony, so too can the Kundalini energy rise and flow.

Embracing these concepts is what will help you better understand the importance of breath in the Kundalini awakening experience. You can incorporate them into your own Kundalini practice. Take a deep breath through your nose, let it out through your mouth, and get ready to learn some Kundalini breathing exercises.

Breathing Exercises for Kundalini Awakening

It is time to practice Pranayama. Your breathing exercises are vital to your overall energy, health, peace of mind, focus and overall well-being.

If you feel, or know you are already on the journey of awakening, you can use the techniques to bring balance to your already awakened Kundalini.

The Sushumna breath exercise, referred to as Anuloma Viloma Pranayama, is what will help you prepare your whole system for awakening the chakras, clearing the energy channels, awakening the Kundalini, and giving you the benefit of calming the mind.

Instructions:

- Sit on the ground with legs crossed comfortably. Keep your spine straight and bring your head into alignment with your spine by slightly tucking your chin. Try to get the openings of your ears in alignment with your shoulders.
- With both hands, gesture like you are saying 'OK' by touching your pointer finger and thumb together with the three remaining fingers sticking out. Lay your 'OK' hands palm up on each knee.
- Close your eyes and take a few moments to focus on your breathing, taking five, slow, deep breaths in and out through your nose.
- Bring your right thumb up to your right nostril and press the nostril closed with your thumb. Breath slowly through your open, left nostril while you count to 4.
- Before exhaling the breath, let your thumb release from your right nostril and reach your pinky and ring finger over to close your left nostril.
- With the left nostril now closed, you can exhale through the right nostril, slowly counting to 4.
- Keeping your left nostril plugged, breath in through the right nostril for four counts. At the end of the inhale, bring your thumb back over and plug the right nostril, releasing the fingers from the left.
- Exhale from the left nostril while slowly counting to 4.

You have now achieved one full round of this pranayama. In the beginning, start with five repetitions of this per day and incorporate it into your Kundalini meditation practice. As you progress, increase the number of repetitions by one each day. Continue this increase until you can comfortably accomplish twelve rounds of this pranayama in one meditation. You can get even more advanced by doing up to 24 rounds of this per day, but for now, just start by practicing with the five rounds and very slowly and gradually work your way up.

Now that you have the basic breathing exercise down for opening up your main energy channels, you can now move through the chakras. You can incorporate each of these breathing exercises below with those practices as you begin developing your Kundalini Practice.

Root Chakra: Muladhara Pranayama

Instructions:

- Sit comfortably on the floor with your legs comfortably stretched straight in front of you and your back straight.
- Bring your hands to your shoulders so that your elbows are pointed to the side and in alignment with your shoulders.
- Take a deep, slow breath through your nose. As you inhale, reach your arms overhead and pull your knees up toward you so they are pointing toward the sky. Keep your feet and sacrum 'rooted' in the ground as you reach up.
- As you release your breath, lower your legs back down, straightening them out as you keep your spine long, and bring your hands back to their original position on your shoulders.
- Repeat this motion as you inhale and exhale fifteen to twenty times. Begin slowly and then gradually get faster with your breath and motion.
- Remember to keep your back straight and focus your vision and breath into your root chakra.
- To finish this pranayama, after your last breath out, pull your legs into a cross-legged position and with your eyes closed, bring focus to the sensation created in your root chakra. Sit this way for several moments until you are ready to open your eyes and move forward.

Sacral Chakra: Svadhisthana Pranayama

Instructions:

- From a seated position, draw your knees semi-close to your chest and place your hands on the front of your knees.
- Take a breath in through your nose and allow your hands to support you as you pull your sacrum forward, like a forward pelvic tilt, to make a curve in your lower back.
- As you pull forward and create this spinal curve, open your chest upward to the sky.
- When you breathe the air out, you will reverse this action to push the curve out of your lower back by bringing your navel closer to your spine (like a seated Cat/Cow Pose*).
- Repeat this forward arch and backward arch, breathing in and out slowly for a cycle of ten to twenty times.
- To finish out this pranayama, relax your legs into a cross-legged position and close your eyes. Breathe normally. Focus on the energy created in the sacral chakra and allow meditation on this energy for several moments.

*The Cat Pose occurs with your body positioned on all fours, knees, and palms on the ground. You pull your spine up toward the sky to create an arch in your back, the way a cat looks when scared. The Cow Pose occurs in the same position on all fours, but you let your navel drop to the floor to arch your back in the opposite direction of the Cat Pose.

Solar Plexus Chakra: Manipura Pranayama

Instructions:

- You will place your body in the same position as you did for the Sacral Chakra pose, hands gently on the knees pulled close to your chest, back straight.
- Arch your back to pull your abdomen forward, supporting your back with your hands on your knees.
- Roll your body from this forward belly stance over to the left side and continue all the way around, pulling your navel to your back (seated Cat Pose), and back around to the front (seated Cow Pose). You want to create a smooth and fluid circle roll.
- Repeat this rolling from the front to left side, then the back to right side, ten times.
- Perform this same rolling motion, starting with belly pulled forward (see step 1), to the right. Repeat ten times in this direction
- If you are comfortable with this motion, you can gradually pick up speed, but only do what feels comfortable for your spine.
- It is important during this rolling exercise that you maintain focus on the breath. While doing the rolls, try to inhale in the belly forward position, and exhale as you reach the navel back position. You would inhale from left to side, and exhale from back to right side, inhale front, etc., and vice versa for the rolling to the right.

Heart Chakra: Anahata Pranayama

- Sit with legs crossed and spine lengthened. Like you did in the Root Chakra pose, bring your hands to your shoulders, elbows pointed to the side.
- As you take a slow, deep breath in, twist your body to the right. Lengthen your spine as you twist and keep your abdominal muscles engaged.
- As you slowly breathe out, twist from the right all the way over to the left, keeping your back straight and long, ore muscles engaged and chest open.
- Be sure to keep the breaths nice and slow.
- Repeat this twisting back and forth twelve times, doing six cycles twisting to the right first and six cycles starting from the left first. Consider one time to count as steps 1-3.
- To finish this pranayama, bring your focus back to the center, drop your hands down to your knees, close your eyes and breathe normally.
- Reflect on the energy center of your heart and the energy created there by this exercise.

Throat Chakra: Visshuddhi Pranayama

Instructions:

- Sit with your legs crossed and spine long and straight.
- Interlace your fingers, clasping your hands together and with elbows pointed down, place your woven fingers under your chin.
- Take a long, deep breath in and raise your elbows out to the side, keeping your fingers under the chin and laced together.
- As you let the breath out, simultaneously lift your chin and press your elbows back together keeping your fingers as they were under your chin, opening your mouth and tilting your head back.
- Make some kind of sound as you let the air out. It can be the sound associated with the throat chakra, 'ham', or you can make any sound that feels right for you in this exercise.
- Repeat this cycle of inhaling and exhaling sixteen times.
- To finish this pranayama, bring your head and breath back to normal and rest your hands in your lap, or on your knees. Reflect on the energy pulled into your throat chakra for several moments before moving forward.

Brow Chakra: Ajna Pranayama

Instructions:

- Sit in a comfortable position on the floor with your legs crossed and your eyes closed and bring attention to your breath.
- When you are breathing, envision opening the curtain hanging in front of your third eye to let light in.
- As you breathe in through your nose, reach your hands out in front of you with your fingers stretched wide and open your eyes as wide as you can.
- Hold your breath as you reach your arms to the side, as though you are throwing the curtains open in front of a window. Picture a light, color, or image as you 'open the curtains.
- Then, as you breathe out, pull your hands to your face and cover your eyes with them, holding in your mind's eye, your brow chakra, the image, color, or light that you saw with your arms spread wide.
- Repeat this inhale and exhale visualization ten to twelve times.
- To finish this pranayama, return your breath to normal and return to your original body position. With eyes closed, keep the focus on visualization in your inner eye. Try to see with your eyes closed.

Crown Chakra: Sahasrara Pranayama

Instructions:

- Sit in a comfortable position with legs crossed, spine long and chest open, hands resting on your knees. Focus on your breathing.
- Places your hands, palms together, fingers pointed toward your chin, in front of your heart chakra.

- As you draw in a long, deep breath, reach your arms and fingers up toward the sky, palms still together.
- As you breathe out air, reach your hands out to the sides in alignment with your shoulders.
- Return your hands to their prayer position in front of your heart before beginning your next inhale and starting the next breath cycle.
- Repeat this exercise ten to twenty times.
- To finish this pranayama, return your hands to your lap, or knees and breath normally, spine long, chest open. Sit in quiet reflection as long as you need.

As a reminder to you with all of these exercises, begin slowly and gradually, increasing your repetitions and speed, where indicated, so that you can build your breath strength. Using your breath for the awakening of your Kundalini will become an ongoing practice. Take a deep breath, and carry on!

Muladhara

Since the element associated with this root, or base, chakra is earth, it represents mooladhara (base support) as a life force that supports and energizes your entire body or life/living functions. This chakra is known to be the basis of life. Much like earth, itself holds and feeds all forms of life inhabiting it.

Here is a guided meditation for activating the Kundalini or root chakra, which features vivid imagery to help you unwind the energy.

- Take a gradual, long, and intense breath. As you breathe out, shift attention to the lower tip of your spine. Visualize a bright red chakra casting an incandescent and almost ethereal glow in the region. It is illuminating the base of your spine like a bright red ruby. This warm and positive red glowing chakra relaxes you and offers you a sense of safety and serenity.
- You experience a feeling of being secure, unshakable, and deeply grounded. Think of yourself as a big, powerful, and unshakable boulder closely held by the earth. Nothing can break or destroy your force. You are grounded, safe, and hugged by the earth.
- Next, visualize standing at the tip of a huge snow-covered mountain soaring loftily towards the sky; just before you is a massive cave opening! There are bright red flowers warmly basking and growing in the glory of the sun's ray at the entrance of the cave. The red flowers sway happily as the gentle breeze kisses them, and the warm glow of the sun envelops them. The warm rays of the sun slowly tricking into the cave are welcoming you to enter the cave.
- You step ahead and enter the cave. Looking around and taking in its breathtaking visuals, you observe that the cave features a very high ceiling. The warm breeze entering this cave makes you feel all comfortable, secure, and cozy. You walk further while taking in your surroundings.
- The path you are walking on opens into a huge, circular space with a large rectangle stone smack in the middle of the room. There is a tiny crack in the stone, and a warm, gentle glow of sunlight enters the stone through the crack. A warm glow envelops the stone.

- You walk further in the direction of the stone and take in its magnificence when standing next to it. You sit cross-legged on the rectangle stone which comes easily to you.
- Slowly, you begin to feel a sense of oneness with the mountain. Now, you are deeply grounded and rooted with the earth. You experience a feeling of complete safety and security. Nothing can move or shake you because the earth cradles you. The entire earth is holding and nurturing your being.
- Observe your first chakra spinning and acquiring momentum. As it keeps spinning more and more rapidly, a bright red light envelopes you and penetrates every pore, cell, and tissue of your body. It goes into every part of the body filling the part with increased energy and vitality. As it enters every cell, tissue, and muscle, you feel them infused with intense energy.
- Breathe slowly and deeply while feeling the force of energy moving to the base of your spine. Absorb the awareness of this phenomenon completely.
- Slowly rise from the rectangular stone and move out of the circular room traveling through a narrow pathway to move out of the cave. Glance at the mighty mountain and experience a sense of oneness with it. You are a part of it. The mountain, the cave, the snow, and the trees are not distinct from you. You are a part of the universal energy, and the universal energy is a part of you. There is no distinction between you and the universe. Feel a sense of oneness with everything around you.
- Once you are ready, slowly open eyes.

Chapter 7. Improve Energy and Psychic Abilities

The belief behind Kundalini awakening methods is that there are channels for energy along the spinal column. These channels, or Nadis, are the Ida, the Pingala, and the Sushumna in between them. The Kundalini is normally found at the bottom of this canal and wrapped around the tailbone for three and a half turns. When it is awakened, it rises up the channel and burns off the layers that separate the individual from Reality.

Coping With Premature Awakening

The Kundalini may activate even if the person has not done anything or if he/she is not yet ready for it. These are said to trigger such awakenings:

· Extreme situations

· Physical or psychological trauma

· Illnesses

· Pain

· Accidents

· Childbirth

· Near Death Experiences

· Energetic or supernatural influences

· Predestined occurrence

· Spiritual practices done during previous lives

· Overall awakening of humanity

These can help manage unpleasant symptoms:

· Relax the mind and body

· Breathe comfortably

· Imagine the Kundalini as a mild form of energy instead of an intense one

· Direct the kundalini's ascent to the crown by visualizing its smooth passage

· With your imagination, widen the passageway of the Kundalini

· Accept the experiences without rejecting or being terrified by them –these negative emotions create blocks, which will worsen the symptoms

· Do not overthink what is happening

· Talk with people who are knowledgeable with Kundalini

Methods of Awakening

There are several ways to awaken the Kundalini:

Spiritual Transmission

A Master or a guru who has already awakened his/her Kundalini traditionally activates that of another person. In India, you can find ashrams where there are teachers who can activate this energy and guide you in your spiritual development. However, it is said that activating the kundalini this way may only be temporary; the student must diligently keep his/her channels clear to continuously receive its benefits. If the teacher is very powerful though, the Kundalini may remain activated for life.

Meditation

Mediation is associated with Kundalini symptoms and other mystical phenomena. Whatever Kundalini activation method you use, it's highly recommended that you do it in a meditative manner. Also, you will benefit from having a regular meditation practice that you can practice at least once a day.

Statistically, those who meditate are more likely to have extraordinary experiences than those who don't. Also, it is found out that meditation is more likely to lead to Kundalini awakening than yoga or prayers. It is believed that an important ingredient in the awakening is the inward focus of the person – a crucial component in meditation but may be ignored when praying or doing Yoga.

Prayer

Prayer sometimes led to Kundalini syndromes especially if done fervently. According to studies, prayers involving strong positive emotions like gratitude or adoration lead to more mystical experiences, while those done out of penitence, obligation, or supplication results to fewer of these.

Yoga

There are different kinds of yoga. Some are aimed specifically for Kundalini activation, while the rest are dedicated for other purposes. Again, no matter what kind of yoga you do, kundalini energy is more likely to be activated if the yoga is done meditatively.

Yoga has many components: physical action (including certain positions of the body and hands), chanting (as with mantras and prayers), breath control (pranayama), concentration, meditation, and visualization.

It is best to attend a Yoga class with an experienced teacher to know how to perform the steps properly. If it is kundalini, you are after, seek yoga forms that are dedicated for that, such as Kundalini Yoga, Kriya Yoga, and Sahaja Yoga.

Purification

There is a tradition in Hinduism that requires Kundalini practitioners to cleanse their bodies in preparation for the Kundalini's passage. This may involve fasting or not eating for a given period of time or abstaining for eating some food such as meat. Also, partaking in sensual activities are discouraged to make the person focus on his/her spiritual nature.

Preparing the Chakras

The chakras are energy centers that line the channel where the Kundalini will pass through during its ascent. Clearing the chakras is recommended to be done in an order starting from the bottom chakra and proceeding sequentially to the top. A chakra supports the one above it, so if it does not run properly, the one above it will malfunction as well. If the chakra is cleared sequentially, you may avoid having to clear a blocked chakra again.

Clearing the chakras involve resolving issues, keeping one's body and mind healthy, and visualizing energy.

Root Chakra

The Kundalini is stored in the Root Chakra located at the base of the spine. It deals with survival issues and links the individual to material life. Signs of an unbalanced root chakra are insecurity, fear, and feeling out of place on earth, while balance leads to security and acceptance of life.

Physical activities that involve the legs and feet will help take care of this chakra. Jogging, dancing, and meditative walking are some of the things you can do to work with this chakra. Actions done in nature also work well with the root chakra – examples are fishing, hiking, and gardening.

Sacral Chakra

The sacral chakra is found in the lower abdomen close to the reproductive organs. It is associated with sexuality, pleasure, relationships, creativity, and primal emotions. Imbalance in this chakra shows up as a lack or excess of the sex drive, being cold or excessively emotional, and unhealthy relationships. A healthy sacral chakra manifests ad fulfilling relationships, well-managed emotions, and a healthy approach to pleasure.

Activities that support emotional expression and sensuality assist in balancing this chakra. Examples are listening to soft music, receiving loving massages, and having satisfying sex with a partner.

Solar Plexus Chakra

The solar plexus is called as such because it is similar to the sun as the source of power of the body. It is stationed in the abdomen and has effects upon the digestive and metabolic systems. It gives the body energy derived from physical food and non-physical origins. Issues related to this chakra are those that have to do with ego, vitality, self-esteem, and will.

Problems with this chakra have symptoms like uncontrolled anger, poor self-esteem, excessive pride, powerlessness, or power-tripping tendencies. Abnormal eating habits and other digestive problems may also be a side-effect of this. A balanced solar plexus induces a healthy regard for one's self and responsibility with personal power.

Actions that are effortful help maintain this chakra – examples of these are martial arts, competitive sports, and marathons.

Heart Chakra

The heart chakra corresponds to the physical heart in the middle of the chest. As the midpoint, it balances the higher and lower chakras. Just as the sacral chakra deals with the lower, primal emotions, the heart chakra manages loftier emotions like love, compassion, and selflessness.

Issues with the heart chakra are linked with negative emotions, inability to handle feelings well, and a hatred for others. A balanced heart chakra generates positive emotions and a loving disposition.

To cleanse the heart chakra, it is recommended to do selfless tasks that evoke positive feelings – helping others, participating in volunteer work, and spending quality time with friends and family.

Throat Chakra

The throat chakra is associated with sound, communication, and the lower mind (intellect). A diseased throat chakra may be caused by abusive language, poor self-expression, dishonesty, gossiping, over-thinking, or avoidance of intellectual activities. A balanced throat chakra enables the person to express himself/herself well and think clearly

Throat chakra-balancing activities are those that make use of the voice and the intellect – examples are singing, poem or essay recitation, public speaking, problem solving, and the like.

Third Eye Chakra

The third eye chakra is in the middle of the head between and above the two eyebrows. It is ascribed to physical and psychic sight. Issues that deal with this chakra are about the higher mind, imagination, abstract reasoning, psychic faculties, and wisdom. It is also said to embody an individual's connection with his/her higher self.

Blockages in this chakra trigger mental problems, confusion, and lack of intuition. A clear third eye chakra supports enhanced psychic abilities, a strong mind, and a connection to one's higher self. Meditation, dream journaling, and studying mysticism are just some of the things that can purify and energize the third eye chakra.

Crown Chakra

The crown chakra is the last and highest of the main chakras. The Kundalini energy rises towards this charka to link the person with the Universe. It symbolizes liberation from suffering and the attainment of perfection in this earthly life. While the third eye chakra connects one to his/her higher self, the crown chakra unifies the higher self to the ultimate Divine.

Issues that pertain to this chakra are those that relate to divine connection, spiritual progress, and higher consciousness. Imbalance in this chakra can lead to insanity, lack of spirituality, and a destructive attachment to materialism. A balanced crown chakra bestows spiritual fulfilment, bliss, and finding meaning and purpose in life.

Things that balance this top chakra are spiritual acts like deep meditation, contemplation, fervent prayer, serving God, and dedicating oneself to spirituality.

There are several techniques that are geared for chakra development, but remember: in terms of results, what trigger the release of the Kundalini are not the techniques themselves but the attitudes of the person in doing them. You may try these techniques to amplify your efforts, but the best way to open the chakras is resolving the issues related to them.

Activating the Kundalini

The Kundalini may activate on its own when the chakras are unblocked. You can also shake it awake by doing certain techniques. For this, you will need your total attention. Thus, you must not perform the following steps when you are sick, tired, sleepy, drunk, or drugged.

It will use up your energy so you have to be physically and psychologically fit. Refrain from doing things that drain your energy. Avoid draining situations. It is also best if you do not become too attached with something or someone before the activation. You need to dedicate yourself to the task. If you are preoccupied with something, the activation may not work or go as smoothly as it should. Take care of what you need to take care of; if you can't for the moment, plan when you will deal with it and let it go for now.

Keep yourself comfortable so you won't be distracted with discomforts during the activation. It is better to be in a non-polluted environment that is cleansed of energetic impurities (by smoking incense or by ringing a singing bowl, for example).

Be careful with the things you eat and drink. Do not eat a heavy meal before the session. If you have eaten, wait at least 1 hour or ideally 4 hours. Consume nutritious organic food and reduce or avoid processed or junk food. Stay away from caffeine, alcohol, nicotine, and other substances that are not good for the body.

Be prepared for traumatic memories and stressful thoughts and emotions that may surface when the Kundalini passes through your chakras. This is a natural side-effect of the cleansing. The energy may trigger dormant issues; consider this as an opportunity to process these so your subconscious mind will no longer find the need to hold on to them.

Because the old energies will leave your system, you may feel as if you have become someone else. You may become dissociated and aloof. You may lose interest in things you were previously involved in. Do not identify yourself with this condition. This will pass when you have adjusted to the new energies.

Process your experiences by reflecting and examining what you need to learn from them. You may talk with other people who have undergone the activation. Seek counsellors and teachers so they can give you sage advice.

Do not plan to do something that needs your focus after the activation because you may become disoriented for a while. Give yourself plenty of time to cope.

Perform some mild exercises before the ritual. Doing so will help bridge the body and mind, shake energetic blocks loose, and make it more receptive to new energy. You can also get a massage to prepare your energetic channels. A massage therapist who works with energy can help you a lot with this.

Kundalini Activation Techniques

People have created numerous techniques to awaken the kundalini. These vary in terms of beliefs, complexity, requirement, and methods. The following are simplified versions of these steps.

Controlling the Breath

Pranayama Yoga has a collection of breath-control techniques that are designed to control the vital energy in one's body. One way of making the Kundalini rise is to control the breath.

Lie on your back and align your head to the North (some believe that this can facilitate the flow of the Kundalini upwards). Inhale deeply and imagine the Kundalini at the base of your spine glowing brightly. Hold your breath for as long as you can – this is when the energy can slide up. Exhale afterwards, then hold it again for as long as possible to make it move some more.

After some time, you may be able to feel where the Kundalini is by a warm spot along your spine. Persevere with this method until it reaches the top of your head.

Remember to accompany your breaths with visualizations to direct the energy more effectively. The breath is a kind of mechanical push, while the visualization forms the energy according to your instructions.

Back stretches

You can combine this with the previous method or do it as it is. Lie on your back with your knees to your chest. Squeeze your stomach for a couple of seconds. Straighten your legs and lower them down gradually without arching your back. Imagine the energy ascending to your crown.

Enabling Kundalini Release

Sit or lie down with your back straight. Focus on the spot between your genitals and anus – this is where the dormant Kundalini is stored. Tighten this area for about five deep breaths. Release the muscular tension for five deep breaths also. Repeat this three times, then tighten and relax the area rapidly for 10 times.

Using Movement

Moving the body can wake up the sleeping Kundalini. You may dance, spin around, sway or rotate your trunk, or just move at any manner you choose; what matters is that you intend to affect the Kundalini.

Always keep in mind that you must be contemplative when you are moving so that you will not be dissipating the energy outwards, but rather concentrated inwards. Do not be engrossed by what your body is doing, instead, feel what is happening inside you. Mentally direct the physical activity into your tailbone and upwards.

Visualization

Thoughts are subtle energy; thus imagination works in controlling other subtle energies like the vital force (chi) and the Kundalini. With your mind free of other preoccupations, imagine the Kundalini arising from the base of your spine and flowing through the top of your head.

Practitioners say the Kundalini has a reddish orange glow or color. You can use any color for as long as this color represents your idea of Kundalini. If you can mentally perceive the Kundalini and it shows up as a certain color, just work with what you see.

The Kundalini will automatically find its way, but you can guide it by imagining the pathways it will travel. See the Ida, Pingala, and the Sushumna as smooth and free of blockages. You may visualize the Kundalini stirring to life. You may also send energy to the Kundalini reservoir so that it will be energized.

After a while of this, blank your mind and release your control of the energy. It will shoot up on its own. If not, you can imagine it to do so.

Mindful Activity

It is said that whatever you do affects your Kundalini to an extent. This is especially true if you pour your heart and soul in what you are doing. So, whatever it is that you find yourself working on, intend for it to awaken the Kundalini. This way, you can awaken it while being productive with other things.

How to Handle Kundalini Release

You may control the effect of the Kundalini on you by mentally changing the energy. If you find it too hot, use a cooler color such as blue. If it is too overwhelming, picture it as a gentle stream instead. If you want to amplify it, see it as a powerful explosion in your mind.

Let every cell of your body and every part of your soul soak in the Kundalini. Distributing the energy this way makes it less overwhelming.

If you feel pain or uneasiness, zone in that spot. It is possible that there are blockages in there. Clear your mind and try to sense what's causing the discomfort. Try your best to resolve the issue, or at least, be at peace with the sensations.

You may shine a healing light upon your whole body, or just concentrate it onto the areas that are giving you problems. Instruct this light to remove impurities, tell the light to dissolve them or pushing them out of your body.

You may also simply rub the painful part to help the force flow more easily.

You may use the Kundalini itself to break through blocks. Imagine it breaking or burning away the impurities. Allow it to warm up frozen parts of the body so that it can glide through them.

Aside from blockages, abnormal sensations may be caused by the Kundalini itself getting stuck somewhere instead of moving along the spine. Pull it back to its proper path with your imagination.

Dedicate some time (ideally every day) to contemplate on your experiences. This will help you handle the new energies better and process the old energies that were expelled from your system. Periods of contemplation also allows you to be in touch with your deeper mind, where you can gain insights from the spirit which can help you with your life.

If you have trouble going back to normal after activation, remember that the strange feelings you have is just part of the transformation. Just do what you have to do regardless of how unnecessary it is for you at the moment. The aloofness will gradually disappear, but your new and enhanced perspective will remain with you indefinitely.

Chapter 8. Step-By-Step Guide to Mastery

The road to mastery means embracing the teachings and practices in such a way that you make them a way of life. Indeed, this road is also marked by trials and challenges. However, do not let this discourage you. After all, every mountain that is worth climbing always has its own share of risks and obstacles. In fact, if you come to think about it, these obstacles are actually the ones that teach you what you need to learn. Instead of seeing other people's failures as a discouragement, you have to them as a valuable lesson that can help you become a better person.

Now that you are already armed with the right knowledge, I encourage you to choose at least two or three techniques/practices from this book and start practicing them right away. Once again, do not allow failures to discourage you. As long as you keep on doing your best, then you will never lose.

Having knowledge alone is not enough. You need to start right away. The road to mastery is long, so do not waste any more time.

You should also learn how to handle frustrations properly. Even if you possess a strong will, you cannot just advance your spiritual progress as quickly as you want. You will have to spend time learning especially the basics. Also, do not be like the others who compete with other practitioners. Your spiritual path is a path that is for you and you alone. Instead of competing with others, you should draw inspiration from them.

But what does it mean to be a master? A master does not even seek for mastery anymore. Instead, they have turned the techniques into a way of life. A true master is not controlled by power nor do they seek to be more powerful than others. They may have psychic abilities, but they are not a slave to these abilities. As a beginner, you should realize that this spiritual path is one that you should tread with love in your heart.

You cannot be a master if you are enslaved by anger or hatred. In the universe, love remains to be the greatest force. A master knows this little secret and makes sure to always act full of love. Now, this is easy when everything is going your way. But, what if you are met with a difficult situation? Well, this is the time when you will be tested. It is up to you to prove to yourself which side you are really on, whether positive or negative. Just always remember: There is always this great force inside you called love, and you can always choose it above other things, and it is truly more powerful than hatred. Unfortunately, only a few have learned to wield love sincerely.

A word should be said about love. Love is, without a doubt, the greatest force in the whole universe. As you learn the techniques in this book, let love be your guiding light. There is no sense in being able to reach a high level of development if you do not have love in your heart. A common mistake committed by practitioners is becoming too absorbed with themselves. Although it is good to focus on what you are doing, never let it blind you from what is important in life. What good is being able to manipulate all the prana in the world if you do not have people whom you share your love with? Never be blinded by power, and always remember that love should be the foundation of your spirituality.

The key to effective Kundalini awakening is meditation. Meditation allows you to direct your intention and allow energy to rise through each chakra, leading to a profound spiritual awakening and mystical experience. This meditation can be approached either vigorously or passively.

The Vigorous/Active Approach capitalizes on meditation that happens while the body is in motion. This approach combines breathing practice, visualization and meditation with physical motion. Many yogi's/guides borrow skills from different active yoga practices such as Kriya yoga and Sahaja yoga. In fact there is a particular yoga that has been conceived specifically to help people interested in awakening the Kundalini safely and is predictably called Kundalini Yoga.

The Passive Approach requires that one expend less physical energy and focus more on the meditation, breathing and visualization components. Many yoga practices fall within this approach including hatha yoga. The awakening is achieved by repeated utterance of a sacred word or chanting a sacred mantra. There have been incidences where a guru/yogi was able to reassign their own energy to an apprentice and trigger the apprentice's Kundalini awakening.

What happens in this instance is that once your expert guru has prepared you and guided you into passive meditation, s/he touches your forehead mid-brow where another one of your chakras, the Adinya-chakra, is found. This touching moves their own energy from their body to yours and triggers your Kundalini to awaken. However, note that this is not common practice and is often done only by gurus who have had many, many years of practice.

Many yogis and apprentices combine both approaches (vigorous and passive) to achieve more a more effective awakening. For instance, they may have sessions of vigorous meditation to increase physical power and passive meditation to encourage intellectual power and control as well as to instill and boost spiritual fortitude.

Regardless of which approach you and your guide choose to go with, please remember that is important to be spiritually, intellectually and physically prepared for the process.

The Step-By-Step Process to Kundalini Awakening
Kundalini awakening is process. The energy doesn't just surge upwards in one big wave but rises from one level to another in a systemic way. When triggered, Kundalini flows through the chakras thereby opening, layer after layer, of the brain's newfound power.

The first step to a successful awakening is meditation. Let's say you're using the active approach, you will begin the motions that you use during the meditation process, going through them one by one until all your attention is turned inwards. If you're using the passive approach, popular practice is to sit in yogic position or lie down very still, turning your attention inwards and urging your own energy to rise.

In both approaches, it is critical for the apprentice to have an open mind. The process of opening the mind and lifting the barriers that we have put up over the years is extremely hard, but with the help of an accomplished yogi, it is quite possible. This phase almost feels like hypnosis and moving into another plane of being where your mind is completely free; unleashed from the barriers that hold it down.

The apprentice focuses on their breathing and the flow of blood within their circulatory system. It is likely that this unfailing focus will lead to the first big wave of energy. This sudden jolt of energy will feel like an electric current emanating from the bottom of your spine and zipping up and down the spine in waves.

This first wave of energy is due to the opening up of the crown chakra and causes a reorganization of your mind and nervous system. Its release comes with symptoms such as extreme sweating, trembling, tingling, itching, sensitivity to sense of touch, insomnia, seeing bursts of light muddled thoughts and absolute mental disconnection from your immediate surroundings. In fact, some people report that when in this phase when they stare in the mirror, they are unable to recognize themselves.

This is where you'll need your guide most because without their help you may not be able to control this energy. An apprentice requires tremendous control to redirect this rampant energy through the various channels and into the other chakras for that spiritual connection.

The second wave of energy is obviously stronger than the first and apart from influencing your mind and spirit, it will also affect your physical body. It is common for your muscles to become limp or to become paralyzed. The reason this happens is because it is at this point that the Kundalini is fusing with your spirit, your physical body and your mind.

This stage is intense and often very overwhelming. In fact, it is during this integration process that many apprentices give up thus compromising their awakening. There is no way to make the experience easier; you have to let it ride because it is just a temporary state. Wholly submit to the process and let your Kundalini integrate with yourself.

The third wave of energy is the strongest. Now that the Kundalini is fused with your old self, it begins to overwhelm it; its objective is to change your whole being and create a new you. This phase is a very strange phase. Where the first two phases were almost painful, this one is euphoric and supernatural. It is almost as if there is someone with a remote control and they are controlling your whole body, reorganizing it.

Once this process has begun, it is impossible to stop. Fortunately, it is a blissful state. By the end of it, the apprentice will acquire a new self; often referred to as a light body. The light body has a refined nervous system, swift and flexible limbs, amplified self-conscious and a shrunken ego.

After the third wave of energy, there will still be waves of energy release, but it will be in smaller volumes than the first three phases and the strength of symptoms of being in the midst of an awakening lessen. These 'little' waves are important to keep you connected to your awakened Kundalini.

Your Kundalini has been Awoken: Now what?
Kundalini Awakening has a profound effect on the mind, body and spirit of the awakened. Immediately after the awakening you will feel an intense feeling of bliss, ecstasy and an out-of-body experience. Your body and mind feel like they have been freed while spiritually you feel more connected to and aware of your diet, yourself and the world around you.

This ecstasy may be accompanied by the physical symptoms that appeared during stage one and stage two of the awakening though at a lesser degree. Such symptoms include intermittent jolts, shudders and spasms, burning and stinging sensations, weak limbs, extreme sweating or shivering, heavy breathing, excessive or diminished sexual desire, migraines, high blood pressure, body pains, sensitivity to touch, light and sound, loss of appetite or the inverse, overeating, liver and gall bladder problems, fibromyalgia, and many more. The energy surges that occurred after the third wave of awakening will continue to pulse through your body as you continue to adapt to your new self.

There will also be mental symptoms including seeing visions, hearing sounds associated with certain chakra, depression or the inverse hypomania, signs of intellectual instability that might be diagnosed as a mental disorder, loss of focus and being semi-conscious as if in a trance, stagnation of time as if the clock has stopped, and an altered perception of the universe where everything around you become more colorful. You might even find yourself travelling to other worlds behind this one for instance the past where you see, hear and speak to heroes of your past. Obviously not all the above symptoms will appear in one individual, but most apprentices report two or more of the above after awakening.

These symptoms are meant to be short term, which means on completion of the awakening you and your guru will begin working on recovery exercises and practice to morph the symptoms into something that is both positive and long-lasting.

The more physical exercise you involve yourself in, the faster you will heal. Start slow; perhaps with the lighter forms of yoga so that limbs that were frozen by the awakening have an opportunity to 'thaw' before you put them through vigorous exercise.

If there was ever a time to change your diet for the better, this is the time. Your body requires proper nutritional sustenance to heal. Some apprentices usually use the initial days after an awakening to conduct detox diets. Detox diets can include days of drinking only healthy fresh juices, or raw food. But a detox diet is not a must.

You can choose to focus on transitioning into a normal but healthy eating lifestyle. This eating lifestyle will have meals made up of whole grains, fruits, vegetables and lean meat (if you're not a vegetarian yet) is best for your body and will leave you feeling like a new person. We're calling it an eating lifestyle because it is your new way of living. Like you're awakening, healthy living does not stop a month from now, or a year from now. It is a lifelong habit.

Also, nurturing and growing relationships is important. The most successful apprentices know that no man is an island and their awakening was a step toward better connection not just with themselves and their spiritual deity but also with the people around them. Strive to repair and/or grow important relationships in your life. If you've been living a solitary existence, then this is the time to start making friends.

Making new friends is as simple as smiling at the person next to you on the bus and starting a conversation. It's as easy as taking the time to talk to your next door neighbor or the saleslady you always see at your local grocery. Join charitable events in your neighborhood like runs, clean-ups, visitations to foster homes etc to meet like-minded friends. Instead of just being an attendant of your place of worship, become a more active participant. You'll find friends gathering next to you even without you noticing.

Avoid any intense tests of control. This is not the time to be fasting or depriving oneself of sleep. You don't want to ruin all the amazing work that you have done so far. Your body is in recovery mode and like a sick person you need to keep your energy up.

Though you're in recovery it doesn't mean that you should stop your reflection and divine activities. If anything meditation and prayer will feel even better now that you have a connection with your deity. And the act of communing with your deity will enhance your healing process. Many yogis advise mediating for at the very least thirty minutes. However, make sure that the kind of meditation you're doing is not intended to reawaken the Kundalini. Once is enough to set you on the path towards self-fulfillment.

Your relationship with your yogi or guru does not end just because your Kundalini has been awakened. If anything, the guru-apprentice relationship should grow and become stronger as a result of it. Your guru will continue to guide your Kundalini so that it continues to operate within the expected bounds and not stray. S/he will help you monitor your symptoms and help you deal with any undesirable side effects. S/he can also help you determine what meditation practices will help to enhance your awakening.

It is also important to join a support group or class of similar minded people; those who have experienced an awakening or are on the path toward spiritual enlightenment. Being around a community of like-minded, encouraging and positive people will help you shelf negative thoughts and any feelings of failure. It will also help you strengthen the desirable symptoms of Kundalini awakening as well as help you deal with the negatives. If you live in an area where it is impossible to join an in-person group, there are many Kundalini forums online that can act as your support group.

The awakening of your Kundalini is not just a process of personal growth. It is also something that you do for your whole community. Remember that during the process you become more connected not just to yourself and to your spiritual deity, but also to your surroundings. It is therefore important to include service to others as part of your after-awakening activities. These services include but are not limited to love, compassion and charity.

Don't hoard this change you have experienced. It is a positive change that can be beneficial to many people and change their lives for the better. Sharing how you started your journey, what you did, who guided you and your whole experience of awakening is important if only to encourage those who are interested on in the process of their own awakening. It doesn't matter whether you do it offline or online, the point is to share.

Continue practice of the above activities will help transform your awakening into a positive life experience filled with spiritual, intellectual and physical enrichment.

Figuring out how to ponder can be basic, and it's probably the best thing you can accomplish for your wellbeing and by and large prosperity. Reflection is a particularly powerful method for stress alleviation since it empowers you to mitigate worry at the time and to make changes in yourself that will assist you with being less receptive to the stressors you face later on. Figuring out how to ruminate can be fun as there are such a significant number of reflection methods that can be powerful—in the event that one style contemplation doesn't feel right, another style will. Figure out how to think a few distinct ways, and see what approach works best for you.

1 Care Meditation

Care reflection might be one of the all the more testing types of contemplation for reflection tenderfoots, yet it is a compensating structure that brings numerous advantages, both for the novice and for the individuals who practice consistently. For those simply figuring out how to ponder, care contemplation requires no props or readiness (no candles to light, mantras to pick, or methods to adapt); long haul practice can bring a more settled personality and less reactivity to push. The key component of care reflection is an attention on the present minute. Instead of concentrating on something outside of oneself, care reflection requires an emphasis on "now." Learn increasingly about care contemplation and careful living.

2 Strolling Meditation

Figuring out how to think with a mobile reflection is basic, and gives a portion of the unwinding advantages of activity just as the standard advantages of contemplation. The way in to a mobile reflection isn't only the strolling itself, obviously, it's the attitude where you walk. Strolling contemplations can be quick or moderate, can be rehearsed with an unmistakable personality or with the guide of music or a mantra. Strolling reflection is particularly valuable for the individuals who like to remain dynamic and may feel worried with the quiet and stillness of a portion of different techniques, similar to care contemplation. Learn contemplation with this straightforward strolling reflection instructional exercise, and adjust your pace or center as you find what feels directly for you.

3 Mantra Meditation

Mantra reflection is another basic system for the individuals who are new to contemplation. On the off chance that keeping your mind totally calm feels like an over the top test, mantra contemplation may be simpler. It joins a portion of the advantages of positive confirmations with the advantages of reflection with the reiteration of a solitary word or sound. A few people feel somewhat awkward with rehashing "om" or murmuring, yet you can utilize whatever mantra you like. Similarly as with strolling contemplation, the key fixing with mantra reflection is the thoughtful state you accomplish and not really the mantra you use, however it's a smart thought to pick a mantra you're OK with. This is a simple one to begin with.

4 Care in Daily Life

While care contemplation normally includes keeping the mind totally clear of considerations and keeping up that state, care can be developed from multiple points of view for the duration of the day. Fundamentally, remaining completely present with whatever you are doing and keeping up an attention on the physical experience of the present minute can enable you to keep up care as you experience your day. There are approaches to develop care, and as you're figuring out how to think, attempt to develop care too—it can enable you to rehearse contemplation all the more effectively, and can fit into a bustling calendar generally effectively.

5 Chocolate Meditation

At the point when you're seeing how to contemplate, here's a moderately brisk and exquisite procedure to attempt. The chocolate reflection is a type of care contemplation that is frequently utilized in care based pressure decrease (MBSR) classes, is basic for fledglings, connects with a few detects, and has a worked in remuneration of making the flavor of chocolate feel progressively exceptional. Utilizing dim chocolate for this activity brings its very own advantages. In case you're searching for something straightforward and new, attempt the chocolate contemplation.

6 Breathing Meditation

Breathing reflection is one of the most prominent types of contemplation as a result of its straightforwardness and effortlessness, just as its accommodation (breathing is continually happening, so it's an advantageous stay for contemplation). The breath gives a characteristic center that is subtle, however consistently there, and makes a characteristic beat to become mixed up in. You can work on breathing reflection for a couple of minutes, or for more, and consistently discover unwinding.

7 Shower Meditation

One relieving strategy for those seeing how to ponder is the shower reflection. A shower contemplation consolidates the standard advantages of reflection with the advantages of an alleviating, hot shower, which can loosen up tired muscles, give a loosening up air, and permit an impermanent sentiment of break from stressors. Being in the water can likewise assist you with staying wakeful, something that is significant yet at times testing in case you're figuring out how to think when tired. Attempt a shower reflection, and be spotless, loose, and prepared for bed (or a low-stress day) when you're done.

8 Smaller than expected Meditations

For the individuals who feel they don't possess energy for full-length reflection sessions (20 minutes is a decent normal measure of time), or for the individuals who might want to encounter a portion of the advantages of contemplation between longer sessions, scaled down (contemplations around 5 minutes long) are an incredible strategy to attempt. Smaller than normal reflections are extremely straightforward and fit in well with even the busiest of timetables. Figure out how to reflect in shorter blasts, and work up to longer sessions, or simply utilize this procedure for fast and helpful pressure alleviation.

Joining Meditation into Your Everyday Life
Attempt to think simultaneously consistently. Planning your contemplation practice for a similar time every day will enable it to turn out to be a piece of your regular daily schedule. On the off chance that you contemplate every day, you'll experience its advantages all the more significantly.

Early morning is a decent time to think since your brain has not yet moved toward becoming overwhelmed by the anxieties and stresses of the day.

It's anything but a smart thought to think legitimately subsequent to eating. In case you're processing a supper, you may feel awkward and less ready to think.

Take a guided reflection class to sharpen your strategies. On the off chance that you need extra direction, consider taking a contemplation class with an accomplished instructor. You can discover a scope of various class types via looking through on the web.

Reasonable MEDITATION TECHNIQUES
These tips aren't planned for helping you to turn into a specialist … they should enable you to begin and continue onward. You don't need to actualize them at the same time — attempt a couple, return to this article, attempt a couple of something else.

1.Sit for only two minutes. This will appear to be strangely simple, to simply ruminate for two minutes. That is impeccable. Start with only two minutes per day for seven days. On the off chance that that goes well, increment by an additional two minutes and do that for seven days. On the off chance that all goes well, by expanding only a little at once, you'll be thinking for 10 minutes every day in the second month, which is stunning! However, start little first.

2.Do it first thing every morning. It's anything but difficult to state, "I'll contemplate each day," however then neglect to do it. Rather, set an update for each morning when you get up, and put a note that says "ruminate" some place where you'll see it.

3.Don't become involved with the how simply do. The vast majority stress over where to sit, how to sit, what pad to utilize … this is all decent, yet it isn't so critical to begin. Start just by sitting on a seat, or on your love seat. Or then again on your bed. In case you're agreeable on the ground, sit leg over leg. It's only for two minutes from the start in any case, so simply sit. Later you can stress over upgrading it so you'll be agreeable for more, however to start with it doesn't make a difference much, simply sit some place peaceful and agreeable.

4.Check in with how you're feeling. As you first subside into your reflection session, basically verify how you're feeling. How does your body feel? What is the nature of your psyche? Occupied? Tired? On edge? See whatever you're bringing to this contemplation session as totally OK.

5.Count your breaths. Since you're settled in, direct your concentration toward your breath. Simply place the consideration on your breath as it comes in, and finish it your nose right down to your lungs. Take a stab at tallying "one" as you take in the main breath, at that point "two" as you inhale out. Rehash this to the tally of 10, at that point start again at one.

6.Come back when you meander. Your mind will meander. This is a practically total conviction. There's no issue with that. At the point when you see your mind meandering, grin, and basically tenderly come back to your breath. Tally "one" once more and begin once again. You may feel a little disappointment, yet it's superbly OK to not remain centered, we as a whole do it. This is the training, and you won't be great at it for a brief period.

7.Develop a cherishing mentality. At the point when you see considerations and sentiments emerging during reflection, as they will, take a gander at them with a benevolent frame of mind. Consider them to be companions, not interlopers or adversaries. They are a piece of you, however not every one of you. Be cordial and not unforgiving.

8.Don't stress a lot of that you're treating it terribly. You will stress you're treating it terribly. That is OK, we as a whole do. You're not treating it terribly. There's no ideal method to do it, simply be cheerful you're doing it.

9.Don't stress over clearing the brain. Heaps of individuals contemplate clearing your psyche or halting all musings. It's definitely not. This can in some cases occur, yet it's not the "objective" of contemplation. On the off chance that you have contemplations, that is ordinary. We as a whole do. Our cerebrums are thought industrial facilities, and we can't simply close them down. Rather, simply attempt to work on concentrating, and practice some more when your mind meanders.

10.Stay with whatever emerges. At the point when contemplations or emotions emerge, and they will, you may have a go at remaining with them temporarily. Truly, I realize I said to come back to the breath, yet after you practice that for seven days, you may likewise take a stab at remaining with an idea or feeling that emerges. We will in general need to keep away from emotions like dissatisfaction, outrage, uneasiness … yet an incredibly valuable reflection practice is to remain with the inclination for some time. Simply remain, and be interested.

11.Get to know yourself. This training isn't just about concentrating, it's tied in with figuring out how your mind functions. What's happening inside there? It's dim, yet by watching your psyche meander, get disappointed, maintain a strategic distance from troublesome emotions … you can begin to get yourself.

12.Become companions with yourself. As you become acquainted with yourself, do it with a cordial mentality rather than one of analysis. You're becoming more acquainted with a companion. Grin and give yourself love.

13.Do a body filter. Something else you can do, when you become somewhat better at following your breath, is concentrate on each body part in turn. Start at the bottoms of your feet — how do those vibe? Gradually move to your toes, the highest points of your feet, your lower legs, right to the highest point of your head.

14.Notice the light, sounds, vitality. Somewhere else to put your consideration, once more, after you've practice with your breath for in any event seven days, is the light surrounding you. Simply keep your eyes on one spot, and notice the light in the room you're in. One more day, simply center around seeing sounds. One more day, attempt to see the vitality in the room surrounding you (counting light and sounds).

15.Really submit yourself. Don't simply say, "Sure, I'll attempt this for several days." Really invest in this. In your brain, be secured, for in any event a month.

16.You can do it anyplace. In case you're voyaging, or something comes up in the first part of the day, you can do contemplation in your office. In the recreation center. During your drive. As you walk some place. Sitting reflection is the best spot to begin, however in truth, you're rehearsing for this sort of care in all your years.

17.Follow guided reflection. In the event that it encourages, you can have a go at following guided reflections to begin with.

18.Check in with companions. While I like contemplating alone, you can do it with your life partner or youngster or a companion. Or on the other hand simply make a dedication with a companion to check in each morning after reflection. It may enable you to stay with it for more.

19.Find a network. Surprisingly better, discover a network of individuals who are thinking and go along with them. This may be a Zen or Tibetan people group close to you (for instance), where you proceed to contemplate with them. Or on the other hand locate an online gathering and check in with them and pose inquiries, get support, empower others.

20.Smile when you're set. At the point when you're done with your two minutes, grin. Be appreciative that you had this uninterrupted alone time, that you stayed with your responsibility, that you demonstrated to yourself that you're dependable, where you set aside the effort to become acquainted with yourself and warm up to yourself. That is an astonishing two minutes of your life.

Reflection isn't in every case simple or even serene. However, it has really astounded advantages, and you can begin today, and proceed for an incredible remainder.

Chapter 9. How to Develop Intuition

Many people are familiar with what the intuition is, but what exactly is the intuition? Some people say that it is the highest form of intelligence. Intuition is the ability to know something without evidence or analysis. It is about knowing. Sometimes, when the phone rings, you simply know who is calling.

The truth is that the intuition is very common. Unfortunately, today, people do not recognize it. Many people do not take notice of the messages from their intuition and only rely on logic or the use of reasons. Hence, they fail to listen to what the intuition tells them. Once they get used to shutting down their intuition, then they reach the point where they can no longer hear or notice it. The good news is that it is never too late to learn to listen to your intuition again.

How to develop your intuition

The best way to develop the intuition is simply by using it. If you have not paid attention to your intuition for too long, then now is the time for you to make some changes and start listening to your intuition again. Learn to listen to how you feel. A good approach is to recognize your emotion or "gut feeling" and then use reasons to justify it instead of relying on reasons alone.

It is also worth noting that the practice of meditation is a natural and effective way to develop the intuition. All the meditation techniques in this book will develop your intuition. Here is another interesting exercise that can enhance your intuition:

Use your intuition in your daily life. For example, when the phone rings, try to "guess" who is calling. When you are at the supermarket or when driving, visualize the first person whom you will see before you take a turn. There are many other ways to put your intuition into work. The important thing is to make use of it regularly. Do not be discouraged if you commit mistakes. The more times that you use your intuition, the more you will get good at it.

Finding the appropriate lessons to exercise your psychic awareness can be challenging. There is plenty of misinformation on the world wide web, and sometimes the resources found in books are hard to find. There are, however, the right sources of information and it is up to you to follow the trail of breadcrumbs.

Step 1: Let the Information Come to You

I realize the idea of waiting for the information you need to find you sound a bit wacky, and if you are feeling any impatience to get started, untimely. Often, when we are opening our psychic awareness, it involves working with the energies of the Universe to be a guide to the right source. Has someone ever given you a book out of the blue and said they thought you just needed to have it? Have you been looking for something and it shows up out of nowhere in your email or conversations?

When you are on the awakened path and you are cultivating your psychic awareness, it is important to allow the information to come to you. The Universe knows what you are searching for, and indeed, what you are ready for next on your journey. So just practice openness so you can be aware when these things pop up. Your intuition will confirm you are on the right track. Trust it.

Another way this can manifest is in the way of Clair cognizance, clairsentience, and clairaudience. Pay attention to the message you are receiving from other realms, dreams, and your own intuition and inner knowing. Your psychic abilities will develop in tandem with you looking for ways to practice them.

Step 2: Clair-Anything Means Clear Energy

If you are going to work on nurturing your emerging psychic senses, it is important that you remain energetically clear so that you don't misread or misinterpret messages, or emotions. Throughout this book, there have been several levels of energy clearing methods and techniques, without which Kundalini awakening and enlightenment would not be possible. Energy is key. If your channels are blocked from your own, or other people's negative vibrations, you will have a harder time giving and receiving psychically.

Developing an energy clearing ritual for everyday use can be very beneficial. This could be as simple as using sage, or incense to smudge or cleanse your home and body after several people have been around you and brought their own negative vibrations into your space. This can energetically disrupt your ability to clearly 'see'. Salty baths can be very helpful, as well as spending time alone in nature to recharge and ground your energy.

You can do these things before you engage with any exercises to develop your psychic awareness, or just in general, to keep your vibration elevated for your awakening process. Incorporate some of the yoga postures and breathing exercises to help keep your channels clear too.

Step 3: Trust Your Own Knowing

It seems like magic, to go from being unweakened and in no way psychic, to being enlightened, full of love and light and able to tap into the energies of all existence through clairsentience and other means. When these things start opening up inside of you and manifesting in your reality, since you have never felt it before, it might feel odd, uncomfortable, or scary. Many people can be ostracized by our society and called crazy, or schizophrenic because they can hear, or see what no one else can. Imagine if those abilities were nurtured instead of medicated and cut off.

No one will have a Kundalini awakening experience quite like yours. The journey will bring you closer to humanity and the whole Universe, but it will be your soul's road to travel. Self-trust is invaluable along this path. Your quest as an awakened soul is to know and trust your divine truth and honor your creative power.

Opening your psychic sense or sixth sense as it is often called demands your trust. Trust your visions and projections. They are your reality. Trust your sense of something. Trust your connection to otherworldly beings and energies. They are here to help you and offer guidance. Do not ignore it when you hear it, see it, sense it, feel it, know it. That is your gift and it is yours to share with the good intention of all.

A word of caution on opening these abilities into your life: check your ego at the gate. This is nothing to brag about. Anyone can do this, especially when they release their Kundalini energy and experience awakening. There is little room for big heads in using your psychic light. You need to have plenty of space in that head to help others in need.

Step 4: Collaborate with the Cosmos

Enlightenment is free. Transcendence is for everyone. It crosses time and space and all realities. There isn't a person alive on this Earth who does not share your ability to know this truth. Awakening comes to all those who seek it and answer its call. Connecting to the other realms of life, forces of nature and cosmic beings is an answer to your soul's desire to know all.

Believe you are known by all that is, by the Universe. Ask to know and you shall receive knowledge. Speak to your knowledge, speak to your energy, tap into your light and primal force. It is always talking and when you speak, listen, and then you will hear the answer.

The Third Eye

In order to fully awaken your Kundalini and to work on your psychic abilities, you have to trust your intuition. As you already know, the third eye chakra is the seat of your intuition. The third eye chakra is what allows you to be able to see the spirit world.

As you develop your third eye chakra, you will find that your intuition will strengthen as well. A developed third eye chakra will allow you to see prana as well.

Everybody has some form of intuition. Most commonly, people will know who is calling before they check their phone. There are plenty of other forms and practical uses of intuition, like avoiding danger or knowing the best course of action to take in different situations.

The pineal gland is an endocrine system organ that regulates your sleep schedule. The third eye is closely connected with the pineal gland. That's why we are going to look at how to activate and clear your pineal gland.

Working with the Pineal Gland

While the third eye chakra holds a lot of power, there are very few people who are able to tap into its power and actually use it. Most people's third eyes are underdeveloped. Luckily, there are plenty of ways to help strengthen your third eye so that you can tap into this power.

Charge with fire

The third eye chakra is related to the element of fire. That means that you can help develop your third eye chakra by charging it with fire. This is a very powerful tool to use, so make sure you follow this carefully.

Get into a relaxed and meditative posture. Shut your eyes and visualize the power and brilliance of the sun.

As you breathe in, feel yourself drawing in the energy of the sun. Allow this energy to charge your third eye. With every inhale, the energy of the sun empowers your third eye.

The more your chakra is charged, the more it will glow its bright indigo light and become more powerful. Believe that with every inhale, you are becoming more intuitive.

Remember that this technique is very powerful. You will automatically know when you do this correctly because you will start feeling pressure in the middle of your forehead. When you are just starting out, try to aim for ten inhales. As you become more used to this technique, you can start adding in more inhalations. Not only should you picture your third eye chakra becoming more powerful, but you should become conscious about the growth of your intuition. Remember, visualization is only as powerful as the intention you set.

Visual screen

This is another great visualization exercise. To create your visual screen, shut your eyes and look up slightly. Basically, you want to look towards your third eye chakra but with your eyes closed. This is where your visual screen is located. You have the ability to project anything that you want onto the screen. This is like an internal mirror. This visual screen is very helpful when it comes to visualization exercises.

Get into a relaxed and meditative position. Look at your visual screen and picture an apple floating there.

Focus on the apple and nothing else. Keep all other thoughts out of your mind. This is a lot like a simple breathing meditation, but instead of focusing on your breath, you will focus on the apple.

When you are finished with your visualization, picture the apple slowly fading and then open your eyes and allow yourself to return to the present.

You can use any image that you want when you do this exercise if you don't want to picture an apple. The important thing about the exercise is that you have something to focus on.

Forehead press

This is a very popular third eye opening technique. That does not mean that it works for everybody, though. This technique allows you to see spots of prana floating around you. They will normally look like dots or some other form of white light.

Lay your pointer finger on the spot between your eyebrows where your chakra is located. Press this spot gently and keep this pressure for about 50 seconds.

Slowly take your finger away from this spot and blink your eyes about five times and then stare at an empty wall. Focus on the wall lightly and try to see things with your peripheral vision.

Are you able to see spots or white light? These spots are prana.

This technique works best when you do it in a dimly lit room. Try to find a wall or something that is of a neutral color.

Who is it?

This is a fun exercise you can do every single time that your phone rings or buzzes. All you have to do is ask yourself, "Who's calling?" Focus on what comes to your mind's eye. Are there any impressions or images? Make sure that you are open to receiving a message. This is a great way to connect with your intuition. Tell yourself that your intuition is strong and that all you need to do is to connect with it. You don't have to limit this to only phone calls or texts. You can also do this if somebody knocks on your door, or if you hear a sound. The main thing is that you connect with your intuition to try and figure out what or who it is.

Even after doing all of these techniques, you have to make sure that you work on all of your chakras. Your crown chakra is especially close to your third eye and can help you to improve your intuition as well.

Chapter 10. Enlightenment

At the point when one who has been illuminated talks, there are things he can say with relative sureness - as much assurance as is conceivable while still in a body in this world. There are different things he can say with significant power, however not with sureness. There are additionally things he might want to have the option to state, yet they are considerably more theoretical - not without worth, however subject to significantly greater contradiction and understanding of importance.

It is very useful if a master recognizes which level of power is connected to articulations that they make. This is especially increasingly significant if the master is in and out of the illuminated state instead of in the edified state pretty much ceaselessly. For the most part, explanations made while in the edified state can be made with relative assurance. Explanations made dependent on recollecting what was seen and known while in the edified state convey huge position, yet not sureness. It is when articulations are made as to strategy and systems for helping other people accomplish edification that even a master talks theoretically, regardless of whether in the illuminated state or not. Nobody, including every single illuminated master, can say with sureness how any other individual can pick up section to the hover of edified creatures.

All illuminated people say the very same thing; they each simply communicate in an alternate language. There are ten stages to pursue to get from where you are to where you need to be. At the point when you arrive you won't have moved an inch.

There is just a single thing. There is just a single issue. There is just a single arrangement. Presently we realize what to do.

1.You become mindful of an aching for something more. You ask yourself: "Is this all there is?" You close: "Most likely there must be something more than this." You have really ventured out.

2.You become mindful of illumination as an idea. It is simply one more thought among the various fascinating thoughts you have in your mind. This is the subsequent advance.

3.You turn a corner and begin to accept that edification is something genuine. This is the third step. You are interested; you need to discover more. You begin to consider illumination. You begin to converse with others about it. You begin to peruse books about illumination.

4.You begin to need edification for yourself. The craving starts to get solid inside, however for the most part inside your head, i.e., you are still simply pondering it. Despite the fact that this is as of now the fourth step, in a way it is the genuine start; the start of the genuine.

5.You start your otherworldly mission. The dynamic quest for illumination starts, however you don't have a clue where to look. You don't have the foggiest idea what it is and you don't have a clue where to discover it. This is the fifth step; it is energizing, yet additionally startling. Your heart joins the pursuit; you become mindful of a profound yearning in your heart to return home. You investigate different otherworldly practices.

6.Your inquiry is basically coordinated into the world, outside of yourself. This is the 6th step. You may start to make changes throughout your life; how you live, where you live, who you live with, your work, and so on., yet nothing you change on the planet contacts your profound aching for something more. You become confounded, disappointed, overpowered; you need to stop and return to your standard life that is progressively well-known and increasingly agreeable.

7.Finally, normally following quite a while of study and looking, you comprehend that the lower can't order the higher; you understand that you have been looking in an inappropriate spot - outside of yourself, and that you can't get illumination going. NO profound practice can get illumination going. You turn your look internal upon yourself. You comprehend that what you are searching for is what is looking. Your mind starts to watch itself. You give up to your high Self; you let go of the inquiry however despite everything you have want, a profound significant, deep longing to wake up. You proceed with your profound hunt, however your training is currently extraordinary. You have chosen one profound practice from the extraordinary buffet of potential outcomes, yet rather than a pursuit, it turns out to be increasingly similar to a supplication of much appreciated, a presenting to God in acknowledgment of your aching to respect him, to recall who you truly are. This is the seventh step.

8.One day, you just wake up. The cover of the dream of detachment lifts. You understand that you are God; you are the one without a second. You see that there is just a single thing, and you are it, every last bit of it. Your clench hand arousing is the eighth step. In any case, it goes on for a brief span, maybe a couple of hours or even less, potentially a couple of days or weeks, however then it retreats and the more common sense of self focused awareness returns. You experience a significant anguish at the loss of this ideal light, love, truth, and knowing. Regardless of this anguish, you have just vanquished passing; you realize that what you truly are can't kick the bucket, just the physical body bites the dust.

9.Your life has now changed. You are living at the time; not the past or what's to come. You proceed with your profound way. Your aching is solid. You remain gave up in a casing of confidence, with an internal realizing that you will come back to that edified state- - regardless of whether it is just right now of your physical passing. You proceed with your internal work of rising above the conscience, recuperating old injuries and consuming gathered karma. Re-arousing is the ninth step- - the illumination returns. Presently you are profoundly certain; not haughty or selfish, no longer terrified of anything- - there is no dread. You simply know, in a way that is steadfast, who you truly are, what everything is, the thing that it isn't, what everything implies, and what you are to do.

10.With the tenth step edification ends up stable. You are there pretty much consistently. Your obligation presently is to help other people stir. School is out. Welcome HOME.

5 Steps to Become Enlightened

1.Shaktipat: The initial step to wind up illuminated is shaktipat. Otherwise called Kundalini Shakti, Deeksha or Grace, shaktipat is the profound vitality that stirs you to illumination. Albeit profound practice and reflection is significant on the off chance that you need to wind up illuminated, at last it is this otherworldly vitality that stirs you to edification. At the point when this Shaktipat winds up stirred in you, you may feel this vitality as ecstasy, or love or harmony. Essentially by enabling your thoughtfulness regarding stay in that delight, the Shakti sanitizes your vitality channels and stirs you into your characteristic edified state.

The principal way you get shaktipat is through an edified ace, one who has arrived at such a high condition of illumination that they emanate shaktipat. Just by sitting with them, this otherworldly vitality is stirred in you and illumination occurs.

However, there is likewise a way you can get shaktipat through sound which we will discuss toward the finish of this article.

2.Purification: The subsequent advance in getting to be edified is refinement. Legitimate eating routine and exercise is generally significant. You need to bring your body into an extremely adjusted and unadulterated state. In the event that you are drinking liquor, consuming medications, eating low quality nourishment, your body will be occupied with battling these poisons and will stay lopsided. You need to eat unadulterated nourishments, heaps of crisp leafy foods, nourishment that sustains the body and psyche.

3.Spiritual Practice: The third means to end up edified is otherworldly practice. Some type of contemplation is typically the fundamental practice, yet prana (breathing) works out, reciting, yoga can likewise be very helpful. It is essential to keep a receptive outlook, to attempt the changed otherworldly practices that are discussed by different edified educators and see what works for you.

4.Discipline: The fourth means to wind up illuminated is discipline: to locate the profound practices that you find advantageous and do them consistently. It does them simultaneously consistently too. I like to rise early, go for a run, do yoga, prana works out, puja and reciting and afterward think before I do whatever else. And afterward I ruminate again before supper and again before I head to sleep.

You ought to pursue what works for you, however keeping a taught routine forms the vitality. In the event that you need to wind up edified it is critical to construct this vitality and not let yourself fall into apathy and interruptions. I would say the possibility of simply "doing whatever you want to do" doesn't work. It just prompts misery and awkwardness. Unquestionably, you ought to have the opportunity to have a fabulous time. Be that as it may, keeping this control will help keep you in an illuminated condition of mindfulness.

5.Surrender: The last advance to end up illuminated is give up. Once, through decontamination, shaktipat and reflection that profound vitality current is effectively traveling through you, all that is left is give up, to enable your experience to be for what it's worth. To acknowledge yourself as you are and enable yourself to feel what is here, to feel it as sensation. In spite of the fact that control is significant, you get to the heart of the matter where you need to give up attempting to do illumination, it is the shaktipat that stirs you to edification. When you feel the shakti as a consistent in your life, you give up to it, you enable it to do its work. You enable yourself to break down into ecstasy.

Conclusion

Thanks for making it through to the end of this book. I hope it was informative and able to provide you with all of the tools you need to achieve your goals whatever they may be.

The next step is to apply everything that you have learned and start practicing the techniques. So, what are you waiting for? Start testing out the techniques in this book and choose the one that you want to master. Always keep in mind that continuous practice is a very important element of success, so be sure to make time and efforts for your practices.

Do not rush the learning process. Instead, you should enjoy it, and learn as much as you can from them. Indeed, this book is more than a collection of texts that reveal ancient secrets and wisdom. Rather, this book is an invitation to a life-changing journey. May this book be a guide like a shining star that leads you to the true path of spirituality. Just the fact that you have read this book only means that you have some kind of spiritual hunger inside you. Once again, knowledge and actual application are necessary to satisfy and make progress in your spiritual life. Feel free to review the pages of this book and be sure that you understand all of the teachings and instructions. With regard to the practices, you are allowed to make some adjustments or changes according to your preference as you deem best and suitable for you. Always remember to always do your best and never give up.

Indeed, so many people have been searching for the right instructions that can help them awaken the kundalini, develop psychic abilities, or even at least to make some progress in their spiritual life, but in vain. Now, this book has given you the keys to power, happiness, and a beautiful life. It is up to you to put this new-found knowledge into actual and continuous practice. Last but not least, remember to use everything that you have learned from this book only for good.

I am glad that you have reached this part of the book. I really hope that you enjoyed the read. If you truly desire to advance in your spiritual life, then know that it is possible, but you need to put in the time and efforts to make it a reality. You can do it as long as you continue to do your best.

BOOK 4

Introduction

Your chakras are an integral part of your daily life. While many people don't realize what is going on in their bodies, most of the time your chakras are the parts that control this. When things seem to be wrong in the body, like you feel overwhelmed or have trouble talking to other people, your chakras may be the reason that you are dealing with this. On the other hand, when you feel really good about your life, you feel like you are able to talk to other people, love other people and you don't feel like things are wrong, your chakras are most likely aligned together.

Knowledge of the chakras and how you can strengthen them is vital to your overall physical, mental and spiritual health. Chakras are typically defined as the (sometimes) invisible force fields around you, which emanate positive or negative energies depending on your mood, emotions and health status.

The history of chakras goes back a long way. Starting in the 7th century BCE, the Hindus produced texts linking the deities, religious canon and the knowledge of these psychic force fields. During this time, the Hindus recorded and wrote the Upanishads – the tome of sacred texts that contained the beliefs of Hindus. Aside from learning about karma and reincarnation, practitioners and then readers of the Upanishads knew that the body had various energy points. Moreover, it claimed that the soul settled in different parts of the body.

Understanding Chakras will have you going back to the beginning of time. It is said that the real birthplace of the human race was in Tanzania, and a certain Mount Meru, also known as a mystical mountain is located here. Mount Meru is believed to be where the Goddess Shri Lalita, who was the main source of the nine interlocking triangles—or chakras—used to reside. She represents the union of the masculine and feminine and also symbolizes the intersection of power from different parts of the body.

The chakras are so important to your body. Even if just one of the chakras is badly aligned, you will notice that all of them can become blocked and not working that well. All of the chakras need to have energy flowing through them properly so if one of the chakras doesn't allow the energy to flow through, there are going to be some big problems that arise. You need to learn how to let the energy flow through the chakras to help them to feel better and this can be done in no time at all.

When the chakras are opened up, you will notice that you feel so much better than ever before. Opened chakras allow you to talk to others, open up your heart to others, feel grounded in the world around you, and even to have a connection to a higher power. All of these can be important to live a happy and healthy life. In many cases, our modern world makes it really difficult to keep the chakras working as well as you would like them to. We are too stressed out, we are worried about keeping our jobs and we may not have much of a chance to open up to some other people. It does take some active work to help keep the chakras as open up as possible.

When the chakras are closed up, you will quickly notice that there can be issues that arise as a result of this. You may feel shy when you are with other people. You may not be able to show or share the love with some of the other people in your life, or you may not be able to stay grounded in the life that you have. There are so many elements of your life that can go wrong when you are dealing with your chakras not working properly and if one of the chakras is out of order, and not letting through the energy that you need, all of them can begin to fail pretty quickly.

Another problem that you may have is that a chakra will allow in too much energy compared to what it should. For example, if your throat chakra is open too much, you may blurt out anything that comes into your head, even if it isn't necessary or will cause a lot of pain to someone else when you don't need to do this. When the throat chakra is working properly, you will find that it works well to help you show honesty and speak up properly, so you don't want it to let in too much and say a lot of things that are not necessary and could cause issues with other people.

Working on the chakras is one of the best things that you can do for your overall health. It allows you to improve your life better than ever before because you get the chance to understand how all of the chakras work together and how they influence the different parts of your life. When you are able to get them to work together well, you will notice a huge improvement in your life in no time.

Mount Meru also signifies one's journey from the start or bottom of his life, all the way to the top, which shows where chakras and the energy system began.

Chapter 1. What Are Chakras?

Over the years, a number of misconceptions have trailed the concept, nature, origin and purpose(s) of the chakras. I have come in contact with lots of individuals who have been misled by information thwarted either simply as a result of insufficient knowledge, or for the purpose of intentionally misleading the 'new world' about the chakras. There are tons of questions on the lips and in the hearts of millions of people about chakras, some of which are:

- What actually does chakra mean?
- Are there four, six or seven chakras in all?
- What are the known chakras?
- What culture do the chakras originate from?
- Are the chakras related to any particular religion?
- What is the significance of chakras to the body, mind, soul and spirit?
- Is there a relationship between the chakras and yoga?

If you are reading this book, or at least, hoping to do so, you are most definitely interested in chakras or seeking answers to your questions about them, which may or may not have been included in the list provided above. Rest assured that what you have in your hand is a detailed book of answers, thoroughly researched and well packaged to make you realize, understand and appreciate the value of chakras to the all-round development of your soul, mind and body. In this section, I provide basic facts about chakras that will usher you into a deeper understanding in the subsequent parts of the book. You are in for a fulfilling journey. You had better brace up for interesting discoveries.

Meaning of Chakra

Chakra (plural Chakras) is alternatively known as 'Çakra'. It refers to any of the wheels of energy naturally located along the spine of the human body. It is believed that the health of an individual chakra is significantly related to the physical, mental, as well as emotional wellbeing of a person. Chakras form the centers from which we derive the energy for meditation. They are way beyond mere spinning physical discs, but significantly placed to hold a lot of influence on the human body in its multi-dimensions. However, although they are located in the human physical body, they reach farther into the psychological and spiritual domains of an individual.

How many chakras are there exactly?

There has been a little difficulty in the chakras scholarship to identify the exact number of chakras in the entire human body, depending on how traditional you are willing to go. While some scholars hold that there are as many as 88,000 chakras in the human body, some others are of the belief that there are only 112. Despite the divergent positions, there is a consensual agreement across scholarship that there are seven major chakras, with six of them situated along the spine, and the last one just above the skull. Each of the seven major chakras is associated to a unique color as follows:

- Maludhara Chakra — Red
- Swadhisthana chakra — Orange

- Manipura Chakra — Yellow
- Anahata Chakra — Green
- Vishuddhi Chakra — Blue
- Ajna Chakra — Indigo
- Sahasrara Chakra — Violet

You would have noticed that the colors of the chakras are exactly the same as the colors of the rainbow, and are arranged precisely in the same order from red to violet. This is rather too significant to be a coincidence. In addition to the beautiful colors they possess, the chakras come in a variety of shapes; associated with one deity or another; have their individual natural elements as well as special mantra. Despite their differences, chakras are heavily interconnected. As a matter of fact, a successful interrelationship between the chakras is what brings about pure bliss, contentment and happiness in all the domains of an individual — spirit, soul, mind and body.

The Origins of Chakra

Chakras have continued to gain increasing popularity in the New Age especially as it is now linked with the modern world yoga. While this appears to be a positive stride in advancing the concept and tradition of chakras, the downside to it is that a lot of misleading information is continually spread through the populace, especially by yogis who themselves have not had the privilege of discovering the true nature, origin and the historical facts about chakras. Based on this, unveiling the true historical roots of chakras has required painstaking efforts by historians. In this section, I discuss the valid and veritable historical reports of trusted historians on the topic of chakras, carefully sifting out Western or New Age conjectures which have grown in popularity over time to be accepted as the truth.

Cultural Origin

The chakra system has been culturally traced to an Indian text identified as Vedas, dating as far back as 1500 and 500 BC. According to Anodea Judith, the Vedas writings were records derived from the oral traditions of the Brahmins, descendants of the Aryans, who are believed to have immigrated into India from the North. The word 'chakra' was originally spelt 'çakra' (with the initial sound pronounced as ch) and believed to be a symbolic representation of the sun as it spans across the entire world and determines the time. Further earlier than this, around 600 BC, chakra was mentioned as the center of consciousness in the Yoga Upanishads and later in 200 BC in the Yoga Sutras of Patanjal.

Beyond mere mentions in these early resources, the chakra system was said to have actually started in the Tantric tradition sometime in the second half of the first millennium but definitely not in the system which holds that there are seven main chakras, as we know them to be today. As a matter of fact, the seven-chakras system came into wide popularity as a result of a 1577 text titled the Ṣaṭ-chakra-nirūpaṇa or 'Description of and Investigation into the Six Bodily Centres' written in Sanskrit by a certain Pūrṇānanda Yati, and later roughly translated into English by one John Woodroffe, better known by his pseudonym, Arthur Avalon, in 1919. This text formed the main vehicle by which the seven Chakras system reached a larger part of the world, including the West, and has formed the basis of many yogic beliefs. However, I should be quick to mention that Pūrṇānanda Yati cannot be credited with the creation of the chakras system in use today. As a matter of fact, a certain thirteenth century small text titled Śāradā-tilaka already mentions the existence of the seven Chakras system, but duly admits that there are other systems that include more chakras, as in the twelve, fourteen and sixteen chakras systems.

Religious Origin

As it has turned out, the chakra system may be difficult to pigeonhole as an exclusive reserve of a particular religion because it has come to be accepted and adopted, although in varying degrees, as a practice in many religions of the world. This assertion, notwithstanding, it can be said with a measure of confidence that Chakras are more originally associated with a couple of religions, specifically Hinduism and Buddhism.

To start with, the term 'chakras' appeared first in the Vedic records, which are believed to be the most reputable authoritative go-to books of Hinduism. More so, the Vedic texts, which formed the historical evidence of the chakra system, were documented in Sanskrit, the operational language of both Hinduism and Buddhism. According to Georg Feuerstein, the early Upanishads of Hinduism, which date as far back as the first millennium BCE, make mention of chakras as energy centers, even though they are not described as full energy theories as we have in yoga and kundalini, for example, today. Also, in the 8th century BCE, Buddhist texts made reference to energy centers, identifying them as four, and were called by different names including cakka, padma and pitha, and Hinduism later established the systems of more than four chakras in the medieval era. Going by these historical references, the assertion that Hinduism must have been at the forefront of the chakra system right from the onset and that Buddhism largely contributed to it definitely holds sway.

The Religious Expansion of Chakra Theories

It is already established that Hinduism and Buddhism are the two most impactful and historically significant religions as far as the origin of the chakra system is concerned, but all that is history! Virtually all religions of the world are implicitly connected to the belief system of chakra, especially with regards to its significance to the spirit, mind, soul and body of an individual. Whereas some religions do not openly declare their adoption of the chakra system, as in the Hindu practice of Yoga, there exists a link, notwithstanding, between their beliefs and practices on one hand, and the chakra theories on the other. In this section, I provide a succinct discussion of some religions of the world and how chakra theories have been discovered and incorporated over time.

Hinduism and the Solar Plexus Chakra

For Hinduism, the solar plexus chakra, or manipura, is the symbolic chakra that represents the principles of the religion. Hinduism believes in the ability of humans to influence their own lives as well as events and situations concerning them using their Agni fires. It is believed that every individual possesses what it requires for them to influence and direct their own lives through their actions and reactions. In other words, we are in control of our individual lives, and can control or transform it into whatever we desire. This would of course demand that every individual understand their self-worth, inmate abilities, and value. The purpose of this chakra in relation to Hinduism is to keep your fire ignited, and to make sure you have enough courage to undertake the proper actions that will set your life on course and help you actualize your dreams.

Taoism and the Sacral Chakra

The sacral chakra, or Swadhisthana chakra, represents the Taoist belief in harmony. Taoism holds that life is a continual balance or harmony of two opposites — Yin (the earth) and Yang (the sky). In the same vein, Taoism is of the belief that life is built on a system of duality: right and wrong, good and evil, success and failure, strength and weakness, etc. As humans, we tend to live on two opposite sides at every juncture of our lives. A perfect balance of the opposite sides is necessary to live a satisfactory life. The sacral chakra is therefore believed to be the energy force driving the harmony of these two sides, ensuring a perfect harmony, and avoiding an undue shift to either side of the symbiotic relationship.

Buddhism and the Heart Chakra

Buddhism relates closely to the heart chakra known as Anahata. The heart is specifically symbolic of love, and for Buddha, the most important love is love for oneself. This is the foundation of all other kinds of love, ranging from agape to romantic to familial love. We cannot open ourselves to love others or be loved by them if we have not first loved ourselves. Buddhism preaches that we are all we need for a blissful life. It also acknowledges the existence and inevitability of hardship and suffering in a person's lifetime. And further points that all that we need to sail through life difficulties is already within us, hence it emphasizes that we should always look into the heart for strength and guidance. Buddhism summarizes this as the four noble truths of life, which can be overcome only by towing the eightfold path. To achieve this, the heart chakra needs to be kept open and healthy.

Islam and Crown Chakra

The crown chakra is in tandem with the 'dreams' of Islam. Dreams are avenues by which we connect to the spiritual realms. Islam is said to have been built on the spiritual encounter of Prophet Muhammad (SAW) with Angel Gabriel, the archangel who took him on a spiritual visit to the heavens on a winged horse where he acquired knowledge. Based on this, Islam believes that we can seek and acquire knowledge via a connection to the divine. What is more important is to be able to secure a steady rewarding connection with the divine realm. To do this, one would need the Sahasrara, or crown chakra, and it has to be active and clear enough.

Judaism and the Throat Chakra

Judaism is founded on Abraham and the belief that he was called to neglect the other deities and accept one God. It is the belief in Judaism that the throat chakra embodies the foundation of the religion. Judaism holds the principle of revealing the inner person within us. The patriarchs on whom the religion was founded all heard a voice which formed the basis of their belief. The throat chakra Vishudda likewise emphasizes self-expression, and helps to energize the inner voice in every individual. Within us, there is a voice that constantly speaks to us, revealing the inner self to help determine and shape the course of our lives. Based on this, Judaism believes that everyone has a story, truth and wisdom within them to share to the world, and that we need to strengthen the Vishudda to energize that voice to grow stronger.

Christianity and the Third Eye Chakra

Christianity believes strongly in light as an avenue for unveiling the truth and displacing darkness. To appreciate and value light, the eyes are needed, hence the need for the third eye chakra, otherwise known as Anna. The religion is founded on Jesus of Nazareth, who is believed to be the light by which his followers see, or the light of the world. It is with the help of the light that we see through darkness, deceit and falsehood. The light also helps to seek true valid spiritual knowledge. We therefore need third eye chakra to enable us see through illusions, darkness and falsehood, to see, appreciate and explore the light and wisdom entrapped within us.

The discussion of the world religions and their relationship with the chakras could go on and on since there are many religions across the world. One basic truth that underlies them all is that, as I have already established, they, either implicitly or explicitly, operate in relation to one chakra or the other. This foundational truth is to help you understand and value chakras for their importance to the universe as a whole, and to you as an individual. As you 'journey' further into this book, you will find a detailed exposition of the seven chakras of the modern world, and how they differ from the Vedic culture; the relationship between Yoga and the chakras; an analysis of the chakras, and how they could help you live a blissful life, among other salient revelations. This is definitely going to be a worthy ride. Brace up for it!

Chapter 2. How Chakras Work, The System

We all have a physical body and we also have an energy body. Our energy body contains our auras and meridian lines. Auras are non-physical energy fields that surround a person. Your aura reveals your thoughts, dreams, and feelings. The colors of your aura may vary and they are usually seen by people who have special training in the healing arts.

A meridian line, on the other hand, is a path where the life energy called "qi" or "chi" passes through. It is a typically used in Chinese medicine. If you go to an acupuncturist or a spiritual healer, you'll hear these terms often.

When you cut the body open, you won't see these auras and meridian lines, but you know that they are there. When you are familiar with auras, you'd know that they are affected by certain vibrations – good or bad. So, if you get a good vibe or bad vibe from someone, you may be feeling his aura. You get certain feelings when you talk with someone because these vibrations are contained in their energy.

Like the auras and meridian lines, the chakras are part of the body's energy anatomy. They operate like a ball of energy and they spin like a wheel to distribute your energy evenly throughout your body.

You can't see these chakras through an X-ray because they are not part of the physical body. They are part of our consciousness and they interact with the physical body through the different organs in the body. Each chakra is associated with one endocrine gland and a group of nerves called plexus.

Are some chakras more important than others? The answer is no. All chakras are equally important. To live a good life, you should balance all the chakras in your body.

The grounding function of the root chakra is just as important as the spiritual function of the crown chakra and the transcendent quality of the heart chakra.

To optimize your mental and bodily functions, you have to balance all your chakras and address your basic, relational, creative, safety, belongingness, and self-actualization needs.

The Chakras and Your Physical Body

We are all made of pure energy. So, if your energy centers are blocked, you'll experience various illnesses. When one or two of your chakras are not spinning, the energy is not evenly distributed throughout your body, resulting to some of organs may not functioning well.

For example, your heart chakra is in your chest area, and it covers the heart, and the respiratory system. So, if your heart chakra is not spinning, you'll experience heart and circulation problems. You are also susceptible to respiratory diseases and allergies.

The throat chakra governs the throat and mouth area of your body. So, if it's not functioning well, you'll experience mouth ulcers, sore throats, and thyroid problems.

Many Western medical practitioners do not believe this, but your chakras can affect your body functions. Balanced chakras can optimize your health and vitality while unbalanced chakras can wreak havoc in your life.

Chakras and Emotions
Chakras do not only represent your physical body, but also your emotions and parts of your consciousness. When there is tension in your consciousness, you'll feel it in the chakra that's linked to that part of your consciousness.

For example, if your boyfriend leaves you, you'll feel the pain in your heart or chest area. You'll feel like you can't breathe. When you are nervous about something, your bladder becomes weak and your legs tremble.

When the tension persists, it can result to physical symptoms.

The Chakras and The Quality of Life
The chakras do not only affect your physical body, but they also affect your mental health and the overall quality of your life. So, if one part of your life seems off or something in your life is not working, then one of your chakras may be blocked.

When one or two of your chakras are blocked, some parts of your life may be doing well while other parts of your life may not be doing well at all. For example, your career may be doing well, but you have difficulty maintaining healthy relationships.

If you are a spiritual, kind, and compassionate person, but you have a hard time paying your bills, you may also have blocked chakras.

When your chakras are not functioning the way, they should, you feel there is an imbalance. Your subconscious tells you that something is amiss.

The chakras represent who you are – your intellect, emotions, creativity, spirituality, sexuality, careers, principles, and your belief system. So, if your chakras are not balanced, you'll lose sight of one part of your life. You'll likely develop psychological problems such as depression, anxiety, delusions, and even nervous breakdown.

What Causes Chakra Blockages
Chakra blockages are caused by several factors – belief system, career, living situation, financial situation and relationships. Traumatic experiences such as abuse, accident, and loss of a loved one may also cause chakra blockages. Negative emotions such as anxiety, anger, stress, and fear may also put your chakras out of balance.

For example, being physically and emotionally abused by a former partner may cause heart chakra imbalance. You might have ended up closing yourself out to potential romantic partners. You may also tend to feel empty most of the time.

Your root chakra represents the foundation of your being. So, if your parents do not have enough money when you were growing up and they failed to provide enough for you, you'll most likely experience root chakra blockage. You may constantly fear that you do not have enough. You may also constantly worry about money.

Opening and Closing the Chakras

The opening and closing of your chakras work a lot like an energetic defense system. When you experience something traumatic or negative, the associated chakra will close itself to keep the negative energy out. If you are clinging to low frequency feelings such as anger, guilt, or blame, you'll experience chakra blockage.

Holding on to the following low frequency emotions for a long period can cause chakra blockage:

- Anger
- Pain
- Resentment
- Jealousy
- Covert hostility
- Grief
- Apathy
- Hopelessness
- Sadness
- Apathy
- Regret
- Pessimism
- Worry
- Blame
- Discouragement
- Shame
- Powerlessness
- Depression
- Disappointment
- Frustration
- Despair
- Guilt

The following positive or high frequency emotions can raise your vibrations and help open your chakras:

- Love
- Joy
- Acceptance
- Eagerness
- Optimism
- Passion
- Hopefulness
- Contentment
- Faith
- Belief

So, to keep your chakras balanced, you must let go of egoism. You must choose to act with love. You should also consider trying various chakra healing tools which will be discussed later in this book.

Chakras and Empaths

Many people have open chakras. These people are called empaths. They are highly sensitive people. They easily pick up other people's energy, so they find public places overwhelming. They also know when someone is not being honest with them. They are creative and they have a strong need for solitude. They feel weak when they are exposed to toxic people.

Empaths should keep their chakras guarded and balanced. They should carry protective stones such as rose quartz, black tourmaline, amethyst, and malachite. These stones help balance emotions and remove anxieties and negative energy.

The theoretical understanding of these relationships and the foundation on which practical knowledge is based on each of the individual chakras described in this book.

The writings that tradition has bequeathed to us mention a high number of chakras: 88,000. This means that in the human body there is hardly any point other than a sensitive organ for the reception, transformation, and retransmission of energies.

But nevertheless, most of these chakras are very small and play a subordinate role in the energy system there are approximately 40 love chakras to which it is assigned a greater importance. The most important of them are in the spleen area, in the neck, on the palms of the hands and on the soles of the feet. The different main chakras, located along a vertical axis next to the anterior half of the body, are so crucial for the functioning of the most basic and important parts of the body, the spirit, and the human soul. You can see what specific spiritual qualities are related to each of the chakras, what body areas are subject to their influence, how the blockages of each of the chakra's impact, and much more.

Here we would like to first describe those characteristics that are common to all the main chakras they truly settle in the etheric body of man. They resemble funnel-shaped floral chalices and a varied number of petals. Thus, in the cultural field of the East, they are often also called lotus flowers. Subdivisions of the flowers in independent petals represent the nadis or the energy channels through which energies flow and penetrate the chakras and through which the energy is transmitted from the chakras to non-material bodies. Their number varies from four channels in the radical center to almost a thousand energy channels in the center of the crown.

From the concavity located in the center of each chalice part a channel, as a petiole of the chakra flower, which reaches the spine and splices directly with it. This channel joins the chakras with the main energy channel, called Sushumna, which ascends through the inside of the spine and continues in the head to the crown.

The chakras are in permanent circular motion. To this quality, they owe their name of «chakra», which in Sanskrit means «wheel». The rotating movement of these wheels causes energy to be attracted into the chakras. If the sense of turn changes, the energy is radiated from the chakras. The chakras can turn right or left. Here you can recognize a contrasted principle in men and women, or a compliment in the expression of the energies of different "species" since the same chakras that in man revolve clockwise (clockwise), in the woman, turn left, and vice versa. Every turn to the right has a peculiarity a predominance of masculine quality, an accentuation of yang according to Chinese doctrine; that is, it represents will and activity, and in its negative form of manifestation, also aggressiveness and violence. All left turn has predominance of yin and represents sensitivity and agreement, and in its negative aspect, weakness.

The direction of rotation changes from one chakra to another. Thus, the basal chakra of man turns towards the right, and more actively expresses the qualities of this center: in the sense of conquest and mastery in the material and sexual field. On the other hand, the first chakra of women makes sense turning to the left, which makes it more sensitive for the life-giving force and engendering the earth, which flows through the radical center. In the love chakra, the signs are reversed: the sense of right turn in women indicates greater active energy in the expression of feelings; the sense of rotation to the left of man can be interpreted here preferably as the receptive, often even as a passive attitude and so on.

Direction of Rotation of the Chakras in Women
The continuous line that ascends undulating symbolizes Pingala, solar energy, and the line of points represent Ida, the lunar force.

Direction of Rotation of the Chakras in Man

The continuous line that ascends undulating symbolizes Pingala, and the dotted line symbolizes going right and left successively and characterizes man differently and women, which leads to a complement of energy in each of the areas of life.

Knowing the direction of rotation of the chakras allows incorporating them into some forms of therapy. For example, in aromatherapy, you can apply the aromas with a circulating movement in the corresponding direction, or also draw with the precious stones turning in the same sense as the energy centers.

The chakras of most people have an approximate average length of 10 centimeters. In each of the energy centers, there are all chromatic vibrations, although a certain color always dominates, which matches the function corresponding main chakra. In a superior development of man, the chakras

They continue to spread and increase their vibration frequency. Also, its colors are clearer and radiant.

The size and number of vibrations (frequency) of the chakras determine the amount and the quality of the energies they absorb from the most varied sources. It is about of energies that come to us from the cosmos, from the stars, from nature, from the radiation of all things and all the people in our environment, of our different non-material bodies, and also of the original unmanifested reason of every being. Those energies reach the chakras, in part, through the nadis, and, in part, flow to them directly inside. The two most significant and key types of vitality are retained through the extreme focus and the coronal focus. Between these two chakras runs Sushumna, to which all energy centers are linked through their "petioles" and that feeds all of the life force. It is the channel through which the called Kundalini energy, which rests, "rolled up like a snake", at the end inferior of the spine, and whose entrance door is the radical center. Kundalini energy represents the cosmic energy of creation, which in Indian wisdom is also called Shakti or the feminine manifestation of God. This active aspect of the divine being it causes all manifestations of creation. Its opposite pole is the pure appearance, amorphous and self-inherent of the divine being, which we will discuss in more detail later.

In most people, Kundalini energy only flows through Sushumna in low proportion as you wake up by a growing development of the consciousness, ascends through the channel of the spine in a flow always growing, and activating the different chakras. This activation produces an extension of the energy centers and an acceleration of their frequencies. Kundalini energy feeds the chakras with the energetic vibration that empowers men to open gradually in the course of its evolution all the faculties and energies that act in the different energy and material planes of creation, in order to integrate these energies in your life.

During its ascent, Kundalini energy is transformed into a different vibration in each chakra, corresponding to the functions of the respective chakra. This vibration is minimal in the radical center and finds its maximum expression in the coronal center. Vibrations transformed are relayed to the different non-material bodies or to the physical body, and they are perceived as feelings, ideas, and physical sensations.

The degree to which a person allows the action of Kundalini energy depends on the degree of awareness that you have in the different areas of life represented by the chakras, and to the extent that stress and unprocessed experiences have caused blockages in the chakras the more conscious a person is, the more open and active their chakras, so that Kundalini energy can flow to them with more intensity; and when the more intense this energy flow, the more active the chakras will become, which, in turn, arouses greater awareness. In this way, a permanent cycle of mutual influence emerges, as soon as we begin to eliminate our blockages and walk a path of the development of consciousness.

In addition to the Kundalini energy, there is another force that flows into each of the chakras through the Sushumna canal of the spine. It is the energy of the divine being pure, of the unmanifest aspect of God. It enters through the coronal chakra and makes the man knows in all planes of life the existential amorphous aspect of God as the original reason, immutable and that everything penetrates, of that manifestation. This energy is particularly suitable for removing blockages of the chakras. In Indian wisdom, it is called Shiva, divinity, who is the great destroyer of ignorance and who with his mere presence unleashes a transformation towards the divine.

This representation of the chakras from Nepal is approximately 350 years old. All the main chakras can be recognized, represented by Lotus flowers. Each of these chakra flowers represents a plane of consciousness, starting with the lower ones and ending with the upper ones at the top. They can also recognize the main energy channels, Sushumna, Ida and Pingala. (Gouache over paper) Thus, Shiva and Shakti work side by side in the integral development of the person, in which we have integrated into our lives both the divine and all planes of relative being.

Next to the Sushumna, there are two other energy channels that play a role particularly important in the energy system: in Sanskrit they are called Ida and

Pingala, Pingala acts as a carrier of solar energy, full of ardor and strength. This channel starts to the right of the radical chakra and ends at the top of the right nostril Ida is the bearer of the lunar energy that cools and calms. It begins to the left of the radical chakra and ends in the left nostril. In its way from the radical center to the nose, both nadis squirm around Sushumna

Ida and Pingala have the power to absorb prana directly from the air through the breathing, and expelling poisonous substances in exhalation. Together with the Sushumna, they constitute the three main channels of the energy system. In addition, there is a large number from other nadis that give the energies of the chakras from the lower chakras and of non-material bodies, and that retransmit that energy to energy bodies neighbors.

But the chakras also directly absorb environmental vibrations, vibrations that they correspond to their frequencies. Thus, through its different forms of functioning, they unite us with the events of our environment, of nature and of the universe, serving as antennas for the full range of energy vibrations.

We can also call the non-material sensory organs to the chakras. Our physical body, along with its senses, is a vehicle adapted to the laws of life of our planet, and with whose help we manage in the external realm of life, but with which simultaneously we can also realize on earth our values and internal knowledge the chakras serve as receivers for all energy vibrations and information that come from the physical field. They are the openings that unite us with the unlimited world of the most subtle energies.

The chakras also radiate energy directly to the environment, thereby modifying the atmosphere around us. Through the chakras we can emit healing vibrations and messages, conscious and unconscious, influencing both positively and negatively about people, situations and even matter.

To experience an inner fullness, and energy, creativity, knowledge, love, and blessing associated with it, all chakras must be open and work in mutual harmony, However, this circumstance occurs in very few people. In general, the different chakras have a different degree of activation. And many times, they are only the two lower chakras activated. In people who hold a social outstanding position, or that somehow exert a great influence, it is common that, in addition, the solar plexus chakra is disproportionately active. it's possible that there is any combination of open, locked or marked one-way concrete chakras. In addition, these degrees oscillate throughout a life, since at times

Different topics may become different. Therefore, knowledge of the chakras can give you invaluable help for the self-knowledge, and guide you on your way to discover all innate faculties, giving you a life of maximum fulfillment and joy.

Chapter 3. Chakras and Human Consciousness

The Upanishads began the teachings of chakras that are still being used and adhered to up to today, which are often called the Centers of Consciousness. This started in 600 BC, and the teachings were adopted by the Yoga Sutras of Patanjali in 200 BC.

Chakras are known to be the centers of consciousness mostly because they say a lot about how you feel, how your day will be, and how your emotions are going to play a role in your life.

Chakras in Patanjali were said to interpret:

- Pure Consciousness (Purusha)
- Prima Materia of the World (Prakriti)

They believed that by doing yoga, one can awaken his chakras, and rise above plain consciousness, in order to realize pure consciousness. This way, the mind will not fluctuate just because of emotions, especially anger and loneliness. This will also invoke a higher and much deeper kind of synthesis for you.

The 1900s to Today

In 1919, the first manuscript that's believed to explain chakras was introduced to the West by a man named Arthur Avalon. This book was entitled The Serpent Power. In the said book, he was able to explain various practices that people did—and can do—to awaken the chakras, including the ways one has to meditate in order to tap into various chakras. This is called Gorakshashatakam, which is now deemed as the precursor of today's Chakra theory, together with Tantric Sex, and Kundalini Yoga.

Chapter 4. The Seven Chakra's System

The Root Chakra

One of the very first major chakras found within the body is the root chakra. This chakra is also known as Muladhara, 'Mula' signifying root and 'Dhara' meaning support or base. Together, they make up the importance behind the root chakra which is to provide balance or support. The root chakra is responsible for a sense of emotional safety and security when it comes to ones day to day activities.

It is all about survival and grounding oneself.

This chakra works by connecting your very own energy to the earth's energy through the practice of grounding oneself with the power of visualization. The root chakra makes sure that you feel at ease when it comes to things such as love, goals, money, and security. This chakra represents the color red that is associated with love, strength, security, energy, desire, and power. It can be found in the lower abdomen, where the tailbone of the spine is located. It makes you feel alive and brings awareness that you are being on this planet living your own life with nothing controlling you.

An imbalanced root chakra can not only damage the mind but the body too. Physically, this chakra is associated with problems and diseases inside the spine, nerve system, the lower abdomen, kidney, hemorrhoids, and sleep disorders. One may also suffer from pain, bladder issues, digestion problems, ovarian cysts, and lower back pains. When emotionally imbalanced, one will live their life worrying about almost anything every single day. Negative feelings like anxiety, insecurity, impatience, and stress will resurface causing other mental illnesses such as depression.

Since the flow of energy is blocked, that energy will not properly reach the legs causing one to always feel exhausted after walking. When your root chakra is balanced, you will live a life free of worries, situations that refer to your survival requirements won't stress you, and you will be able to react to different circumstances with a calm mindset. The trust is found within yourself, you believe that you can get through any obstacles without it interfering with your mental health. Physically, when this chakra is balanced, the body is healthy and energized.

There are no difficulties relating to the lower abdomen. Emotionally, this chakra deals with anxiety and stress so when it is in balance, those feelings simply fade away. With a positive mindset, no negative thoughts, and the root chakra can help achieve a mental balance as well as balancing other chakras such as the sacral and the heart by getting rid of negative emotions. The reaction to obstacles and problems will improve without a panic state of mind state. Chakras can also be either overactive or underactive, meaning that its either too open which can affect one not in a good way or it's not open enough.

When the root chakra is overactive, the root chakra can also create 'threats' inside your mind, making you believe in it when in reality there is nothing that can harm you. These threats will cause paranoia, leading to jittery and anxious. You will also find yourself getting aggressive, annoyed, and angry all the time.

The slightest provocation will tick you off. This type of person always tries to control others for their greedy deeds.

They often resist higher authority, change, and are known to obsess over feeling secure. When the root chakra is underactive, then it means that one has taken care of the survival needs but not in a healthy manner. It is not 'open enough' meaning that one still feels disconnected or insecure when it comes to the outside world. They easily feel nervous, anxious, afraid, and find it hard to finish daily tasks on time.In order to balance this chakra, one must also consider changing daily habits to help assist in the opening of this chakra.

A change in diet can strongly influence the mind, body, and root chakra. A healthy and well-balanced diet can help achieve mental clarity, provide health for the body, and even help balance the root chakra. Try to consume healthy foods and drink a lot of water, it is not only beneficial for the root chakra but can even help to prevent any unwanted diseases within the body. Especially eating red foods such as tomatoes, strawberries, red peppers, and many others can help assist in the opening of the root chakra. Exercising like jogging, hiking, or yoga can help the body's health and the root chakra.

An open root chakra will make you feel grounded and more confident in yourself. Meditation is known to be one of the best ways to awaken and open the root chakra, but before beginning with this meditation, one should ground themselves first. Grounding can help the person connect to the earth more which is what this chakra is all about. A perfect way to ground oneself is by walking barefooted in nature, the beach, or the forest.

Walking barefooted at home can also help. Another popular way is to use the power of visualization by imagining yourself as an energy tree by extending your arms upwards. Visualize roots below you, sinking deeper into the ground, and the branches above you, extending from your hands. This is a brief visualization exercise, and it can help ground you. It shouldn't take longer than two to three minutes, it can also help calm the mind before you get into the meditation state.

Meditation For the Root Chakra

Begin by getting comfortable in the meditation sacred place of your choosing. This time, instead of laying down, you will be sitting with your legs crossed. Make sure that your spine and shoulders are straight and tall which will be more effective when healing the lower abdomen and the root chakra. Allow for your hands to rest on your knees, with the palms facing up. Form your hands into the mudra hand position by forming a circle using your thumb and your index finger, it can also be interpreted as an okay hand gesture.

Begin to breathe deeply, inhale and hold the breath for three seconds before exhaling it and dragging it out for another three seconds. Make sure that when you are breathing in and out that you use your chest, rather than breathing in through your stomach. When you are using the chest, the spine extends and moves along with the breathing, this will enable the relaxation of the body even when you are sitting up.Take a few minutes to simply relax your muscles and the body as you breathe in. Bring your attention to your breathing as you inhale and exhale to help calm the mind. Try your best to not listen to your thoughts and the mental clutter that is going on inside your head.

Instead, bring your focus to yourself as a being in this big universe. Don't think about anything else that you have to do or things that might be bothering, instead focus on breathing through your chest, making the lungs expand as you breathe in.

Take some time to bring your attention to different parts of your body, relaxing them in the process.

Think of your face muscles, relaxing as they tingle with your life force energy that you always have within you.

Then bring your attention to your arms, legs, belly, and other parts of your body that you might feel some tension in.

Allow yourself to feel the different tingling sensations all throughout as you let your body go numb and relax.

Gradually bring your attention back to your breathing, notice how your chest rises and falls every time you inhale or exhale.

Allow your eyes to lightly close, as if you are slowly falling into a deep slumber.

Create a breathing pattern, it is often related to how you would breathe normally.

Slow down your breathing by holding it in and extending it one or two seconds longer when you breathe out.

When you take a deep breath in, notice how the air travels down into your lower belly and then back up through your nose as you exhale.

Deeply breathe in and out a few times before bringing your awareness to the location of the root chakra, the base of your spine where your tailbone is.

Focus on your breathing and don't let your mind slip away as you allow for your energy to awaken.

Begin to resurface the energy within you by visualizing your body glowing white, the white that represents your pure energy that is deeply in connection with your soul.

The white begins to surround your body, circulating and connecting with your aura.

Rest in that sensation for another minute or two before concentrating and directing that energy into the palms of your hands.

Center the flow of energy into your palms, by imagining it all flowing to your hands as it travels from different parts of your body, like arms and legs.

Let yourself feel any tingling sensations or warmth.

Allow it to rest there, forming a white ball of light in each of your hands.

Lift your hands up and place them down on your lower abdomen.

Imagine the light and energy that you have gathered begin to change color, from a pure white into a red while allowing it to enter through the lower abdomen and into the root chakra.

Red is associated with the root chakra and using this color can help not only open the chakra but also direct the energy into that specific area.

Visualize that red light enters your chakra point and the healing energy that is being sent with it.

Inhale and contract the muscles between the pubic bone and the tailbone as the light enters, engaging the Mula Bandha that can help to further activate your energy and release the root chakra energy.

You are drawing the perineum towards the root chakra.

Bring your attention to how the Mula Bandha feels as you breathe flows in and your muscles contract.

Hold your breath for one to two seconds before releasing the Mula Bandha and relaxing your muscles.

Repeat again by tightening and contracting the muscles once again, feel how your spine becomes taller, pulling you up while pushing your legs and feet down.

Let go after one or two seconds and let your muscles relax again.

Repeat for at least two to three minutes or however long you seem it fit.

As you release the contract, the root chakra energy increases.

Visualize the energy intercepting with that of the root chakra, connecting and expanding further.

Allow for your body to fall into a state of relaxation, you might find it even more relaxing than when you started your meditation.

Let that energy simply travel around the lower abdomen.

You might feel some tingling sensations or warmth down your spine or throughout your body, this indicates that your chakra is being opened and the body is experiencing high energies.

Let that red light circulate in the lower abdomen, cleansing out all of the negative energy within that area.

Then, continue the healing process by imagining that red light traveling down your crossed legs as you are sitting up, connecting with the muscles and relaxing any tensions that you might have.

Allow for it to travel back up into the lower abdomen, resting there and releasing all the tensions before allowing it to travel back down again.

This time, as it makes its way all the way down to the souls of your feet, imagine that energy leaving your body through the bottom of where you are located.

If you are sitting on a bed, or on the floor, imagine that energy reaching out into the ground, as if you are a tree and the red energy is your roots.

Let it rest in that sensation, grounding you and connecting with the energy from the earth's element.

Feel the earth's energy connect with your own, intercepting and becoming one before allowing your red root energies to return back to your through the souls of your feet.

Let that magnified energy to travel back up to your lower abdomen, letting it rest there as you take notice of any tensions within your lower abdomen or your legs.

If you feel any tensions or tingling, then allow for that energy to go there.

Let the energy rest in that area while you imagine healing and banishment of any tensions or negativity.

If there are any other tensions within the root chakra area, then allow for the energy to travel there.

The glow is expanding, making you feel warm and relaxed.

Feel the root chakra, feel any sensations, warmth, or tingling in the tailbone area.

Gently rest in the sensations for a few minutes as you breathe in deeply.

Once you feel relaxed and good about your healing, return the energy to the lower abdomen.

Bring your attention back to your breathing as you bring your awareness back into your body.

Take a minute to simply breathe and stay present at this moment.

Allow for your eyes to slowly open, adjusting them to the light and the physical world around you.

Consider laying down somewhere or continue sitting up if you wish, but take some time to reflect and think back to your meditation before proceeding with your day.

When you are done, thank the universe for guiding you and for helping you heal yourself.

Take some time to relax after the healing process, don't push yourself to do anything.

Stay at home, relax, take a hot bath, and let your body heal itself while the energy within your body is still present.

Sacral Chakra
The second major chakra is the sacral chakra.

It is also known as Svadhishana which signifies 'the place of the self'.

In context, this chakra is all about making you feel like you belong in this world.

It gives you the feelings and emotions that make you enjoy your life, as well as living with creative energy that makes up your persona.

This chakra provides the feeling of satisfaction and survival which comes from the root chakra.

The sacral chakra is responsible for one's inner feelings that make up the happiness, it is also responsible for all of the emotional aspect of a person.

It represents connection, intimacy, pleasure, and sensuality.

The sacral chakra is associated with the color orange which represents creativity, joy, success, and self-respect.

The location of this chakra is below the belly button in the lower abdomen region which mostly affects that specific region within the body.

When imbalanced, a person will experience extreme difficulties when it comes to both the mind and body.

Physically, one will suffer from problems within the reproductive system, kidney infections, urinary problems, prostate problems, constipation, hormonal imbalance, gynecological problems, abnormal menstruation in females, and problems within the sexual organs.

This chakra is also the cause of one's negative addictions and emotions.

In order to be healthy, one must first realize that negative actions have negative consequences.

Ask yourself if what you are doing is good for your health.

Change starts from within the mind by drawing the energy away from what you are addicted to.

Emotionally, one will suffer from negative feelings, weakness, insecurity, and fear, which will then affect the root chakra and its feelings of security.

One will also find themselves to be enjoying things that shouldn't be the main cause of one's happiness.

New addictions will resurface as well as lack of motivation, restlessness, emotional confusion, and feelings of unimportance.

However, when this chakra is balanced, it lets one stay and live in the moment, experiencing all the wonderful feelings that come with it.

The sacral chakra let's one understand the things that life offers and that everything happens for a reason.

Physically, the lower abandonment region such as the reproductive organs, bladder, and stomach suffer no physical pain.

The energy within the body is also well balanced, meaning one will never feel tired or exhausted.

Emotionally, one will be able to express themselves easily since this chakra is linked to the feelings and emotions of the mind.

The emotional state will be well-balanced meaning that when situations will get heated, you will not overreact which is known to often cause more stress.

When this chakra is overactive, the sacral may be experiencing too much energy causes an imbalance to the sacral chakra region.

When it happens, the overall well-being of a person is affected.

One will experience conflict, drama, and unhealthy relationships as well as constant overwhelming feelings.

The emotions will be expressed more deeply, they will also be heightened.

Moodswings, a strong dependence on others, attachment, aggression, anxiety, and emotional imbalance are common side effects of an overactive sacral chakra.

When the sacral chakra is underactive, then one is most likely experiencing a disturbance in the flow of energy.

You will begin to suffer from losing control, feelings of uncertainty, and inability to cope with changes and obstacles in your life.

It often affects the environment and personal relationships with friends, family, and lovers.

You will feel detached from your emotions causing drastic changes for yourself and others.

Changing your diet, adding yoga, and meditation into your daily routine can only help if you let it.

Keeping an open mindset can also be of use to make sure that all the little things that one does will help in healing the sacral chakra.

One must first welcome change into their lives in order to be healed completely.

The sacral chakra is often associated with water meaning that drinking plenty of water and/or herbal teas especially fruity ones can help heal and balance this chakra point.

Eating orange foods such as oranges, melons, coconuts, and other sweet fruits can be beneficial in aiding to balance this chakra.

Foods that are orange in color can also be of help.

Specific practices such as yoga and particular yoga pose that involve opening the hips like open-angle pose, bound angle pose, and upavistha konasana are not only good for the body but can help open the sacral chakra.

Meditation For the Sacral Chakra

Find a comfortable position while you are laying down preferably in the area that can become your meditational sacred place.

When you lay down, make sure to place a pillow under your head so you will not fall asleep, and another pillow, rolled-up preferably, under your knees to support your legs.

Your body will notice that it is not your usual sleeping position which will make you stay awake.

Turn off your phone and lock your doors to ensure that you will not get distracted.

When you lay down, strengthen your body, facing up and begin by breathing deeply. Keep your hands on your sides, with the palms facing upwards.

Start off by focusing your attention on the way your body moves as you inhale or exhale.

Relax your arms, legs, belly, and other parts of your body where you feel most tension in.

Gradually let your eyes close themselves, slowly and not forcefully.

Make sure to maintain balanced breathing, smooth, deep and slow.

Slowly begin to close your eyes gently, not forcefully.

Allow for your body to feel as if it's entering the deepest state of relaxation while the mind and the soul are wide awake.

Continue to breathe in and out, focusing on the way your chest rises and falls with every breath you take in.

If you find your mind wandering around, simply bring it back to your body and your attention to your breathing.

Take a couple of minutes to silence your mind, getting rid of any mental clutter and bringing the mind to a state of relaxation and meditation.

Once you relax your body, bring your awareness to how your stomach and organs expand as you breath in and out.

Feel any sensations or tingling inside where your sacral chakra is located at the lower abdomen, in your pelvic region.

Breathe slowly and deeply and try to notice any changes in the area of your focus.

Can you feel your pelvic organs pulsating or tingling as you breathe?

Continue to breathe deeply, relaxing your body in the process and observing your lower abdomen.

Bring your attention to the way you breathe in, as your organs are expanding and changing their shape when you inhale or exhale.

Imagine your kidneys, and other organs moving in your body slightly as if swaying from side to side.

Begin to call out to the universe and ask to resurface the life force energy from within you.

Ask for guidance and support while setting your intention to achieve constant healing within the sacral area, the gut, and the stomach.

Allow for that energy to resurface while imagining yourself glowing white color.

Feel the flow of energy throughout your body, resurfacing, recharging the body, and getting rid of any impurities.

Thank the energy within you as it constantly moves and tries its best to heal you physically, emotionally, and spiritually.

Form a Gassho with your hands and place them in front of you where your heart is.

Focus on centering the energy into your hands as you ask for guidance and healing from the Universe.

Once you've gathered energy white and pure energy within your hands, proceed by pressing them down onto your sacrum, the lower abdomen stomach area, that is a couple of inches below the belly button.

This is where the Sacral chakra resigns.

Allow that energy to hover in the sacral chakra, opening it and freeing its own energy.

Place your hands on the lower abdomen, skin to skin, and feel any sensations or movements through your hands.

Visualize the warmth radiating from both sides of the skin, picture an orange glow lighting up and warming up your hands.

You will start to feel tingling and movements in your lower abdomen.

Let it move all throughout your stomach and gut area, visualize receiving healing, improving your digestion, or even increasing your intuition, the gut feeling.

Lift your hands up and place them on your mind.

Visualize sending the healing energy into the mind, imagine opening it and balancing your emotions.

Think of all the negative energy simply letting go and moving on.

Replace those negative feelings that are letting themselves leave your body with those of happiness by thinking back to your happiest memories or about things that make you happy.

This will let the body experience its 'true' and happy state.

Imagine the light evolving and glowing brighter and brighter, radiating from your hands with the feeling of warmth and tingling sensations around that area whether you have physical contact with the skin or are simply allowing your hands to hover above.

Remove your hands and place them back on your lower stomach, the region that connects to feelings of enjoyment of living and happiness.

Allow for yourself to enjoy and live in this moment, notice the butterflies and the joyous feelings they give out in your stomach.

Each time you deeply inhale, bring that orange glow a tiny bit brighter and bigger.

Feel the creative and inspirational energy run through your veins.

Lay in that feeling for a few minutes before gently opening your eyes.

Breathe in the air around you and look around as you still feel that strong and bright energy.

Clear this area for about two to three minutes before placing one of your hands on your back, with the palms facing downwards.

Proceed to visualize further healing and opening of this chakra.

Allow for the energy to travel all around, to any tensions within the area and banishing any impurities.

Visualize cleansing and purifying the mind by healing and opening the Sacral chakra.

Hold your hands there for two to three minutes at most, resting your mind as you breathe in deeply and slowly.

Consider taking some time to gently massage the area to promote a healthy flow of energy, relaxation, and freedom of any tension.

If you choose to massage the area then make sure you do it clockwise for women and anticlockwise for men, or whichever way feels right to you.

Gently press three fingers, the index finger, the middle finger, and the ring finger against your exposes stomach.

Begin by gently applying pressure before massaging it in a circular way.

Proceed by breathing in deeply, holding in the breath for three seconds before letting go as you massage it.

Continue to visualize the orange healing energy swimming within the area that you touch, healing it in the process.

Slowly bring your attention back to your breathing, allowing for the energy to evenly spread back throughout your body while cleansing it and removing any impurities.

Rest for a minute before gently opening your eyes.

Allow yourself to lay in the feeling of being aware of your surroundings for a couple of minutes while reminding yourself of your pure intentions of healing yourself while cleansing the body with the energy.

Reflect on your meditation.

Did you receive any sensations or visions?

Often times during meditations especially with healing, the universe might speak through visions to hint something else that might be needed for healing, either physical or mental.

Breathe in the air around you and look around as you might be filled with strong and bright energy.

This new found energy might overwhelm you with a strong urge to create, so allow it to guide you in releasing the energy through creating some with inspiration.

Solar Plexus Chakra
The third chakra point is the solar plexus, it is also referred to as Manipura which means 'lustrous gem' and 'resplendent gem'.

Since the chakra is located in the upper abdomen, just a couple of inches above your belly button, it is known as chakra of intuition, or 'gut feeling' due to its location.

This chakra is the representation of one's willpower and the strong desire to achieve success.

It is also associated with wisdom, confidence, and the perception of who you are as a person.

The solar plexus is the origin of one's self-discipline and self-esteem that makes up a person as a whole.

It turns thoughts and goals into actions through willpower.

This chakra is associated with the color yellow which means energetic, cheerful, happiness, intellect, and encouragement.

When the solar plexus is imbalanced, the energy is either directed too much on the body or mind.

Physically, the solar plexus is responsible for the problems found within the muscular system, the cellular respiration, the nervous system, digestive system, blood sugar problems, hypertension, and gallbladder.

When this chakra is imbalanced emotionally, one will always suffer from migraines, changes in attitude, mood imbalance, and lack of motivation.

You will also begin to feel powerless in situations within your life, like losing control of everything that happens around you.

This will cause you to always be angry or lashing out to surrounding people, applying negative energy to the environment and influencing other people negatively.

Life will become a hassle rather than being filled with joy and living it to the fullest.

When balanced, one feels as if they have the power to accomplish any of their goals, this strong feeling is able to turn the thoughts into actions.

The balanced solar plexus chakra makes you feel full of energy, lively and gives you the ability to accomplish challenges.

You are confident in yourself and your power to follow through the difficulties that life throws at you while making sure that the mind stays in a calm, cheerful, and confident state.

Physically, the body is healthy and fit due to the fact that the solar plexus has all the control over the cellular respiration system within the body.

This makes sure that the body is in great condition and health.

The flow of energy throughout the body is balanced and strong, also aiding in the healing process of the body.

Emotionally, this chakra can ease the worries of the mind as well as releasing it and other negative feelings, maintaining the mind clear, healthy and well-balanced along with the body.

A balance in the solar plexus promotes strength, motivation, courage, and happiness in the body, mind, and soul, thus enabling this chakra to balance out the other major chakras.

When the solar plexus is underactive, it will disturb the flow of energy within the body.

You may start to experience a lack of control as well as a loss of purpose in life.

This often leads to a lot of emotional problems, self-destructive behavior, and self-doubt.

Underactive solar plexus makes one feel helpless, indecisive, grants a low-esteem, and a lack of confidence.

When the solar plexus is overactive, it means that the solar plexus has way too much energy in the region compared to other chakras.

You will experience issues in controlling people, yourself, and your environment.

Having control over your own life is good as long as it is not going overboard which an overactive solar plexus does.

When it is overactive, you will feel overwhelmed in energy that can overstimulate the system and tire the body out.

One will also become stubborn, aggressive, judgmental, and overcritical.

This chakra is best to be opened with meditation but adding certain changes in diet can also help greatly.

Eating yellow-based foods such as grains, yellow peppers, bananas, and corn, as well as other complex carbohydrate foods that are able to give you plenty of energy can help in the opening of the solar plexus.

However, you must avoid too many sugary foods seeing as the glucose is not natural.

Make sure to drink plenty of chamomile tea which is known to help clear the blockage of this chakra.

Decorating one's house with yellow flowers or wearing yellow clothing can help stimulate the solar plexus visually.

Meditation For The Solar Plexus Chakra

Begin with a light stretch, too relax the muscles for your meditation.

Stand up, and lift your hands up into the air as if you are reaching up to touch the sky.

Reach as far as you can while you take a deep breath in, holding the position and your breath for two seconds.

As you exhale, drop your hands to your sides, pulling the breath for another two seconds.

Lift your hands up again as you breathe in and drop them to your sides as you exhale.

Repeat at least three times before proceeding with the meditation.

Sit up in a comfortable position on the floor or on a chair in the room of your sacral chakra meditation healing practice.

Cross your legs, as you extend your spine nice and straight.

Lift your head up, as if you are balancing a book right on top.

Place your hands on your knees with the palms facing upwards.

Get rid of any distraction, by closing the windows, turning off your phone, and locking the doors.

Start off your meditation by breathing slowly and deeply while staring off into space.

Take as long as you need to relax your body, muscles, and adjust your mind from wandering around and gently allow for your eyes to slowly close.

Further bring your body to relaxation by focusing on and relaxing different parts of your body such as legs, stomach, chest, arms, shoulders, neck and head, as you move your focus along your body from top to bottom.

Take a couple of seconds to hold the image of yourself sitting up, while you are relaxing your body.

You can also direct your focus to how your chest and body rise taller as you breathe in or falls shorter as you breathe out.

Hold your attention on your breathing to ensure that your mind won't slip away.

By bringing your focus somewhere else except your mind, you are able to clear your thoughts from any worries of troubles.

Now that your body is close to its relaxed state and so is your mind, change the way you breathe to fit the opening of the solar plexus area.

Since the location of the chakra is on the lower part of your ribs, you will be using your chest to breath.

Inhale the air and expand your lungs, hold the breath for at least four seconds before exhaling through your mouth.

Visualize releasing any negativity through your exhale as your spine expands higher every time you breathe.

Focus on the way your chest rises and falls and don't let your mind wander away.

If it does, then gently bring your attention back to your attention to the movement of the spine.

Just like any other healing treatments, call on the Universe and ask to heal your solar plexus chakra.

Visualize channeling your energy and centering it on the palm of your hands.

Allow for the energy to resurface your body, as a white pure life force healing energy.

Let it hover all throughout your body for a minute, energizing it and gathering its strength.

Place your hands on the area above your belly button but below your heart.

You will be touching the lower part of your ribs.

You should place your hands next to each other and not overlapping each other.

Concentrate on making the energy flow through your hands and to the solar plexus.

Visualize it healing the chakra, clearing it of any blockage and releasing the negative emotions or negative tensions that could possibly affect the physical health of the body, imagine anything negative leaving through your mouth as you exhale.

When you are sitting down, start to connect and feel the coldness or warmth of the floor, the bed, or the ground beneath you.

Visualize the energy from the ground traveling up through your body, through your toes.

Imagine sucking in that energy that belongs to the earth.

Focus on this energy as it's moving up towards the location of the solar plexus which is in between your belly button and the bottom of your rib cage, also known as the upper abdomen.

With your hands still on the upper abdomen, imagine yellow glow forming and expanding in that area as all the energy begin connecting, rotating clockwise and getting larger every time you take a breath in.

Feel the warmth and sensation that the yellow light is providing and how it makes you feel emotional.

Keep your hands on that area for at least two to three minutes before moving on and placing your hands on the top of your knees, forming a mudra by touching both the thumb and the index finger together.

If you'd like, you can keep cleansing the area for longer than three minutes, however long you feel is necessary for your upper abdomen to heal.

Begin to imagine that you are sitting on top of a grassy hill, sitting right below the sun that is shinning right back down on you.

Your eyes are closed as your own sacral chakra begins to glow and react with the sun.

The energy tingling within your upper abdomen, experiencing healing and cleansing.

Focus your attention on the part of your body that you imagine is the warmest from the sun, such as the top of your head.

Yellow stimulates the feelings of joy and it also represents the solar plexus.

Feel and appreciate the warmth that you are receiving and accept the tingling sensations that are spreading through your body.

Then start to bring your attention inwards, notice how the ground beneath you feels like, is it cold or warm?

Can you feel any tingling or pulses through it?

What about the space above your head?

Does it feel like a whole universe is right above you just by feeling a little pressure on your head?

Freely lift your arms up towards the sky as you inhale and feel the astral world above you.

Picture a bright yellow flame at the tip of your fingers, feel as it connects through your hands and travels down to your upper abandonment where the solar plexus is located.

Breath out and lower your arms down to the ground.

Place your hands on the ground and feel the earth beneath you and the perfect balance of life and energy around you.

Inhale once more, raising your hands up towards the sky as if connecting your energy with the one with the sun.

Let the yellow glow travel down to you upper abandonment, clearing and opening that chakra point.

Notice what you are feeling during this moment, are you feel calm, balanced and happy?

Repeat the hand motions for a few minutes or however long you wish.

Place your hands back down on your knees, forming the mudra. Use the mantra 'ram' by saying it out loud physically.

This specific mantra vibrates the body and helps the negative energies flow out of the chakra and out of the body while leaving only positive and pure healing forces.

Mantras are just words that are said during meditations but it can also be used in practices to ensure that the body is cleared effectively.

Place one of your hands on your back, with the palm facing outwards while you repeat the same process of visualizing the yellow energy healing moving and releasing any tensions in the upper abdomen.

Take a minute to rest in the healing sensations.

To finish, place your hands back to the ground.

Breath in deeply with an open mind for a minute while bringing your awareness back to the physical world.

Imagine the room that you are in to help get back to your consciousness and the body.

Make an intention to express utmost gratitude to the Universe for guidance, your energy for healing you, and opening your solar plexus chakra.

Take another minute to simply breathe in deeply, in through your nose and out through your mouth.

Open your eyes slowly but do not move your body.

Look around you, take in the details of your room, stay in the moment for a few minutes while reflecting on the healing that you just achieved.

Heart Chakra

The fourth major chakra point is the heart chakra, also known as Anahata chakra that means 'unhurt'.

The context of the meaning connected to the heart chakra, when it is healthy and in balance, the heart and mind are not hurt.

The heart chakra connects to the mind, it is also the source of the deepest emotions such as unconditional love, compassion, passion, and joy.

The feelings of the heart are able to be expressed through the throat chakra and the mind, those deep feelings that are sometimes very hard to express verbally come from the heart.

Since the heart is the middle chakra, it connects the chakras below it and to the chakras above it.

The heart chakra is associated with the color green which represents prosperity, wealth in any aspect of one's life, health, and abundance.

This chakra can help heal both mental and physical issues.

The location of the heart chakra is right in the middle of the chest area.

When imbalanced, the heart experiences many negative emotions and negative energy in the body, mind, and the physical environment due to the fact that low vibrations attract other low vibration.

Negative thoughts and emotions can also cause the proper function of the body to fail.

Physically, the heart chakra is responsible for the problems found in the immune system, the circulatory system, respiratory system, muscle, and diaphragm.

Illnesses such as breast cancer, lung diseases, heart disease, allergies, asthma, high blood pressure, and other health problems revolving the heart chakra region.

Emotionally, this chakra deals with very deep emotions such as grief, anxiety, jealousy, hatred, loneliness, fear, and isolation, especially when the heart chakra is imbalanced.

You will always feel like you are stuck in the past or constantly thinking about the future, unable to focus on the present and what is really important at this time.

Negative feelings can cloud one's judgment, making one feel like they must always protect themselves when in fact there is no danger.

Negative emotions can also strongly impact the physical environment, causing separation, abandonment, and emotional abuse.

When in balance, you feel comfortable and healthy both physically, mentally, and spiritually.

When it is in balance, the body and mind are also at an equal with no worries, which satisfies one spiritually.

You are able to find forgiveness in your heart to those who hurt you in the past, which is also a great way to move on from that situation that left a mark on your heart.

Being stuck in the past doesn't help one focus on the present which is all life is about, enjoying and living in the moment.

The heart chakra grants compassion, peace, comfort, and gratitude for every little thing you have.

Physically, the heart is located within the heart chakra.

The heart is healthy, as well as the surrounding areas such as breasts, lungs, and ribs when the heart chakra is in balance.

It is also responsible for keeping us alive by promoting the beat of the heart and the blood circulation.

Emotionally, the heart chakra is known to be quite vulnerable but when it is in balance, one is able to experience the true meaning of happiness and what it is like to live their life filled with love and acceptance.

The mind is known to be in a very calm, confident, loving, and cheerful state.

However, that can also be the heart chakras undoing, being too cheerful and loving can sometimes backfire if it is given to the wrong people.

The underactive heart chakra revolves around the unhealthy distribution of the flow of energy within the body.

You will begin to experience an inability to forgive, forget, and move on with your life which will cause you to always be stuck in the past.

It can also prevent you from creating new relationships and opening your heart to more people.

This detaches you from the outside love as well as leaving you feeling withdrawn, isolated, critical of yourself and others.

The overactive heart chakra is distributing way too much energy, meaning that one can be giving away too much love and not leaving any for themselves.

This can leave you feeling emotionally drained and can affect your physical health.

An overactive heart chakra can lead you to feel a lack of discernment, especially in relationships as well as leave you feeling like you overexert yourself in terms of your personal life, this can make your relationships become toxic.

You will also find yourself feeling under control of your emotions and create a dependence on the personal relationships that you have with people rather than relying on yourself to be happy.

The overactive heart chakra can also cause a loss in personal boundaries, loss of identity, neglect, and always saying yes, even to things that can bring you pain.

Many times the main problems of having a blocked heart chakra revolve around a question, 'are you giving the same amount of love to yourself that you give to others' or 'are you putting yourself and your needs before anyone else'.

Many of those who have a blocked heart chakra either put other people before themselves or block their own heart from receiving love.

In order to open the heart chakra, one has to practice self-love and putting themselves before anyone else.

Your feelings and your own happiness are what matters most in the end.

Take some time to relax and gather your thoughts, follow the path which makes you the happiest self rather than pleasing and doing what other people want you to do.

Eating plenty of nutritious foods, especially those that are of green color, can help encourage the healing of the heart chakra.

Performing small acts of kindness such as smiling at a stranger or complimenting them can not only give out love but receive in the process.

No matter how much loved one gives out, it will always find its way back to them in different shapes or sizes.

Opening your heart chakra will make you feel hopeful for the future, your relationships will strengthen with the people that you love, and you will be able to attract more people into your life so place the stone above your heart or wear it as a necklace.

Meditation For the Heart Chakra

The key to healing the heart and chest area is through music.

Begin by picking a soft melody with gentle beats and sounds, no lyrics so you won't be able to sing along in your head.

It is scientifically proven that the right music can make you feel happier so make sure you find something that you feel a certain connection to.

Turn it on by a few bars that are soft enough to hear but not that loud, for example, 1/4 of the music bars.

Make sure that the melody is longer than ten minutes or on repeat.

Begin by laying down and relaxing comfortably.

Place a pillow under your head, and another under your knees for utmost comfort.

Leave your hands laying next to your body with the palms facing up.

Take a minute to focus and clear your mind by breathing in deeply.

Breathe in from your nose, hold the breath for two seconds and exhale through your mouth.

Continue this easy and simple breathing technique for a minute.

Inhale through the nose, and exhale through the mouth while setting a mental intention to relax your body as much as you can.

Proceed by gently closing your eyes and giving all of your attention to your chest area.

Use your lungs when you are breathing, instead of your stomach.

This means that when you breathe in, allow for your lungs to expand, moving around, filling up with oxygen.

Make sure that all of your attention is centered on your chest and the way it rises and falls or the way your body stretches upwards as you breathe in or shrinks as you breathe out.

Imagine that with every breath you take, you clear out the negativity within the chest, releasing it through the mouth, and allowing for yourself to let go of any tensions or impurities.

As you allow for your body to relax further and as you become more familiar with the deep breathing rhythm of your body, begin to listen carefully to the different tunes that you hear and try to focus on a specific one that stands out to you.

For example, if it's the sound of the bells you hear, then bring your focus there.

Try to push away any thoughts that might be emerging to the back of your head and relax while listening to that soft and quiet sound.

Take a moment to appreciate the music that you are hearing.

Observe how that melody makes you feel emotionally, are you feeling happiness and love in your heart, if so then continue by visualizing your heart fluttering as if it is opening up to love.

Think of flower petals emerging through your heart, floating around you ready to travel to your loved ones.

Keep in touch with your own emotion of love and connect it to the flower petals.

Think of a person close to you, a friend, a lover, or a family member, think of sending them those pink or green glowing petals filled with your love and empathy.

Wish them happiness and abundance through their life.

Picture those petals flowing to wherever they are now and connecting with their hearts.

Do this with two or three other people that you hold close to your heart.

Feel the warmth and tingling as more petals leave your heart and travel to your loved ones.

Let the energy gathered within your heart be released through your body, spread love throughout it and feel it within you.

Let the energy run freely up and down your spine through all the chakras, uniting them and growing your spiritual growth.

Proceed by making an intention to resurface the energy and asking the universe for guidance in this practice.

Focus on the white auric field surrounding your body, making you feel safe and comfortable.

You will begin to feel tingling sensations and warmth in different parts of your body.

Let the healing energy take its time resurfacing within your body and allow for it to center exactly where the heart is.

As you preformed the petal release exercise, the heart became more pure and positive, allowing for the energy to access it easier.

Place an intention to receive protection from anything negative in your life, negative events, negative emotions, and negative people.

This will help you feel safer and at ease from negativity.

Place another intention of receiving self-healing energy targeting the specific part of your body, the chest.

Allow for that energy to move from the heart to the shoulders and down to the palms of your hands, all connecting with one another.

Channel your energy and concentrate on centering it on your hands.

Allow the flow of white energy to resurface in your palms and glow a white and pure color.

Take a minute to just let all of the energy to catch up and gather in that area, healing the hands along the way.

Lift both of your hands and place them on your heart, one over the other.

Allow the energy to sink into your heart chakra and visualize the white-colored light changing into a bright green which is associated with the heart chakra.

Focus on feeling the beat of your heart against your hands, feel the pulsing vibrations underneath.

Rest in the moment as that green light sink in deeper into your chest.

Allow the energy to circulate and explore the chest area, going exactly where tensions are present.

Feel the tingling sensations throughout your body, smell the air around you as you take in deep breaths, hear the soft melody echoing in the room or against your ears, taste the freedom and the love life gives you and finally, although your eyes are closed, notice the glowing green light emerging through your heart.

Visualize the color glowing brighter and brighter as it opens your heart chakra to all the love and happiness that you deserve.

Think of the people who you care deeply for, imagine sending them your love and blessing to ensure that they are safe and happy with their life.

Think of different times when love was expressed and given to you, even the small things that made you happy still count!

Open yourself to healing within your heart.

Use the mantra 'yam' to help you open this chakra further.

Spend some time to opening your chakra, don't rush through the process but let your body heal its heart, either physically or emotionally.

Finish up by deeply breathing in and out through your mouth for a few minutes, just focusing on the music and the emotional feelings you receive from it.

The point of this meditation is to make you feel love to live, love for others around you, especially for yourself, and healing your chest area with positive and pure energy.

When you think you have finished, take some time for the energy to settle in within your body for a minute or two.

Allow for your eyes to slowly open, adjusting them to the light and the physical world around you.

Make sure to reflect on the meditation that you have just performed and the healing that you have received.

Proceed by doing something that makes you happy or something that you love.

Take some time to relax after the healing process, don't push yourself to do anything.

Stay at home, relax, take a hot bath, and let your body heal itself while the energy within your body is still present.

Throat Chakra

The fifth major chakra is the throat chakra that is also called Vishuddha.

Vishuddha means purification or very pure, and it signifies one having a pure mindset.

This connects to the throat chakra because, in order to have a pure mind, one must first be able to release the emotions and thoughts that happen within their mind through their throat chakra.

If the person is unable to find a way to release all the emotions, they can become bottled up in the mind, polluting it in the process.

The throat chakra is your ability to express yourself, the feelings inside the heart, and the thoughts inside the mind.

It is located within your thought region, representing the color blue which is associated with healing, peace, calmness, and content.

When the throat chakra is balanced, you are able to speak freely without no one or nothing stopping or preventing you.

You are able to express yourself and who you truly are, saying whatever is on your mind.

Those who are able to express themselves are also able to inspire others around them by speaking up and sharing their own opinion.

You know that people listen to you and are able to understand you.

Not holding or suppressing emotions and thoughts back will be able to clear your mind, returning it to its 'pure' state.

Physically, the area of the throat is healthy and in balance with the rest of the body.

Both the mental and psychological aspect of one's life is also in balance.

The throat chakra is accountable for the maturity and development of your body, especially the mouth, jaws teeth, vocal cords, throat, nose, and voice.

Emotionally, this chakra is associated with self-expression, letting go of the feelings that you were holding up from past situations that left a mark on your heart and mind.

Letting go and expressing yourself can be done through crafting, music, writing, and in many other ways.

It is important to let go and share your feelings instead of bottling them up inside of you.

When the throat chakra is blocked, you will have trouble expressing what it is that you think and feel, this will turn you into an isolated and shy person.

Physically, the throat chakra causes problems within the endocrine system, the metabolic system, sore throats, the hormones in the body, and the thyroid gland.

This chakra also causes many diseases such as hypothyroidism, laryngitis, chronic throat defects, autoimmune thyroiditis, and many others relating to the body's growth and throat area.

When this chakra is out of balance emotionally, you will suffer from feelings of low self-esteem, restriction, low self-love, isolation, and no self-expression, as well as feeling like no one is here to listen to what you have to say.

This can cause depression and anxiety.

An underactive throat chakra revolves around insecurity, introversion, and timidity, meaning that when the throat is blocked, one will struggle with speaking up and sharing their opinion which will detach them from their true selves.

Other factors such as fear of speaking, introversion, and small voice are the causes of an underactive throat chakra.

If the throat chakra is overactive, one will find themselves experiencing a lack of control over their own speech, meaning they will talk too much and say whatever is on their mind without considering the consequences of their speech.

Those with an overactive throat chakra will experience talking too much, criticizing yourself and others, struggles in relationships and feeling like no one understands what they are saying.

Other factors such as gossiping, arrogance, rudeness, condescending, and overly criticality is caused by the overactive throat chakra.

Since the color blue is associated with the throat chakra, drinking plenty of water can help open and balance the throat chakra.

Especially drinking warm water or warm herbal tea which can help release tensions within the throat and clear out negative energies.

Singing your favorite songs or humming to a tune is also considered as a way of speaking, speaking can help awaken and balance the chakra as well as releasing any negative energies or tensions within that area.

It is also scientifically proven that singing can raise up one's mood, meaning it can help heighten your vibrations.

Specific yoga poses that involve you stretching the muscles can also help balance out not only the throat chakra but other chakras too.

Consider leaving some spare time out to practice different yoga poses that relate to different chakras, it will help ensure that your chakras will become balanced and healthy.

An open throat chakra will make you speak clearly and will help you express yourself more freely.

Meditation For The Throat Chakra

Comfort is key, it is important to get comfortable when meditating so both your mind and body can relax and not disturb you through this process.

Start your meditation by getting comfortable, sit down with your legs crossed, your spine straight and reaching out as high as possible.

Make sure your head is not sulking, but nice straight and tall.

Your head should face the front as the chin is raised, imagine as if you are balancing a book on your head.

Form a mudra with your hands, an 'okay' or 'zero' look-a-like sign by uniting the thumb and the index finger together before placing it on top of your knees, the palm of your hand facing upwards.

Begin by taking a few minutes to relax your body and muscles, focus your attention on your breathing as your chest rises and falls.

Breathe in deeply, inhale through your nose and hold the breath for up to three seconds before exhaling it through the mouth and dragging it out for another three seconds.

Make sure that when you are breathing in and out that you expand your chest, instead of breathing through your stomach.

When you are using the chest, the spine extends and moves along with the breathing, this will enable the relaxation found within the body, as well as the throat region.

Feel the way your lungs expand inside of you as they are filled with the air around you, cleansing you, and getting both your mind and body ready for the pure energy of your life force energy.

The throat region is often linked with your voice, in other words, the awakening of the throat chakra can be used to heal both.

The purpose of this meditation is to take your worries away from your inability to speak up so try not to let the feelings of worry and anxiety take over, this is your time to let go of all the bad thoughts and let you be the person you are meant to be as well as healing the throat and shoulder region.

Take a few minutes to simply relax your muscles and the body as you breathe in.

Bring your attention to your breathing as you inhale and exhale to help calm the mind.

Try your best to not listen to your thoughts and the mental clutter that is going on inside your head.

Instead, bring your focus to yourself as a being in this big universe.

Imagine yourself to be one with the universe as the energy flows through your body.

Don't think about anything else that you have to do or things that might be bothering, instead focus on breathing through your chest, making the lungs expand as you breathe in.

Relax the different parts of your body including your throat and neck.

As you breathe in, feel how the air comes through your nostrils, to your throat, and into your lungs before coming back up.

It is clearing all the negative energy out when you inhale and lets it all go as you exhale.

Breath in deeply, form a rhythm of your body.

Begin the usual energy harnessing by calling out to the Universe, and making an intention to harness your life force energy.

Imagine a white light emitting from within your body, spreading all throughout.

Allow for your mind's goals to be clear by setting an intention to receive healing within the throat area and helping yourself speak up more and become more involved with the community through the healing found within the chakra.

Focus on centering your energy within your hands. Imagine the white light surrounding you, traveling all the way to your hands.

Let the energy catch up and gather there, forming a bright ball of light.

Lift your hands up and place them on your collar bone, one hand over the other.

Visualize the healing energy leaving your hands and sinking deep through your body and making its way to the center of the throat chakra.

While allowing the pure white energy to settle down, begin to visualize the color blue, think of the first emotion or thing that pops into your head.

Feel your body calming down and becoming more stable.

Then picture that color blue evolving through your throat, a gently blue glow expanding every time you inhale, merging together with the energy of the white.

The throat chakra represents the gateway between the heart and mind, you are able to freely speak what is on your mind and in your heart.

But just by thinking about it can bring forth feelings of worry, so imagine all that worry resurfacing and letting it go as you breath out.

This is your voice and your own opinions, you have the right to express what is really in your heart.

This is also a perfect time to release any stress or worries that you might have by simply bringing them back up to the surface and making an intention for the bright blue light to simply purify them.

Let go of anything that might be bothering you.

Feel the tingling and warmth sensations through your neck as they emerge and push you to want to open your mouth and speak whatever is on your mind.

Bring an intention forward to receive a physical healing, through the healing of the mind.

Visualize that glow becoming bigger and brighter for three to five minutes before drawing your attention back to your breathing.

While still holding your hands on that area, use the mantra 'ham' which can create vibrations that have the power to alter the flow of energy within the communication center.

Once you spend at least two to three minutes healing that part of your body, move your hands upward and extend the healing energy to your throat.

Hold your hands there for another brief two to three minutes before rotating and moving them to the back of your neck.

Allow for the white energy to sunk in right around the throat while releasing blue energy of the throat chakra, bringing in healing and relaxation to that area.

Visualize the tensions going away, the muscles relaxing.

Hold your hands against your throat for a minute before moving down towards your shoulders.

Allow for the blue light to intervene with the white, creating a light blue hue.

Let that healing energy work its magic, traveling and releasing any negative tensions within the shoulder area.

Rest that energy against the shoulders for a brief minute.

Allow for the energy to evenly spread throughout your body, returning back to its original state, this time more powerful.

Imagine the body relaxing and energizing itself as your life force energy returns back throughout your body, purifying along the way.

Continue to deeply breathe in and out for about a minute, simply resting in the newfound sensation.

Slowly bring your attention to your body, the way you breathe, or the weight that your body holds against the earth below you.

Open your eyes. Remain seated in complete silence for another minute, allow for the healing energy to further settle in while you take some time to reflect on your meditation.

To finish off the treatment, tell someone what is on your mind or sing your favorite songs before carrying on with your day.

Speaking, reading or singing can help heal the throat region much faster after the chakra healing that you have experienced.

Third Eye Chakra

The sixth major chakra is the third eye chakra, it is also known as Anja which means 'beyond wisdom'.

Just like its translation, the third eye relates to the concept of following your gut feeling, intuition, and the discovery of psychic ability, all of which are able to abandon critical and logical thinking.

The third eye is also known as the sixth sense, it is able to see things that are far beyond what the human five senses notice.

With the third eye, one is able to see into different worlds and see into what people are feeling, something that the physical eyes can't do.

Spiritual gifts emerge through the opening of the third eye since the third eye is known to connect one to the spiritual world and set one on their spiritual journey.

The third eye is located in between one's eyebrows, usually in the middle of the forehead, it is known to be the origin of foresight and intuition.

The third eye is also linked to the color purple which is associated with inner wisdom, power, intuition, and extrasensory perception.

When the third eye chakra is in balance, one has the power to not only see into their own soul and look for what they desire but also look into other people's desires and motives.

It is very hard to trick one with an open and balanced third eye chakra, they are able to see through a person and recognize their true motives due to the heightened intuition ability.

You also achieve a sense of confidence within your life as well as the knowledge of what you are here for the sole purpose of living.

You will also gain a strong sense of inner truth and resolving physical problems that will happen in your environment will become a piece of cake due to your intuition which will guide you through your life.

Since the opening of the third eye grants the person different psychic abilities, it also enables easier communication between higher beings, angels, and spirits as well as seeing into the future and seeing your past lives.

Physically, the body is in great shape and is healthy, everything, as well as the flow of energy, is in balance.

Since the third eye is one of the strongest chakras found within the body, it also can strongly affect the chakras below it, opening and cleansing them, bringing equality within the body.

The area that the third eye is located will function better, eyesight can improve, the brain will receive more knowledge, and many other related functions will increase.

Emotionally, the one who has an open third eye chakra is able to live their life freely and control their emotions to not affect the environment.

Clear thinking, decision making, awareness, seeing past lies, spiritual gifts, and a stable mindset is all thanks to an open third eye.

However, when the third eye chakra is blocked, one will start to doubt their own existence.

The questions of what the purpose of life is will constantly cloud one's judgment, refraining them from living their life to the fullest.

You will become disconnected with yourself, your environment, and other people.

Physically, the third eye is responsible for the endocrine system which affects the person's growth, metabolism, and maturity, it is also responsible for the hormonal imbalance as well as the sleep cycle, fatigue within the body, migraines, and headaches.

Emotionally, the blocked third eye causes anxiety, an emotional imbalance, a lack of understanding of reality, depression, and a feeling of always being lost or lacking something.

An underactive third eye chakra can negatively affect one's thinking, how they process information, concentration, motivation, and inspiration.

You will also become fearful of the things that you do not understand or the unknown.

You may experience a lack of intuition, believing everything people tell you, live in constant fear, and low self-esteem.

An overactive third eye chakra is able to overindulgence your mind and your imagination.

One will constantly be in a daydreaming state, with no focus on what is happening right now in the present moment within their environment.

When the third eye is giving off too much energy, you will start to feel mentally exhausted, and overwhelmed.

You may experience anxiety, become judgemental, overly analytical, experience indecisiveness, clouded vision, and judgment.

Yoga can help open the third eye chakra, specific yoga poses such as the eagle pose and the child pose is programmed to help open and balance this chakra.

Exercising and eating healthy can help all the chakras be balanced due to the release of negative energies, however, specific foods that aid the third eye are foods with high omega-3 fats such as sardines, walnuts, chia seeds, and salmon can help enhance the third eye.

When opening your third eye chakra, you will enhance your intuition and creative inspiration.

Meditation For the Third Eye Chakra

Begin by selecting a place where you will feel comfortable and undisturbed, so lock your doors and turn off your phone.

Put on some loose clothing so you will feel more comfortable and lower the lights if they appear to be too bright for you.

It is recommended that you lay down during this process, but you can sit up if you want to, however, you might find it hard to hold yourself upward in a chair.

When laying down, remember to not place a pillow under your head, only under your knees.

You can use a blanket to keep you warm but make sure to leave your hands by your sides on top of the blanket.

Proceed by slowly closing your eyes, breathing in deeply.

Focus on your breathing, in with the nose and out through the mouth.

Allow yourself to become in tune with the moment that is happening right now.

Feel your arms and legs become more relaxed.

Breathe in once again and this time hold the breath for an instant before you let go through your mouth, feel yourself relax even further.

Each time you breathe in or out, notice how every second your body becomes more and more relaxed.

Bring your attention to whatever is beneath you, if it's the bed or the ground, feel yourself connect to that energy.

Imagine your own energy connecting to the ground, like roots of a tree extending right into it, convincing and intertwining with the energy of the earth.

Embrace it and let it travel through your spine, let go of any anxiety, fear or resistance that you might have.

Allow for the earth's energy to travel upwards, all the way to the top of your head.

Imagine branches and leaves sprouting from the top of your head. You are a tree now, in your visualization.

You are one with the earth and the universe.

Allow for the energy to sprout and grow, for the roots to extend all the way below you and the branches and leaves to grow above you, reaching towards the ceiling.

Allow for your energy to resurface by visualizing a white light emerging from within your body.

Let that light grow, growing brighter with every breath you take.

Center your energy to your palms.

Close your eyes and concentrate on visualizing a white light emerging and entering your palms.

Let the energy rest there for a brief minute, gathering and forming a bright bulb of light. the third eye, immediately lifting your spirits up.

Focus on transmitting the energy and getting rid of any tensions and blockages.

Visualize the third eye-opening, enhancing your intuition and other psychic abilities.

Lift your hands up and place them on your head, each hand on the side of your temples.

Continue breathing deeply and slowly as you focus on releasing that energy into your mind with the intention to achieve healing.

Draw your attention to the middle of your eyebrows, where the third chakra is located.

Feel the energy that has emerged from your temples, making its way into the center of your forehead, feel the tingling as it is opening and radiating indigo light in all directions.

Visualize both lights combining together.

It small and faint at first but it is growing with each deep breath you take.

Let go of any uncertainties as you let the light evolve within your head, healing any tensed areas that you might have.

This experience is natural and completely safe.

Let the indigo light purify your frequency and heighten it, drawing positive feelings and experiences towards you.

Just relax, stay calm, breathe deeply and allow the experience to happen.

Let the indigo light open in your forehead, sending the gently streams of its like in all directions, relaxing you in the process.

You will start to feel the tingling sensations on that point if not already.

Enable to relax your body further and further.

Feel your weight on the floor or the mattress if you are laying down become lighter and lighter as more light flows around and through your body.

Allow your mind to open by itself naturally and on its own, don't force healing to happen otherwise too much energy can backfire and not work.

Let go of any thoughts or worries that can cloud your mind and stop you from continuing with the process.

Don't think too much of what can happen but relax your body further and focus on that warm, tingling sensation between your brows.

Using your index finger place the finger down on the third eye chakra and start to massage it in a clockwise circulation for women and an anticlockwise circulation for males.

Don't stop the light from flowing through your body as you massage your third eye, releasing its energy and letting it join together with the energy of the chakra.

Allow for yourself to feel the energy flow through you as your chakra point is opening.

Breath in deeply and out through your mouth to clear and cleanse any negative feelings or energy within your body, this is only a pure experience.

You might begin to see visions in your mind or hear something calling.

Since this healing practice is located so close to the third eye chakra, it will naturally begin to heal it and opening it.

The third eye is known to see things that can't be seen with your physical eyes, don't stress over the newfound feelings that might erupt in your body.

Simply continue this very pure experience.

It might begin to feel as if your mind just naturally wandered away, or you are having a daydream, but you are not making it all up, that is the energy of the guides that are helping you realize what else needs to be done.

Begin to say the mantra 'Ksham' out loud for another two to three minutes to encourage the healing energy.

Slowly bring your attention to your breathing and make an intention for the energy to fall back evenly throughout your body, purifying and cleansing it in the process.

Make an intention to return your energy and spread it out evenly across your body.

Take some time to simply stay in the feeling of being aware and conscious of your surroundings but at the same time remind yourself of your pure intentions of healing and cleansing your body with the help of the third eye chakra.

When you feel as if you have meditated long enough and that you are done, slowly bring your consciousness back to what is happening right now.

Feel how heavy your body is becoming as you are focusing back on what is happening right now, in this present time.

Become aware of your legs, arms, hands, and body.

Open your mouth and say, 'I am fully present, here and now'.

Your voice might come off as if you haven't spoken in a long time.

Take another and final deep breath, holding it in for a minute before slowly opening your eyes.

Take a minute to simply rest while reflecting on your meditation.

Crown Chakra

The last seventh chakra is known as the crown chakra; it is the hardest one to open and balance.

The crown chakra is also known as Sahasrara which translates to 'thousand-petaled'.

The crown chakra is the conscious chakra, compared to all the other chakras below it.

It revolves around your own personal consciousness and the subconscious part of the person.

This chakra is also responsible for attracting the same level of vibrational beings or things into one's life.

Located at the top of your head, the crown chakra acts like a magnet, pulling things the same vibrational frequency as your body towards you, it also extends upwards towards the universe and connects you to the higher energies.

The color this chakra is associated with indigo which represents devotion, inner wisdom, intuition, self-responsibility, spirituality, and trust.

When the crown chakra is in balance, you will feel a deep connection to the universe, the higher power, and with yourself.

You will also begin to feel as if something or someone is watching over you, making sure that you are going towards the right direction and clearing up your path towards success by making sure you avoid the difficulties and bad things in life, that is if you vibrate on a high level.

This energy is looking after you understand exactly what you desire and is able to help you achieve your goals along the way.

You will begin to feel a deep and strong sense of gratitude towards not only the universe but to yourself as well.

Feelings such as appreciation and love to yourself, your environment, and others around you will feel at peace surrounded by happiness and the feelings of safety.

When good things happen, they are able to affect our emotional states which affect the vibration level and works to attract more good things into our lives.

It is not only important to understand that even if bad things happen, but there is also always a good side to them, a hidden lesson that the universe is teaching you and it is up to you to be able to understand it and connect it to your life.

When this chakra is balanced, you will feel like everything within your life is going by perfectly and smoothly that is because you understand that you control your own life and can shape your own future with the power of thoughts and high vibrations.

There are absolutely no fears, worries, or problems resigning within your mind and even if there is one, you are able to deal with it on a positive level that doesn't even affect your wellbeing, either mentally, physically, emotionally, or spiritually.

Physically, the crown chakra is responsible for not only the mind area of the body but the other chakras too.

The mind is able to not only cause illnesses but heal them too.

When the mind is in balance with the body, the chakras can feel the peace and begin to open up their pure energies.

Emotionally, the crown chakra is aligned with the body, mind, and spirit and promotes a healthy mindset.

When the crown chakra is blocked, then it is able to influence and block other chakras due to this incredible amount of energy found within the crown.

You will begin to feel disconnected from the higher power as well as your spiritual journey.

You will feel as if there are no 'angels' watching over you and that your life is going downhill.

Physically, the body will begin to always feel exhausted, out of energy, minor headaches, trouble in many of the body's systems, organs, and glands.

Many parts of the body like the nervous system, brain, pituitary gland, and many others will be affected by the imbalance. Illnesses like

Illnesses such as brain tumors, amnesia, migraines, and cognitive delusions are caused by the imbalance within the crown chakra.

Emotionally, you will be filled with feelings of isolation, loneliness, insignificance, and a lack of connection.

The feelings of anxiety, stress, depression, hysteria, and other mental illnesses are all the causes of the crown chakra due to its location.

Not only that but negative thoughts and feelings are able to damage the body physically too when there is too much energy, especially negative energy, directed in a specific location, it can not only overflow but temporary stop that part of the body from working.

You will also constantly be afraid of change which can put you in an environment that will cause your unhappiness.

The underactive crown chakra is when the crown is blocked, thus blocking other chakras and the proper function of the body.

When it is underactive, it can limit one's ability to let go of either of the past or any materialistic needs.

It will detach you from the world around you and lead to s spiritual malaise.

Not only that but the relationships that you've built with other people will be strongly influenced the negative way.

Other signs of an underactive crown chakra are mental fog, feeling of greed, lack of motivation, and lack of inspiration.

An overactive crown chakra gathers way too much energy in one place, it can cause a disconnection of the physical body, as well as an overwhelmed feeling due to the energy.

This will affect the physical body, giving headaches and migraines.

Other signs such as superiority, lack of empathy, and a sense of elitism are all caused by the overactive crown chakra.

If you drink many herbal teas, they are guaranteed to help reduce the blockage within the crown chakra by clearing and cleansing the body from negative energy and toxins.

While consuming specific indigo-colored foods such as eggplants or grapes, they are known to help the crown chakra balance itself out.

Once your crown chakra is open, you will feel a spiritual awakening.

This chakra is a pathway to all the other chakras which is why it can be the hardest to open for some people.

Meditation For The Crown Chakra

Begin by getting comfortable by sitting with your legs crossed, spine straight and shoulders back.

Place your hands on top of your knees forming the mudra, an 'okay' or 'zero' look-a-like hand gesture by allowing the index and the thumb finger on each hand touch, or just simply place your palms on your knees, making them face upwards.

You can even meditate outside in nature which can help you feel more connected with the world around you.

Start off by simply breathing deeply, form a rhythm with your breath as you inhale and exhale.

Inhale through your nose, hold the breath anywhere from two to three seconds before letting go through your mouth.

Make sure when exhaling you drag the breath out for another two to three seconds.

Relax your body, each part at a time, like your legs, arms, belly, shoulders, etc.

If you find your mind drifting away, focus on your chest rising with each breath you take and the way it fills and expands your lungs with oxygen, this way your mind will become more relaxed and will prevent unnecessary thoughts from emerging when you get further into the meditation.

Once you feel as if your mind is settled in, then focus on feeling the energy through the ground with each breath you inhale, you can sense it more and more.

Continue by bringing up that energy, make it travel up your spine, through all of the previous regions with your body, purifying and relaxing on the way.

Let it travel up your spine and fill your other chakras in with energy and finally let it travel to the last region, the crown of your head, located slightly above your head.

It signifies your subconscious and conscious mind which can affect the body spiritually, physically, and mentally.

Let that energy gather around like a faint ball of light, floating just above your head.

With the color white to signify purity and spiritual awakening, let that light connect you to the universe.

Picture the bright glow becomes bigger and brighter with each deep breath that you inhale.

Spend some time focusing on this magnificent ball of energy and light, observe how it makes you feel emotionally and physically.

Can you feel overwhelming energy radiating from that ball of light?

Or can you feel tingling sensations or warmth coming from above that area?

At this point in the meditation, you might start to forget about your physical body as you are connecting with that energy on a spiritual level.

Surround yourself with that light, imagine it flowing through your head into your third chakra, then to your throat chakra and so on until it reaches your root chakra.

Let it rest at each point for a few seconds before moving on to the next chakra point.

Make the energy come back up to the crown at the top of your head.

Let it rest there for a few minutes, glowing and warming up your head before it comes back down to the root chakra and then back up to the crown once more.

The energy should travel up and down three times.

Let the energy flow back through your body to the ground through the bottom of your spine or where your body touches the ground.

Observe any emotions that you might be feeling when the energy was moving up and down or when it left and merged with the ground.

Breathe in deeply for a minute, resting in the sensation of having all your chakras united and opened.

Set an intention to resurface the energy that is already there within your body, ready to be called to healing.

Allow the bright light of your energy to resurface, surrounding your body like an auric field.

Let the light warm your body, purifying your soul and removing any negative impurities that are the cause of all of your troubles and pains.

Center all of that energy into the palms of your hands.

Allow the energy to form a ball of bright and pure light.

Lift your hands upright in front of your chest and form them into a Gassho position, the national praying and gratitude gesture.

Draw your life force energy further into your hands and ask the Universe for guidance to be able to heal your mind, getting rid of any bad habits that need to be healed.

Channel the energy in your hands.

Lift your hands up as high as you can while still maintaining the Gassho position.

Hold the position for a couple of seconds before lowering your hands and placing them one over the other on top of your head, where the crown is.

Feel the tingling sensations and make an intention to open this chakra.

Hold the position for about three minutes before beginning to massage your head with your hands in a circular clockwise motion.

Visualize giving more healing energy to the crown and your subconscious while concentrating on opening the crown and healing the mind, body, and soul.

Get rid of any negative emotions that do not belong within your mind by simply making at the intention for them to vanish.

Breathe in through your nose and out through your mouth.

Move your attention to your breathing and imagine that with every breath that you take, the air inside your lungs travels to all different parts of your body that the mind controls, purifying it and granting it the energy it needs to do its day to day activities.

Proceed to heal for another three minutes.

As the energy heals the body, keep on breathing deeply as you begin to lightly say the mantra 'ohm' to help further intensify the healing energy.

Proceed to carry your attention back to the top of your head before slightly moving your hands lower to your temples, engaging with the third eye region for a minute while stimulating the flow of energy.

Return the energy to all of the body, cleansing and purifying it with its powerful energy.

With your eyes still closed, take a deep breath, hold it for five seconds before letting it go with your mouth.

Give your chest the attention that it needs to ensure that the mind is aware of what is going on around it.

Take a minute to let the energy settle down as you meditate normally, keeping your mind from slipping away.

Slowly begin to bring your awareness back into your body by noticing the weight that you have against the physical world before you open your eyes and stay put for another minute.

When the crown chakra is being opened, you might feel like your head is going to explode.

You might get some headaches because the energies are being drawn to you and everything else that is not important is being let go.

When the energy is released, you will feel tingling sensations throughout your body, as well as heat, electricity, and sparks.

Raise your vibrations by doing something that you enjoy and love deeply after the meditation.

Consider taking some time off to relax while letting the energy that you just experienced settle in and continue healing you and the body.

Chapter 5. Awaken Your Seven Chakras Through Guided Meditation

Meditation for the Root Chakra

Meditation is going to be the most important tool for healing the chakras. There are some variations on mediation that can be used, but in this book for beginners, we are going to focus on the most standard method of meditation. This involves the visualization of a spinning wheel of energy that has the appropriate color for the given chakra that we are working with.

Before you begin meditation, the first thing to consider is where you are going to meditate, when, and how long. You can meditate once or twice per day. At a minimum, you should meditate for 15 minutes per session. If you have the time, meditating for 30 minutes is acceptable, as well.

Don't worry if you have trouble meditating in the beginning. If you are new to meditation, it may take time to train your mind to focus. Being able to focus and rid the mind of thought is one of the important aspects of meditation. People have active minds, you are probably always wondering about something, having conversations with yourself, or maybe your mind is filled with worry. Certainly, if you have a blocked root chakra, you are going to have an overactive mind filled with worry, thinking about how you are going to pay your bills or wishing you could move or other issues. When meditating, your aim is to completely calm the mind, so you shouldn't have any inner voices or ideas flowing through your head.

The space where you meditate should be comfortable and quiet, and if you live with others or have children in the house, you need to ensure that you are going to be able to meditate without being disturbed. You can include soft Indian, Chinese, or Japanese music in the room if desired, or you can meditate in silence.

The position used for meditation is called the easy pose, which is called Sukhasana in Sanskrit. This is basically sitting on the floor with your legs crossed in front of you. If you feel uncomfortable, you can sit on a pillow. When you are beginning, you can also sit against a wall or other object to give yourself some back support.

To begin the meditation process, close your eyes, and breathe slowly and deeply. Spend a few minutes concentrating on your breath, clearing your mind of any thoughts. To help yourself clear your mind, focus on the breath. Breathe naturally, or if it makes you feel more relaxed, you can breathe in through your nose and then exhale through the mouth.

Now, begin to visualize a completely black space. It should be the darkest black you can imagine, an inky dark blackness. Now see a distant red light. Slowly imagine this red light, which can be either a slowly spinning disk or a spinning lotus flower with four petals.

See it slowly getting larger and larger as it comes closer to you. Now, imagine it entering your body, slowly rising up to the location at the base of your spine where the root chakra is. As it gets closer, see it get larger and larger. When you visualize it entering your root chakra, see it spinning faster. Now, when you inhale, see the disk of light or flower grow in size, and then see it shrink when you exhale. Keep up this exercise until you have reached your time limit for meditating.

You can also say the LAM mantra while meditating to help set the right energy level.

Affirmations for the Root Chakra

Affirmations are statements that we can say to ourselves in order to help train our subconscious mind. A lot of the blockage in a chakra can be due to beliefs that are held in the subconscious. They were programmed in there by caregivers and experiences that may have been with us long ago. As a result, you may not even be fully aware of the belief systems that are governing your life. Saying affirmations every day can help to reverse these thought patterns.

Here are some examples that can be used to help heal the root chakra:

I am safe.

I am protected.

I am able to take care of my needs.

Mother Earth will care for me and protect me.

I am safe at home.

I feel safe and secure.

You can say these affirmations and hold a crystal in your hand to help enhance the energy. Say the affirmations as often as needed, but at least once a day. Saying them prior to going to bed is a good way to ensure that they enter into the subconscious mind.

Meditation for the Sacral Chakra

Meditation is going to be an important component for healing the sacral chakra. When you need to heal the sacral chakra, fill the meditation space with bright orange colors. If you can meditate during the day, especially in the morning hours, have open windows that allow a lot of sunlight into the room. Meditation for the sacral chakra will follow the basic pathway. Begin by sitting in easy pose position and close your eyes, breathing deeply and regularly. When meditating for the sacral chakra, tuck your chin down a little bit to help open up the spine to increase energy flow. Some people even advise meditating nude or with little clothing when working on healing the sacral chakra so that you can feel the sensuality throughout the body. If you feel comfortable doing this and have the privacy to do so, it can really heighten the experience.

Begin by imagining a glowing white disk in front of you. Hold your breath for three to five seconds as you breathe. Start to see the disk rotating, slowly at first. As it rotates, see the disk gradually assume an orange color. Visualize the orange color gradually filling up the disk as it spins faster with time, generating more energy. Now, feel the ball of light enter your body, rising slowly and assuming a deeper and brighter orange color as it moves up to your root chakra. Keep visualizing it, and imagine the glowing disk fully assume a deep, bright, and energetic orange color. Now, visualize it moving to your sacral chakra region, below the navel.

Concentrate on your sacral chakra region and genital area. Be consciously aware of all the sensations, and in particular, feel sensations of heat as they arise. You can also visualize warming, glowing orange energy covering the area of the breasts. Do not be shy; healthy sexuality enjoys it to the fullest while maintaining natural control. The mediations will help you to arrive at this place in your life.

Now, imagine the orange disk rising into your brain. This will help elevate your creativity and have healthy fantasies that are not destructive and don't become obsessions. You can end the meditation at this point.

Affirmations for the Sacral Chakra

Using affirmations can help with the sacral chakra to help you achieve a healthy balance and to undo negative programming related to sexuality and sensuality.

I strongly feel my emotions, but I am not overwhelmed by them.

My emotions are strong and balanced.

I feel relaxed and at peace.

I am gifted with creativity.

I experience creativity and am happy to share it with others.

I allow my feelings to move through every pore in my body.

I am comfortable with my body.

I feel sensuality in my body.

Sex is safe and allows me to form sacred connections.

I am safe while enjoying sex.

I radiate sexuality and sensuality.

I allow myself to feel comfortable.

I can enjoy pleasure without guilt.

I am able to feel and enjoy all the pleasures life has to offer.

My ability to enjoy good meals is heightened and intense.

I attract like-minded people who are healthy in their sexuality.

I can express my sexuality in healthy ways.

I enjoy the passions life has to offer, without being overwhelmed by them.

Meditation for the Solar Plexus Chakra

To meditate for the solar plexus chakra, assume the easy pose position and close your eyes, breathing deeply. Meditating in the morning hours or at sunset can be very helpful for the solar plexus chakra, especially if you can meditate outside or by a window where you can sit in the sunlight. The sun's energy is yellow, so it is highly attuned to the solar plexus chakra. But don't worry if meditating in the sun isn't practical for you.

During the meditation, see a spinning wheel of bright yellow light. While meditating for the solar plexus chakra, you will want this disk of light to pass through the root and sacral chakras on its journey. Try to see the disk of light grow brighter and more energetic as it rises up into the location of the solar plexus chakra. When you breathe in, see the disk expand in size, and then see it shrink as you breathe out. Meditate on this chakra for about 15 minutes per day.

If you are able to meditate in the sun during the morning hours or toward sunset, this can be very helpful. You can feel and absorb the warming energy of the sun's yellow light as you meditate.

Affirmations for the Solar Plexus Chakra

So much that is associated with the solar plexus chakra takes place on a subconscious level; daily affirmations can be especially helpful in this case. Use the following to help you get started.

I am strong and confident.

I will finish anything that I start.

I am a leader, and I am comfortable setting the direction of others.

I deserve to have my ideas heard.

I am a creative being, and I can turn my visions into reality.

I feel awakened by the sun's powerful yellow energy.

I will channel the powerful yellow energy of the sun into a creative purpose.

I rejoice at my ability to make things happen.

I believe in my own abilities and feel strong and independent.

My body is full of the energy I need to complete all my projects.

I can establish plans and turn them into reality.

I am full of personal power.

I am smart and have clear judgment.

I can express my will without harming others.

I am able to accurately evaluate any situation.

I am a leader and a decision-maker.

I am a master of my own life.

I am attracting wealth and abundance.

Meditation for the Heart Chakra

The meditation for the heart chakra will focus on green colors. As usual, assume the easy pose position. Imagine a green ball of light coming toward you. See it growing large, getting as large as you are, and positioned right in front of you. Now, each time you breathe in, see the green light enter through your nose and fill your entire chest energy. When you do this, feel the energy of love, connection, trust, and empathy that the green energy carries with it. See yourself breathing in the green light for 15-20 minutes. Each time, hold your breath for a count of five seconds.

Affirmations for the Heart Chakra

Affirmations for the heart chakra can help you to restore your proper sense of self and the confidence to enter into healthy, loving relationships.

I feel love and connection with other human beings.

I trust others, but they must earn my trust.

I deserve to be loved and respected.

I love socializing and being with family and friends.

I will give freely to others without expecting anything in return.

I will help others but not at the expense of causing me pain.

The love I feel for all life is boundless and filled with joy.

I am open to giving love to others.

I forgive myself for the mistakes I have made.

I love myself unconditionally.

I am open to receiving love.

I forgive others completely and unconditionally.

I am compassionate for others and the suffering they may be experiencing.

I will devote a portion of my life to helping others after I have met my own needs first.

Meditation for the Throat Chakra

The throat chakra is associated with energy levels that are in the blue part of the spectrum, so you will imagine blue lights when you do your basic meditations. Wear blue colors while doing your meditation, and you can fill your meditation space with items that are blue-colored such as pillows, rugs, and drapes. The energy of a room with blue colored carpet can be soft and comforting.

Sit on in the easy pose position. You might want to slightly tilt your head back during this meditation to open up the throat area. I have found it also helps to sit on a blue cushion while doing throat chakra meditations. The addition of a blue cushion helps to bring more blue light energy to the meditation while also helping to elevate the spine a little bit, helping to open the throat chakra.

Close your eyes and begin breathing calmly. See a blue ball of light against the inky blackness of space, and imagine it slowly approaching you. As the ball of light moves through space, see the shades of blue change, starting from a light shade of baby blue, progressing through turquoise colors, and gradually darkening into the rich blue colors of lapis lazuli stones. Then, see it gradually lighten and have it repeat the color sequence.

See this ball of light come closer and closer, until it is right in front of you, bathing your body in soft blue light. Begin inhaling deeply, and see the light energy enter your lungs, passing through the throat area and healing the larynx. Then see the blue light energy filling your entire body and then exhale, and see the blue light gradually leave the body.

Keep repeating this exercise for 15-30 minutes, with the color of the light changing gradually so that you can inhale the light of different energy levels. This will help you to heal all aspects of the throat chakra, from having insecurity about speaking your own truth to being able to listen to others and heal them.

I have found that when meditating on the spiritual chakras, using guided meditations can be helpful. These can be found in mobile apps or free of charge on YouTube. They can help you with the appropriate colors of light, pleasing music and meditative sounds, and also with mantras. You can spend two to three weeks meditating on the throat chakra, and vary your meditations using multiple methods and techniques.

Many aspects of the throat chakra are tied together with the solar plexus and heart chakras. Therefore, you might consider balancing and healing meditation for all three chakras simultaneously. This is how I do it.

Begin by sitting in the easy pose. Breath calmly and naturally. See a spinning disk of yellow light approaching, and let it enter your body, moving up to the root chakra. Have it moving at a constant speed, slowly moving through the sacral chakra and then coming to rest in the solar plexus. Now, see the size and brightness of the disk of light increase, and visualize bright yellow colors. Feel the pleasing and calming effect of the energy as you watch the disk of light spinning. Have it grow when you breathe in, and shrink a bit when you breathe out. Keep it in the solar plexus chakra for about five minutes, and then see it move out of the solar plexus, gradually moving up toward the heart chakra, and becoming green in color. Have it turn deep and bright green when it reaches the chest area, and let it reside in the heart chakra area for another five minutes, concentrating on the light as you breathe in and out, calmly and methodically. Since the heart chakra is higher energy, have the disk spin faster.

Then see the disk exit the heart chakra area and begin moving up toward the throat chakra. Let it gradually take on blues mixing in with the green color to form shades of turquoise and aquamarine. As it settles into the throat chakra area, feel its warmth bathing and soothing your throat. Let the disk spin faster, taking on higher frequencies of spiritual energy, and let it take on darker shades of blue. You can meditate another five minutes or so on the throat chakra and then see the light gradually fade away to close out your mediation. This mediation will not only help heal all three chakras together, but it will also help to properly balance them.

Affirmations for the Throat Chakra

Although the throat chakra is higher energy, spiritually oriented chakra, it can be strongly influenced by the subconscious mind and the programming that you received throughout your younger years. You can use affirmations to reprogram the throat chakra. The more you say affirmations for the throat chakra, the more they will enter your subconscious mind and reprogram it to initiate better behaviors. The subconscious mind is actually dumb as a computer, and it needs to be told what to do, step-by-step. You have the power to control it using daily affirmations.

I am able to speak clearly and with confidence.

I always speak the truth.

I keep my word, and I am reliable.

When I am upset about the way I am being treated, I speak out calmly and confidently about it.

I never get a lump in my throat when I need to speak.

I am comfortable speaking to others.

I enjoy public speaking.

I am a confident speaker.

The words I speak always contain the truth.

I enjoy sharing my ideas with others.

When I communicate through writing, I communicate the truth.

I am not afraid to voice my opinions.

I hold myself accountable for speaking the truth.

I feel safe when speaking my truth to others.

I will not use communication to hurt other people in any way.

I speak the truth freely and without fear.

Meditation for the Third Eye Chakra

When meditating for the third eye, try and focus the energy toward the midpoint of the brow. As always, you can meditate in the easy pose, with eyes closed, and you can use regular breathing. When you begin your meditation, focus your attention on the location of the third eye. As you breathe, become consciously aware of the sensations of pressure, heat, and energy that you may get in the center of the brow region. As you do this, imagine a ball of purple light coming toward you. See it in the dark but extremely fluorescent and vibrant purple colors. Allow the light to come toward you and see it emit a beam of energy. Let the beam of energy connect to the center of your brow at the location of the third eye chakra. Now, see it go all the way through your head, and have it exit at the back of the head. The third eye is often viewed as extending all the way through the brain toward the back of the head, so it is the reason it is useful to see the beam of light go all the way through. Meditate on this for 15 minutes, and then see the beam of light shut off, and the energy ball gradually disappear before your eyes. You may be feeling exhausted by this experience and breathing heavily, so focus on your breath and return to a state of calmness as you end your meditation session.

Some people find that they are able to enhance the energy flow into the third eye by holding their hands in the prayer position during their meditation sessions. You can also try this any time during the day when you need "mini" healing or meditation. Simply close your eyes and put your hands in the prayer position, and then allow the energy to pass through the brow region, concentrating on that area and becoming fully aware of all the sensations that you are experiencing.

Affirmations for the Third Eye Chakra

In this section, we will review some affirmations that are useful for the third eye chakra.

I am trusting and worthy of receiving intuitive knowledge.

I trust my intuition.

I will listen to my inner voice.

I am open to imagination and visualization.

I will receive knowledge that the universe has to give.

I trust my feelings and will listen to them.

I seek inner wisdom and guidance.

I trust in the light of the Universal Consciousness.

I am open and accepting.

I am intuitive.

I accept Higher Truths.

I let my sixth sense guide me to the truth.

Spiritual truth is the realm of unlimited possibilities.

Meditation for the Crown Chakra

For meditation with the crown chakra, I like to do a complete balancing mediation. Use the standard mediation procedure, but have a disk of light go through each of the major chakras, moving up through your body and spinning faster as it gains energy. As it passes through each of the seven major chakras, have it change color as appropriate, moving through red, orange, yellow, green, blue, indigo, and purple. When it exits your body at the top of the head, see it as a white light beaming upward toward heaven, connecting you to the Universal Consciousness.

Affirmations for the Sacral Chakra

I am complete.

I am a spiritual being.

The universe is kind and loving.

I am connected to the universe and to all that is.

I am connected to my Spirit Guides.

I am a light being.

I am perfect as is, and I accept myself as is.

I am loved, and the universe is pure love.

Chapter 6. Guided Meditation to Heal and Balance Your Chakras

How to Balance Your Root Chakra

Restoring balance to your root chakra may not result in money going directly into your bank account, nor will it miraculously solve your professional or personal problems. However, a balanced root chakra will help you to lose the fear associated with constant money worries and the obsession to exert control over every situation. By restoring balance to the root chakra, you will be able to allow the divine order to assume responsibility for controlling events in the world and your life. Your role will be transformed into the much more manageable responsibility of maintaining your sense of well-being and safety. Here are some techniques you can use:

Practice focused chakra meditation.

- Find a quiet, safe, and secluded space.
- Sit it in a cross-legged pose with your back and spine straight, and your shoulders relaxed but held firmly back.
- Rest your hands on your knees, with the palms pointed upward.
- Close your eyes and begin breathing in and out deeply, relaxing all your muscles completely, one by one, as you do so.
- Focus on the region where the root chakra is located at your tailbone. Try to notice any tension and relax.
- The root chakra is associated with the color red, so try to visualize a warm red circle at the base of your spine.
- For the next 3 to 5 minutes, maintain steady breathing, and focus on trying to expand the size and warmth of the red circle.
- Eat "grounding" foods.
- Changing your diet can be a big part of restoring balance throughout your chakras.

The following types of food can help:
Beans, tofu, green peas, and other vegetables and foods rich in protein
Red-colored fruits such as strawberries, cherries, and tomatoes
Root vegetables such as beets, radishes, and potatoes that grow in the earth

- Use affirmations.
- Chants and affirmations are essential for redirecting your energy as you learn to balance your chakras.
- The following are affirmations that have helped many restore balance to the root chakra:

"Wherever I go, I am always safe and secure."

"At this moment, I am stable and grounded."

"I trust that all of my needs for safety and security will be met."

"I am healthy in body and mind, and have abundant life."

"I am anchored to the earth."

"I trust the universe to support and guide me."

"My home is secure and happy."

In many ways, the root chakra is the most important of all chakras. Together with the crown chakra, it represents one of the two points through which prana enters the subtle energy body to provide the nourishing power and life force we need to sustain ourselves—mentally, physically, and spiritually.

More importantly, because the root chakra is associated with essential necessities of life, it will be very difficult to find balance in any other area if there are disruptions or difficulties here. Especially if chakra meditation practice is new for you, taking time to explore the ways in which a balanced root chakra can help you heal and grow can be rewarding and enjoyable.

How to Balance Your Sacral Chakra
If you are suffering from symptoms indicating your sacral chakra is imbalanced or closed, there are proven techniques listed here you can use to restore balance and health.

Focused chakra meditation

- Find a quiet, safe, and secluded space.
- Begin by sitting in a cross-legged pose with your back and spine straight and your shoulders relaxed but held firmly back.
- From here, move into any poses that allow you comfortably to open your hips, and includes rocking motions that increase circulation and movement in the pelvis and hip region.
- Change your diet. A healthy diet is essential to the healthy functioning of the chakras. Healing foods for a blocked sacral chakra include:
- Orange-colored foods, such as carrots, oranges, peaches, apricots, sweet potatoes, or pumpkin.
  Any food rich in Omega-3, such as salmon and other types of seafood or nuts and seeds like flax, almonds, and sesame.
- Practice affirmations
- Repeating affirmations during meditation or throughout the day can help you redirect your energy, which can help to support your other efforts to restore health to the sacral chakra.
- Following are some affirmations that many people have used successfully:

"I love my body, and it brings me joy."

"My senses are open to the present moment."

"I am passionate."

"Each breath fills me with pleasure and abundance."

"I will nourish my body with only healthy food and clean water."

"I respect my body."

"I am open to experiencing pleasure and joy.

"My sexuality is a sacred gift."

"I am at peace."

Especially in the status-conscious world of contemporary popular culture, self-expression is everything. Too often people's lives may descend into a downward spiral of negativity and self-recrimination simply because of imagined, petty social slights and negative self-perception.

By focusing on the health of the sacral chakra, you can find the confidence to feel comfortable in your own skin at the level of social intimacy. Begin with ensuring that your root chakra is attuned and balanced, and once you have addressed your basic needs for survival and safety, you will find that work in this area can help you let down your guard enough to let your inner beauty shine through.

How to Balance Your Solar Plexus Chakra
Bringing your solar plexus chakra back into healthy alignment and openness is possible through a combination of many proven techniques and methods. The following are several suggestions that can help you regain perspective.

Spend time in reflection. When your solar plexus chakra is out of balance, your ability to perceive the worthwhile course of action will be impaired. Especially if you are laboring in a highly competitive environment, you may be spending too much time focusing on goals that are not important. Instead, spend time in quiet reflection. You can write in a journal, plant flowers or vegetables in a garden, or perform some other type of work that restores your ability to perceive what matters and what doesn't.
Meditate. There are many forms of meditation that can help restore the health of this vital chakra.

- **Focused chakra meditation 1:**
Find a quiet, safe, and secluded space.

Begin by sitting in a cross-legged pose with your back and spine straight and your shoulders relaxed but held firmly back.

Raise both arms with the elbows bent at right angles.

On each hand, touch the fingers to the thumbs.

From the waist, rotate the upper body to the left while breathing in.

As you breathe out, rotate the upper body to the right

Repeat this exercise for as long as one minute.

- **Focused chakra meditation 2:**

Find a quiet, safe, and secluded space.

Begin by sitting in a cross-legged pose with your back and spine straight and your shoulders relaxed but held firmly back.

With your eyes closed, visualize a bright yellow sun emanating from your solar plexus throughout your body, healing and strengthening your organs.

As you breathe steadily in and out, intone the vowel sound, "ah." Focus on the vibration at the level of your solar plexus.

- **Affirmations**.

During meditation, we can often be distracted by the worries and concerns of the day. One way to resolve this difficulty is to focus on breathing. This can be easier than trying to suppress all your thoughts. In combination with focused breathing, you can also recite affirmations; together these techniques can help you create the focus you need to restore balance to this chakra. Reciting affirmations can also help you stay focused on the many goals and objectives with which you will engage at the level of your solar plexus chakra to accomplish. Many people have found these affirmations helpful:

I am healthy and strong in body and mind.

I am motivated by my soul's playful and gentle energy.

I am energized by my spirit.

I am fully responsible for all my thoughts and feelings.

On my spiritual journey, I see how everything serves as a lesson.

I am the creator and director of my life's journey.

I am connected to a larger purpose to life around me.

My life itself is valuable as it is.

I am committed to self-acceptance and self-love.

I choose to live according to the dictates of love, light, and healing.

I have the courage to trust my instincts and be genuine.

The gentleness of my soul gives me the power to act.

- **Change your diet.**

Drink beverages that are room temperature or warmer. Avoid iced drinks.

Avoid overeating by limiting yourself to two cupped handfuls of food at a sitting.

Sip small amounts of water while eating, and avoid alcohol, soda, or fruit juices.

Avoid constant snacks between meals so your stomach has an opportunity to digest and eliminate waste.

Too often, we find ourselves convinced that success in the workplace is reserved only for the most popular and the most outgoing. Although there may be some truth to this generalization, remember that genuine professional accomplishments and success are really the result of hard work and dedication.

Knowledge, skills, and abilities can certainly help us achieve this kind of success, but the world is a big place and making any kind of lasting change or impression can be a daunting task. By ensuring the health and vitality of the solar plexus, which in turn requires open and balanced root and sacral chakras, you can give yourself the ability to draw upon the primal forces and drives that can help you succeed in the professional world.

How to Balance Your Heart Chakra

Opening your heart chakra is an important step in ensuring your life stays on a healthy, happy, and successful course. Using a combination of many proven techniques and methods, you can not only achieve a mature state of openness and love but sustain this state throughout your life. The following are several suggestions that can help you achieve balance in this area:

- Reconsider your priorities. The heart chakra represents the successful balance between two seemingly opposite and conflicting forces. The immature view is to satisfy your ego, wants, dreams, hopes, and desires; you must shut out everything else and pursue them relentlessly. This approach may make sense at a very rudimentary level, and many people believe they must give up the pursuit of what is in their hearts to make more money. However, by opening your heart chakra, you will find that the abundance of the universe will more than compensate you for any sacrifice you make to pursue goals that contribute to the world's reservoir of love, understanding, and forgiveness. The power of the heart chakra to restore bounty to your life is infinite—the more love you give, the more you will receive in return.
- Meditate. Seated meditation can also help restore balance to the heart chakra.
- Focused chakra meditation:

Find a quiet, safe, and secluded space.

Begin by sitting in a cross-legged pose with your back and spine straight and your shoulders relaxed but held firmly back.

Move to a position in which you are lying face down, with your arms at your sides.

Move your hands up to your shoulders, and place them, palms down, on either side of your body at shoulder level, with your elbows pointing upward.

Using your hands, lift your head, neck, and shoulders off the mat, with your back arched back, and the tops of your feet on the floor, point toes away from the front of your body.

Push upward with your hands toward your shoulders, relax your necks, and gaze forward

Breathe in and out several times as you maintain this position from 30 to 60 seconds.

- Affirmations. While in meditation, reciting affirmations can help you focus your mind on healing the heart chakra. By giving yourself something to focus on, clearing your mind of distractions will be much easier, and meditation will be more effective. Also, as you go through your day, you will be constantly bombarded by distractions and disruptions; quietly reciting one of the following affirmations can help you stay on track:

I allow myself to be guided by my heart.

I surrender completely.

I will let go of fear and trust my heart.

I will remain open to deep self-love.

I welcome the embrace of universal love.

I will remain open to healthy relationships.

I choose to live according to the dictates of peace.

I forgive myself.

I am grateful for all the good that is part of my life.

I will remain open to the connectedness of everything.

I am loving and compassionate, both with myself and with those around me.

I accept myself as I am.

I accept others as they are.

I have a connection with a greater life purpose.

- Change your diet. As with all chakras, the heart chakra is tied directly to our physicality and paying attention to our diet can contribute significantly to our efforts to restore balance and vitality. The following types of food are generally recommended for restoring the proper function of the heart chakra:

Green vegetables, including broccoli, asparagus spinach, zucchini, kale, Brussels sprouts, and peas

Green fruits, including green grapes or apples, avocado, cucumber, and lime

Herbs such as mint, oregano, parsley, basil, and sage

Green tea and beverages containing wheatgrass, barley grass, and spirulina

The visceral pleasure of surviving and thriving in the outside world of natural and professional competition can bring much satisfaction, especially if the lower chakras are balanced and healthy. But as human beings, we are more than just animals, and if our happiness is to be lasting, it must be sustained by more than just the ability to provide basic necessities.

By caring for the heart chakra, you can give yourself an advantage in an effort not to be swallowed up or consumed by the demands of money and other needs. In addition, the capacity for selflessness fostered by the heart chakra can help all your efforts align with a healthier and saner perspective.

How to Balance Your Throat Chakra

Opening your throat chakra can allow you to express the joy of spiritual maturity and the happiness that is planted in your heart by awakening the lower three chakras. To deny yourself this gift is to deprive yourself of the freedom to grow and experience all the good things in life the universe has in store for you. A combination of reflection, meditation, and behavior changes can help you achieve success in this area.

- Reflect. The modern world values analysis, debate, measurable facts, and analysis; it is very status conscious. It often uses the results of statistical analysis to encourage impulsive and judgmental behavior. A blocked throat chakra may have the result that you are often bothered by conflicted internal dialogs and drives. A balanced throat chakra will help harmonize these polarizing forces. Throughout the day, take some time in quiet reflection to consider your true motives are and whether they represent your actions.
- Keep a journal in which you allow yourself to be completely honest with yourself about whether you are happy, and whether you feel you are true to yourself. By removing the clutter from your internal mind, you lay a successful foundation for healing.
- Meditate. There are many forms of meditation explicitly designed to restore balance to the throat chakra. One such exercise—sometimes called the "cat-cow stretch" is included below as a focused chakra meditation.

Find a quiet, safe, and secluded space.

Begin by sitting in a cross-legged pose with your back and spine straight and your shoulders relaxed but held firmly back.

Move to a position in which you are kneeling, with your upper body bent forward and supported by your hands on the ground, facing forward, parallel with your knees. Your back will resemble a table, with your upper legs and arms acting as the four table legs.

As you inhale deeply, lift your tail upward, drop your belly toward the floor, and stretch your neck as your head looks upward.

As you exhale, tuck your tail under, arch your back upward, and you're your head and neck downward, as you gaze toward your belly button.

Maintain each position from 30 to 60 seconds.

If you feel comfortable, after a few repetitions, you may open your throat further by exhaling forcefully through your mouth, while chanting the Sanskrit syllable, "ham."

- Affirmations. Whereas stones and crystals provide a more passive means of helping you maintain focus on your throat chakra, affirmations can help you replace the clutter in your conscious mind with helpful thoughts. The following are several affirmations many people have found useful:

I communicate easily and confidently.

I can state my needs clearly.

I can speak my truth with ease and comfort.

I am comfortable with silence.

I can be understood easily.

I listen actively and intently.

I vocalize my feelings.

I balanced speaking with listening.

I speak using my true voice.

- Diet. Finally, making some changes to your diet can help you achieve a healthier state of mind-body balance. The following foods are helpful in opening, healing, and balancing the throat chakra:

Liquids can help lubricate and clear the throat, so increasing your intake of fluids is advisable. Try and of the following:

Soup

Warm tea

Cool juice

Water

Avoid dairy-based beverages that can clog and congest the sinuses and throat

Blue food is rare in nature, but there are some exceptions:

Blueberries

Blackberries

Fruit

Apples

Pears

Oranges

Peaches

Apricots

Plums

Especially in the Information Age, the ability to express oneself accurately, articulately, and easily is an invaluable skill and a key to success. We would waste all the gifts of the lower chakras, joined by the heart chakra with the capacity to seek a higher purpose if we could not express their value using an open throat chakra.

The responses of a complex world to all of your efforts must be made with a strong and assured voice. Speaking truthfully and clearly can help not only your personal relationships but can also add depth and meaning to the relationships you form in the professional workplace.

How to Balance Your Third Eye Chakra
More than any of the other chakras discussed so far; the third eye chakra is associated mostly with mental activity. As a result, it may be tempting to assume that the types of activity to restore balance to the lower chakras will be ineffective with this chakra. Although there is certainly a different focus in the combination of practices used to open Ajna, a simple plan of disciplined changes in behavior can work here, as well.

- Develop your capacity for critical thinking. The third eye represents your capacity to develop sharp intellectual insights. As muscles atrophy when we fail to exercise, so our powers of reason and analysis erode when we fail to develop our cognitive skills. The following are two suggestions for keeping the mind active and engaged.
- Learn to learn. Often, when our third eye is blocked, it may be the result of internal or external interference. In such cases, we may not be able to see the forest for the trees and trying to reason our way out of a problem of calcified mental atrophy would be ineffective.
- The current educational environment has spawned new games and activities designed to stimulate learning. If you have children, tune in to their school time activities and see if any of the teaching methods that seem to inspire them can help you out of your doldrums. While your life and professional career are by no means a game, the uncluttered minds of young people serve as a good reminder of how we learn best and making a game of menial work can reinvigorate your spirit.
  ○ Begin study in a field that interests you. Your current state of mental entropy may be caused by boredom, repetition, and overexposure. No matter what area of study you choose to pursue, you will eventually find that is part of the same whole in which you currently spend most of your time. Moreover, the skills of logic, reason, and analysis are transferable and absolute. Gaining insight by studying mathematics, biology, sports statistics, or chakras will help you push past the barriers you encounter in your occupation.
- Meditate. All chakras respond to meditation. If your third eye is currently blocked or impaired, meditation is one of the most effective means of clearing the pathways to allow your capacity for insight to regain sharpness, clarity, and focus.
- Focused chakra meditation:

Find a quiet, safe, and secluded space.

Begin by sitting in a cross-legged pose with your back and spine straight and your shoulders relaxed but held firmly back.

Rest your hands on your knees, with the palms pointed upward.

Close your eyes and begin breathing in and out deeply, relaxing all your muscles completely, one by one, as you do so.

Slowly bring both hands to your face and place the two middle fingers over your eyes.

Let the index fingers rest at the eyebrow line, with the pinky fingers resting just under the cheekbones.

Use your thumbs to plug your ears.

Inhale deeply.

As you exhale, pronounce the syllable "AUM," stressing the final "M" by making a sound like a buzzing bee.

Repeat the exhalation and inhalation for two minutes.

This meditation practice can help relieve tension in the head and begin to awaken the third eye chakra.

- Affirmations. Using affirmations to open a chakra associated with intellectual acuity and insight may seem counterproductive but redirecting your mental focus when you feel stuck and inflexible can be extremely beneficial.

I will listen to my deepest wisdom.

I listen to the wisdom of elders.

I trust my intuition.

I am receptive to the wisdom of the universe.

I seek inspiration and bliss.

- Diet. Paying attention to the color of foods ingredients of foods can help open any of the chakras. The following foods can be especially helpful with this chakra:

Purple foods:

Grapes

Eggplant

Purple kale

Purple yams

Blackberries

Blueberries

The following foods contain ingredients that are useful in restoring mental acuity:

Cacao (contains antioxidants that release serotonin)

Salmon, walnuts, and avocado (contain Omega 3, which helps the brain)

Water (to relieve stagnancy and restore energy).

By meditating on the chakras, we can gain an awareness of our connectedness to the world around us. This important feature of our consciousness allows us to develop ways of living that are responsive to the needs of the world and to others. By avoiding selfishness and unhealthy obsessions, we increase our chances of attaining success and happiness.

Yet, as individuals, we still have desires, needs, and interests. Ignoring these impulses would cause disruptions in the flow of energy, so it is important to consider how to address them. The third-eye chakra is means through which we can insight into how best to approach our own individual intellectual development in such a way that maintains a harmonious relationship with all the other competing needs and interests in our lives.

How to Balance Your Crown Chakra
The crown chakra is the height of the seven-chakra system and the reason for the importance of ensuring the health and vibrancy of the entire system. When this chakra is out of balance, we may feel that the whole purpose of chakra meditation has been defeated. Similarly, impairments in this region can prevent success in opening and maintaining a healthy balance and energy flow throughout the lower chakras. A combination of many behavior changes, exercises, and practices can help you restore health and vitality.

- Expand your horizons. Feelings of depression and futility may result from a belief that there is nothing more to live than what our limited perceptions tell us. Especially in the midst of the "war on education," you may feel pressured to turn your back on learning new things and remaining open to new and different possibilities in your life. A common response is to find comfort within this cocoon familiar misery. I this has happened to you, try taking a different approach by reading books, watching films, or listening to audio broadcasts about self-growth. If you can be honest with yourself about areas in which you are ignorant, maintain bias, or prejudice, learning more can help you combat some of the claustrophobia. In the Information Age, knowledge is power more than ever.
- Meditate. As always, meditation is one of the most important keys to healing impaired chakras. Meditation creates self-awareness, regulates emotional and psychological chaos and disruption, and establishes a foundation of calm and inner peace that can foster your ability to act with purpose. The following technique can be helpful in awakening the energy of the crown chakra:

Focused chakra meditation:
Find a quiet, safe, and secluded space.

Begin by sitting in a cross-legged pose with your back and spine straight and your shoulders relaxed but held firmly back.

Rest your hands on your knees, with the palms pointed upward.

Close your eyes and begin breathing in and out deeply, relaxing all your muscles completely, one by one, as you do so.

With your eyes closed, look inward and visualize a lotus flower at the top of your head, within your skull.

With each breath in and out, visualize the petals of the lotus opening slowly and steadily, illuminated by bright violet light.

Continue breathing and imagine the energy traveling from the base of your spine toward the lotus, sending energy and life through the center and outward toward the tips of each of the thousand petals, as they continue to open and spread outward, beneath the surface of your skull at the crown of your head.

When the lotus is fully open, visualize the warmth and vitality traveling back down the chakras, giving warmth and life throughout your neck, shoulders, and back; through your heart and chest; down into your belly, and all the way to the base at your root chakra.

Maintain this breathing for five to ten minutes before slowly opening your eyes.

Sit quietly for a few minutes until you feel ready to resume your activities.

Affirmations. Often, we may adjust to routine actions, thoughts, and behavior patterns that may be familiar and comfortable, but that cause considerable harm. Reciting affirmations—either silently to yourself, or in groups where you share spiritual healing and growth goals—can help redirect your mental focus and help support your efforts in other areas. For the crown chakra, you may find these affirmations helpful:

I am an intricate part of the divine universe.

I respect and honor the divine within myself.

I seek understanding from my experiences in life.

I cherish and value my spiritual energy.

I value and seek universal wisdom.

I trust my intuition.

I am willing to let go of my attachments to the physical.

I live in the present.

I am grateful, humbled, and thankful for all that is good.

I am at peace.

- Diet. Ensuring you eat a healthy and balanced diet is essential not only to your physical health, but also your emotional, psychological, and spiritual health. The following foods may helpful:

Purple or violet foods:

Grapes

Eggplant

Passionfruit

Red cabbage

Purple kale

Ginger

Herbal teas

Water

The crown chakra represents the other end of the spectrum of the chakras system from the root chakra. From here, we receive direction for all of our highest callings. Especially in the modern world, thoughts about our ultimate destiny can lead to depression and despair, so it is important to ensure the health of your crown chakra. When this chakra is in balance, your entire chakra system will be more aligned and attuned, and you will be more receptive to the joy and happiness that crown chakra meditation can bring to your life.

Chapter 7. Heal Yourself with Chakras Meditations

Meditation gives you the power to transform your mind. It is meant to help positively change your emotions, improve your concentration, and bring you a sense of calm. Through different meditation practices, you can train your mind to new patterns. With chakra meditations, you will be focusing your mind on your chakras to help clear them of blocked energies.

Root Chakra Meditation

This mediation is a tried-and-true method of creating a connection with your root chakra.

Find a comfortable position, either laying down or sitting, and take in three deep and slow breaths. With each inhale, imagine the breath sending energy to your perineum; this is the space between your anus and genitals. With every exhale, release whatever you are holding in this area. This could be pain or fears. It could even be what you think you should be feeling while in this meditation.

Begin to gently tap at the top of your pubic bone or on either side of the lower parts of your hips. This will wake up the connection you have with your root chakra.

As you continue to breathe in and out through your nose, direct your breath to your chakra. Picture a red glowing light growing and pulsing in your lower pubic area. For people who identify mostly as male, the light should spin clockwise. For people who identify mostly as female, the light should spin counterclockwise.

As you fall further into your meditative state, talk to your root chakra to see what it needs. Take some more breaths to notice if you get any feedback. This feedback could be a word, intuition, color, image, song, sound, or feeling. Act upon the feedback you receive. If nothing comes up, you don't need to worry about it. You will get something as you continue to practice.

If you didn't receive a message but you start to feel a new awareness in your root chakra, something like a pulsating in the lower hips and down through your feet, you have made a connection to your root chakra.

As your meditation comes to a close, take three deep and slow breaths. Direct your inhales towards your feet so that you are grounded, and then slowly open your eyes.

Make sure you take things slowly as you start. This will take some time and practice so be patient. If you end up feeling any sort of pain in your legs or lower back, you are trying too hard. Take a break and go back to it later. Remember that even seasoned meditators will sometimes find it hard to shut off their mind. Take this moment to observe these thoughts without judging them; let them go and gently refocus your mind.

Sacral Chakra Meditation

Find a comfortable position, either laying down or sitting. Take in three deep and slow breaths. With each inhale, imagine the breath sending energy to the space right below your bellybutton. With every exhale, release whatever you are holding in this area. This could be pain or fears. It could even be what you think you should be feeling while in this meditation. You can place your hand on this area while you meditate if you would like.

Begin to gently tap the area below your bellybutton with two fingers. You can also gently massage the area in a circular motion.

As you continue to breathe in and out through your nose, direct your breath to your chakra. Picture an orange glowing light growing and pulsing in your lower abdomen area. For people who identify mostly as male, the light should spin clockwise. For people who identify mostly as female, the light should spin counterclockwise.

As you fall further into your meditative state, talk to your sacral chakra to see what it needs. Take some more breaths to notice if you get any feedback. This feedback could be a word, intuition, color, image, song, sound, or feeling. Act upon the feedback you receive. If nothing comes up, you don't need to worry about it. You will get something as you continue to practice.

If you didn't receive a message but you start to feel a new awareness in your sacral chakra, something like a pulsating in this area, you have made a connection to your sacral chakra.

As your meditation comes to a close, take three deep and slow breaths. Direct your inhales towards your feet so that you are grounded, and then slowly open your eyes.

Make sure you take things slowly as you start. This will take some time and practice so be patient. If you end up feeling any sort of pain in your lower abdomen, you are trying too hard. Take a break and go back to it later.

Solar Plexus Chakra Meditations

Find a comfortable position, either laying down or sitting. Take in three deep and slow breaths. With each inhale, imagine the breath sending energy to the space right above your belly button. With every exhale, release whatever you are holding in this area. This could be pain or fears. It could even be what you think you should be feeling while in this meditation. You can place your hand on this area while you meditate if you would like.

Begin to gently tap the area above your belly button with two fingers. You can also gently massage the area in a circular motion.

As you continue to breathe in and out through your nose, direct your breath to your chakra. Picture a yellow glowing light growing and pulsing in your upper abdomen area. For people who identify mostly as male, the light should spin clockwise. For people who identify mostly as female, the light should spin counterclockwise.

As you fall further into your meditative state, talk to your solar plexus chakra to see what it needs. Take some more breaths to notice if you get any feedback. This feedback could be a word, intuition, color, image, song, sound, or feeling. Act upon the feedback you receive. If nothing comes up, you don't need to worry about it. You will get something as you continue to practice.

If you didn't receive a message but you start to feel a new awareness in your solar plexus chakra, something like a pulsating in this area, you have made a connection to your solar plexus chakra.

As your meditation comes to a close, take three deep and slow breaths. Direct your inhales towards your feet so that you are grounded, and then slowly open your eyes.

Make sure you take things slowly as you start. This will take some time and practice so be patient. If you end up feeling any sort of pain in your upper abdomen, you are trying too hard. Take a break and go back to it later.

Heart Chakra Meditation

Find a comfortable position, either laying down or sitting. Take in three deep and slow breaths. With each inhale, imagine the breath sending energy to the center of your chest. With every exhale, release whatever you are holding in this area. This could be pain or fears. It could even be what you think you should be feeling while in this meditation. You can place your hand on this area while you meditate if you would like.

Begin to gently tap your chest with two fingers. You can also gently massage the area in a circular motion.

As you continue to breathe in and out through your nose, direct your breath to your chakra. Picture a green glowing light growing and pulsing in your chest. For people who identify mostly as male, the light should spin clockwise. For people who identify mostly as female, the light should spin counterclockwise.

As you fall further into your meditative state, talk to your heart chakra to see what it needs. Take some more breaths to notice if you get any feedback. This feedback could be a word, intuition, color, image, song, sound, or feeling. Act upon the feedback you receive. If nothing comes up, you don't need to worry about it. You will get something as you continue to practice.

If you didn't receive a message but you start to feel a new awareness in your heart chakra, something like a pulsating in this area, you have made a connection to your heart chakra.

As your meditation comes to a close, take three deep and slow breaths. Direct your inhales towards your feet so that you are grounded, and then slowly open your eyes.

Make sure you take things slowly as you start. This will take some time and practice so be patient. If you end up noticing your heart is racing uncomfortably, you are trying too hard. Take a break and go back to it later.

Throat Chakra Meditation

Find a comfortable position, either laying down or sitting. Take in three deep and slow breaths. With each inhale, imagine the breath sending energy to the notch of your throat. With every exhale, release whatever you are holding in this area. This could be pain or fears. It could even be what you think you should be feeling while in this meditation.

Begin to gently tap the bone at the notch of your throat with two fingers. You can also gently massage the area in a circular motion.

As you continue to breathe in and out through your nose, direct your breath to your chakra. Picture a blue glowing light growing and pulsing in your throat. For people who identify mostly as male, the light should spin clockwise. For people who identify mostly as female, the light should spin counterclockwise.

As you fall further into your meditative state, talk to your throat chakra to see what it needs. Take some more breaths to notice if you get any feedback. This feedback could be a word, intuition, color, image, song, sound, or feeling. Act upon the feedback you receive. If nothing comes up, you don't need to worry about it. You will get something as you continue to practice.

If you didn't receive a message but you start to feel a new awareness in your throat chakra, something like a pulsating in this area, you have made a connection to your throat chakra.

As your meditation comes to a close, take three deep and slow breaths. Direct your inhales towards your feet so that you are grounded, and then slowly open your eyes.

Make sure you take things slowly as you start. This will take some time and practice so be patient. If you end up feeling any sort of pain in your neck, you are trying too hard. Take a break and go back to it later.

Third Eye Chakra Meditation

Find a comfortable position, either laying down or sitting. Take in three deep and slow breaths. With each inhale, imagine the breath sending energy to the space between your brows. With every exhale, release whatever you are holding in this area. This could be pain or fears. It could even be what you think you should be feeling while in this meditation.

Begin to gently tap the area between your eyebrows with two fingers. You can also gently massage the area in a circular motion.

As you continue to breathe in and out through your nose, direct your breath to your chakra. Picture an indigo glowing light growing and pulsing in the area between your brows. For people who identify mostly as male, the light should spin clockwise. For people who identify mostly as female, the light should spin counterclockwise.

As you fall further into your meditative state, talk to your third eye chakra to see what it needs. Take some more breaths to notice if you get any feedback. This feedback could be a word, intuition, color, image, song, sound, or feeling. Act upon the feedback you receive. If nothing comes up, you don't need to worry about it. You will get something as you continue to practice.

If you didn't receive a message but you start to feel a new awareness in your third eye chakra, something like a pulsating in this area, you have made a connection to your third eye chakra.

As your meditation comes to a close, take three deep and slow breaths. Direct your inhales towards your feet so that you are grounded, and then slowly open your eyes.

Make sure you take things slowly as you start. This will take some time and practice so be patient. If you end up feeling like your getting a headache at the front of your head, you are trying too hard. Take a break and go back to it later.

Crown Chakra Meditation

Find a comfortable position, either laying down or sitting. Take in three deep and slow breaths. With each inhale, imagine the breath sending energy to the top of your head. With every exhale, release whatever you are holding in this area. This could be pain or fears. It could even be what you think you should be feeling while in this meditation.

Begin to gently tap the top of your head two fingers. You can also gently massage the area in a circular motion.

As you continue to breathe in and out through your nose, direct your breath to your chakra. Picture a purple glowing light growing and pulsing in the top of your head. For people who identify mostly as male, the light should spin clockwise. For people who identify mostly as female, the light should spin counterclockwise.

As you fall further into your meditative state, talk to your crown chakra to see what it needs. Take some more breaths to notice if you get any feedback. This feedback could be a word, intuition, color, image, song, sound, or feeling. Act upon the feedback you receive. If nothing comes up, you don't need to worry about it. You will get something as you continue to practice.

If you didn't receive a message but you start to feel a new awareness in your crown chakra, something like a pulsating in this area, you have made a connection to your crown chakra.

As your meditation comes to a close, take three deep and slow breaths. Direct your inhales towards your feet so that you are grounded, and then slowly open your eyes.

Make sure you take things slowly as you start. This will take some time and practice so be patient. If you end up feeling any sort of pain in your head, you are trying too hard. Take a break and go back to it later.

Conclusion

Blockages to your chakras are common and they can result in a variety of physical and mental ailments. When we start to dedicate ourselves to a healthy chakra system, we can heal pretty much everything that is wrong with us. Energy is everywhere and controlling the energy inside is pivotal to our lives.

Spending the time to look for blocked chakras is also important. Through meditation, yoga, and other practices, clearing blockages can become easy. It does take research and dedication to ensure you are living the best life that you can. This can be done through balancing chakras and allowing positive energy to pass through your system fluidly.

While our chakra system is quite complex, it is also very simple to focus on. There are practices and rituals that can help you on your way to true enlightenment. Opening your third eye and allowing your energy to flow all the way to your crown chakra is going to take time; however, once you have, you will understand why the dedication you put forth was totally worth it.

BOOK 5

Introduction

Like other religions, Buddhism strives to help you find the answers to more in-depth questions in life, like Who am I? How will I be happy? But the wonderful thing about Buddhism is that it doesn't just ask you to do this and that, take the Buddha's word for it and then leave you to try to make sense of it all. Instead, Buddhism invites you to experience the nature of reality for yourself.

Once you are awakened or enlightened, you will experience your internal reality and external reality. That inner reality is that part of you that remains constant and untouched by the outer world. Think of it as your anchor, which will keep you steady despite the chaos of the world around you. Think of it like the lotus, which will remain untainted even as you float along a polluted pond.

Buddhism's ultimate goal is to enable you to experience the awakening in the same way as the Buddha.

If Buddhists don't worship a Supreme being, who was Buddha, then?

To get straight to the point, Buddha was a man who lived in the 5th century BCE. Nevertheless, he was immortalized in his disciples' memory because of the extraordinary life that he had lived.

He was part of the Shakya royal family clan in what is known today as Nepal. Although he was able to experience all the sensual delights that the world had to offer, Prince Siddhartha, as he was then called, had deep compassion for his suffering brethren. Even when surrounded by luxuries, he understood the universality of sorrow. At age 29, he abandoned his wealth and all worldly pleasures. At the prime of his life, he chose to lead an austere existence. He wore a simple yellow garment and roamed the world in a quest for Peace, Truth, and Freedom from Suffering without a penny to his name.

For six years straight, he prayed and performed self-mortification. He tormented his body in an attempt to nourish the soul. He did this until he reached the point of emaciation. He ascertained that self-mortification only weakened the body and, consequently, exhaust the spirit through his personal experience. He then used this experience to form an independent path. It is when he found the Majjhima Patipada, also known as the Middle Path.

Buddhist philosophy sharply diverged from another new religion that came up through similar circumstances and methods: Jainism. It is also an ancient Indian religion that persists today and is often compared to Buddhism due to the many similarities and overlaps in the teachings they preach. Unlike Buddhism, however, Jainism does espouse the virtues of asceticism through fasting and various other forms of penance. Jains also retain a belief in the soul, which they believe is found in every living creature on Earth.

That different view on asceticism is usually one of the most relevant factors for newcomers to these religions. Jainism can be significantly more challenging for some individuals to get into because of it. Buddhism is usually much more accessible and more comfortable to introduce into regular, contemporary life, giving it a significant advantage in the western hemisphere.

And much like Buddhism, Jainism sought to reform the faith and introduce new philosophy to the followers. These religions also mention a few similar principles and ideas, such as Reincarnation, Karma, and other vital beliefs.

However, despite the common origins and common ground, Buddhism received much more official support than Jainism, which was probably the primary factor that allowed Buddhist teachings to spread much further. It's also interesting that, just like the Buddha, Mahavir, who was one of the key figures in Jainism's creation, was also of noble birth.

Enlightenment came to him as he was meditating under the Bodhi tree. It was at this moment that he awakened to Buddhahood. From then on, he became known as Shakyamuni Buddha or "the awakened wise man of the Shakya clan." He did this all on his own, as a man with no supernatural powers.

For the next 45 years of his existence, the Buddha dedicated his life to preaching all over the North Indian subcontinent. He taught whoever was interested in living a life free from suffering.

He was 80 years old when he died. The Buddha was mortal, and yet he was godlike in every respect. However, although he had plenty of followers who revered him, he was never so arrogant to refer to himself as a divine being.

The bottom line is that the Buddha was human, much like you and me. And like him, we, too, can achieve awakening. Like him, we again can become Buddhas. As a Bodhisatta (an aspiring Buddha), you also can follow that path which the Buddha has led and, in so doing, find Truth, Peace, and Freedom from Suffering. The Buddha pointed out that we shall find salvation only by relying on ourselves, our capabilities, and our efforts. Simply put, you are your savior.

A significant portion of the Buddha's journey, tribulations, and spiritual growth was a story of trial and error. It was a man who exercised his thoughts frequently while trying to fine-tune his philosophy before teaching others. His arrival at the Middle Way is the right course due to that trial and error and Siddhartha's ability to be self-critical and think for himself. As you can see, the Buddhist affinity for critical thinking and their encouragement of skepticism is a direct reflection of how the Buddha himself traversed our troubled world and, as such, he led by example.

This emphasis on how one lives instead of adopting strictly defined beliefs will become even more evident later in this book. Buddhism is practical to the point of making numerous scholars and theologians not even recognize it as an organized, mainstream religion. There are different schools and traditions that it is sometimes challenging to lump into this one all-encompassing religion. Apart from just the official sects and denominations, the openness to interpretation and personalized adoption by new adherents adds even more to Buddhism's versatility and diversity. Above all, Buddhism puts excellent faith into the individual and supports their natural inclination to think and question matters independently. It could be argued that some other religions go the opposite, dogmatic route, where they strive to hardcode beliefs into the followers and do most of their thinking for them.

Buddhism recognizes that human beings possess the capacity to distinguish between good and evil. Simply put, Buddhism promotes the use of human intelligence as well as your freedom to choose. You are encouraged to possess an open mind and an open heart. However, you are also encouraged to employ skepticism when it is necessary. The Dalai Lama of Tibet couldn't have said it better: If the teachings suit you, then incorporate them into your life using the best of your capabilities. If, however, the instructions don't work for you, then leave them be.

Buddha told his followers not to embrace everything he says merely because he said it. He advised them to test his teachings as though examining the authenticity of gold. If, after a thorough examination, his teachings proved to be accurate, then the followers may put them to practice.

This lack of aggressive indoctrination is why many argue that Buddhism is a scientific religion if you will. The Three Marks of Existence, which form the core of the Buddhist way of perceiving the world, are subject to the scientific method and analysis. One can look into the concepts of impermanence, no-self, and even suffering and observe that they are indeed based in reality and are very difficult to disprove. Unlike the assertions made by some of the other major religions, these claims are not hard to disprove because they are an unfalsifiable hypothesis. Instead, their sturdiness and plausibility stem from the fact that they result from a thorough analysis of the real world.

It has long been a powerful talking point of critics of religion that significant, monotheistic faiths make use of unfalsifiable hypotheses to solidify their claims for God's existence. It means making a proposition that cannot be disproven through logic or any scientific method by giving your request supernatural attributes that prevent it from being observed in nature. It is evident in Abrahamic religions, where God is described as impossible to hear, see, or feel, making it impossible to debunk His existence. Buddhism doesn't make use of this concept. Everything that Buddhist teachings assert about our reality's circumstances is based on that reality, and anything that goes beyond that can and should be taken with a grain of salt. There is no punishment in Buddhism for not believing in other realms and similar propositions to the letter.

You can now see the appeal of Buddhism as a religion. It doesn't command. It doesn't demand. Buddhism doesn't provide you with the illusion that you were born free and then enslave you with set rules in stone. More importantly, it does not mean you are loved and frightens you with eternal damnation ideas.

Instead, Buddhism encourages you to become the best version of yourself, utilize your inborn capacities as a human being, and maximize these potentials to create a better world than the one you have found.

It's also essential that Buddhism doesn't seek to deliver you from the suffering of this life utilizing fear and by barring you from temptation and possible sources of corruption through strict rules and notions of sin. Buddhist teachings don't teach their layperson followers that acquiring luxuries, pleasure, or enjoying life in other ways is an inherently terrible thing. Instead, Buddhists are taught how not to attach themselves to transient possessions and sensory pleasures so that their happiness and fulfillment don't depend solely on these things. A Buddhist can thus acquire material gains, but he will know better than to equate these gains with existential fulfillment. Therefore, if these things are lost, this will create no void or a deep sense of loss in a person. No matter what we do and have in life, we should look within ourselves if we value spiritual growth and true satisfaction – this is the core message of wisdom.

Christianity is also one of three religions (the other two are Judaism and Islam) that exist within the "Abrahamic tradition," They trace elements of their beliefs to Abraham, father of Isaac and chosen by God as the father of nations. Abraham's story is among the most moving episodes of the Old Testament and has provided grist for innumerable scholars and exegetes over the centuries. But the specifically Christian tradition begins with the coming of Jesus of Nazareth.

The Man and the Christ

We know about Jesus from the four gospels written by Mark, Matthew, Luke, and John (mostly from the first three, known as the Synoptic Gospels).

According to tradition, he was born in humble circumstances: son of a carpenter, born in a stable as his parents Joseph and Mary journeyed to Bethlehem to participate in the Roman census.

Chapter 1. What is Buddhism, The First Buddha, and His Teachings

What is Buddhism?

What is Buddhism? Many consider Buddhism a religion, though some deny it because Buddhism teaches no worship of the gods. They say that Buddhism is a philosophy or merely a way of life. This distinction between religion and philosophy has arisen among Western commentators since a difference between the two in Asia originated is not clear. According to some sources, it has around 500 million followers, making it the third-largest religion globally (if we could call it that).

The name Buddhism derives from the title given by its followers Siddharta Gautama. They called him the Buddha, meaning "the awakened" or "the enlightened one." Siddhartha Gautama lived around 500 BC. In northern India. The exact date of birth is unknown. He is commonly known in the Buddhist world as Shakyamuni, "the sage of the Shakya." These are the only historical facts we have about the Buddha. To learn about his teachings and his life, we must now look at him with Buddhist eyes.

His father had overprotected him. He saw no pain or suffering during his life in the castle. However, at this time in this life, he experienced the human condition's misery for the first time. He saw a sick person, an older man, and a corpse. He asked his servant about it, and he said that we are all destined to suffer that.

I'm talking about all this because we must understand what questions Buddhism is trying to answer. The Buddha found the origin and solution of suffering. Then he told me this suffering arises because we are attached to things. This attachment comes from our ignorance and deception.

Then he talked about the solution to this suffering. He said that Nirvana is the solution. Nirvana means to blow out. It merely is the extinction of all our desires that causes our lives to continue in a painful cycle. It's hard to think of Nirvana as a favorable destination from a Western perspective, but it's very desirable for Buddhists.

So, the Buddha tried to end human suffering. He answered no questions about the ultimate source of reality or our connection with the gods but only decided to solve a real problem he had in life. If you look at Buddhism from this perspective, it is difficult to talk about it as a religion. It is more of a philosophy or even shares aspects with modern psychology.

Mahayana Buddhists have fundamentally changed the beliefs and practices of traditional Buddhism. Some varieties of Mahayana worship heavenly Bodhisattvas and Buddhas. These are beings who have attained Enlightenment or are advanced practitioners of the path. They can intervene in this world and save people as if they were gods.

So, Buddhism is a very complicated tradition. It could be considered a religion or something else, depending on how we look at it.

Who is the Founder of Buddhism?

The basic practices of Buddhism are focused on meditation. But the methods of Zen Buddhism go even further.

"Zen" originates from the Sanskrit word for contemplation. Everything can change into "zazen," which is the name of a Zen Buddhist contemplation method. Regular everyday practice is critical.

Buddhists from Monaco invest a great deal of energy pondering, and the part of Rinzai-Zen mostly utilizes the reflection on the koan. All professionals of Zen Buddhism look for illumination. Even though the thought is a fundamental piece of the activity, including different systems, it can help accomplish that objective.

Buddhism is religion dependent on the lessons of the Buddha known as the Dharma. The individuals who practice Buddhism are looking for a condition of complete edification known as nirvana.

This religion concentrated on Buddha's lessons by helping the sangha (meditator) in reflection to prepare the brain, dispense with affliction, and achieve nirvana.

Mahayana Buddhism is practiced mainly in China, Korea, and Japan and includes mysticism and cosmology elements. Mahayana Buddhism is divided into two variants. Zen Buddhism, which focuses more on internalizing the spiritual journey and self-esteem, and the Pure Land, which teaches devotion to the Buddha Amitabha, are needed to reach nirvana.

Although Mahayana Buddhism heavily influences Tibetan Buddhism or Vajrayana, it forms another major discipline of the Buddhist faith. Tantric Buddhism, Vajrayana contains both text and writing, including Theraveda Mahayana Buddhism and Buddhist Tantra.

The Story of Siddhartha Gautama

Siddhartha Gautama was born below the Himalayan foothills in approximately 567 B.C.E. into the clan of Shakya, of which his father was chief. The story says that when Siddhartha Gautama was about 12 years old, the brahmins – members of the highest Hindu class, who were priests, teachers, and overall protectors of sacred learning – gave the prophecy that Siddhartha Gautama would either be a collective ruler or a celebrated holy man. His father kept him confined with the palace walls, where Siddhartha Gautama grew up in luxury. He was held within the castle walls to prevent him from becoming a holy man, also known as an ascetic. An ascetic one who practices self-denial to the extreme, leading a simple life while pursuing spiritual goals. It was not the life his father wanted for him, so he shielded his son from the outside world in hopes that Siddhartha Gautama would grow to be a great ruler.

Siddhartha Gautama was trained to swim and wrestle and train in archery and as a swordsman. Siddhartha Gautama eventually married his cousin, and they soon had a child, a son. It was not uncommon for royal families to marry among themselves because no other people were considered equal; they wanted to keep the royal line pure. Siddhartha Gautama's life was full and rich – in today's world, he would be one of those who have everything – wealth, luxury, a wife, and a child. With all of this happiness and luxury, what possible reason was there for Siddhartha Gautama to feel unsatisfied?

There was a longing inside of Siddhartha Gautama, a need to know more, a feeling of dissatisfaction with the life surrounding him. This longing led him to explore the world outside of the palace walls. In Kapilavastu, he came across three things: an older adult, a sick man, and a dead body being taken to the grounds for burning.

Siddhartha Gautama had never seen such things before during his sheltered existence – he was not prepared; he did not understand what was happening before him. His chariot driver simplified it for him – every living being gets older, faces sickness, and eventually dies. This information caused great worry and uneasiness inside of Siddhartha Gautama.

He saw an ascetic dressed in a robe and carrying a bowl of a sadhu or a holy man on the way back to the palace. It was then that Siddhartha Gautama vowed to leave his life of luxury in the castle, as well as his wife and child, to find the solution to all of the suffering in the world. He never woke his wife and son up to bid them goodbye; instead, he said his goodbyes under cover of darkness, and he disappeared into the woods. Siddhartha Gautama used his sword to cut his long hair and donned a simple robe – an ascetic robe.

When Siddhartha Gautama decided to leave behind his royal life for that of an ascetic, he joined an entire group of men who had also left their lives behind. All of these men, including Siddhartha Gautama, were searching for blissful deliverance from individuality and suffering from the cycle of life – birth to death. Arada Kalama was his first teacher. Arada Kalama had more than 300 disciples learning his philosophy. He taught Siddhartha Gautama to train his mind to enter a state of emptiness, of nothingness. It took great discipline to reach this level of mindful peace. However, Siddhartha Gautama knew that this was not the liberation, the deliverance that he sought, so he left Arada Kalama's teachings, and he moved on to Udraka Ramaputra. Here, he was taught to enter a realm of his mind through concentration, a not conscious or unconscious kingdom. But again, he was dissatisfied with what he learned because he knew it was not true liberation.

They no longer have to sit through what Buddhists believe to be an endless cycle of suffering known as life.

The path of Enlightenment has a few principles that are the foundation of Buddha's teachings. These principles are divided into three categories, which are prajna, sila, and samadhi.

Prajna

One of the first principles of the Buddhist path is prajna, also known as wisdom. Prajna is regarded as Enlightenment, which is the main focus of Buddhism. When it comes to prajna, understanding is a lot different than knowledge. Knowledge is what you know, a collection of facts. Wisdom comes out when you are most calm and pure. It's obtained through meditation and cultivation and comes at the end of your path.

Sila

The word sila translates to moral values and is essential in the path's progress as it's the foundation of qualities. There are two principles that sila is based on, and these are the principles of reciprocity and equality. When Buddhists talk about the direction of equality, they are speaking about the equality of all living things, including the equality of security and happiness.

Samadhi

Samadhi translates to mediation. As a Buddhist, you want to obtain pure freedom, which you can do through mental development. You need to purify the mind, and the only way to do this is through meditation or samadhi.

When you hear the word suffering, you may have images of pain and anger come into your mind, but they believe that all life is suffering in Buddhism. As humans, we feel the pain of loss, the emotions of sadness, happiness, disappointment, and so on. These emotions are manifestations of our mind, and they do not come from our inner selves. Because they do not come from our true selves, they are thought of as suffering. These are false feelings created by the meat of our brains, programmed into us by what our societal view has taught us. The way forward was through following the Noble Eightfold Path, which allowed people to be closer to Enlightenment's potential.

Currently, Buddhism is increasingly becoming a popular way of life for millions of people worldwide. Even those in the Western countries seek to follow The Middle Path because they find that it speaks to their heart. There is also the fact that traditional medicines do very little for the status quo. For example, if you are depressed or unable to deal with your feelings, scientists have established that the Buddhist way offers you a better and more permanent solution to your problems. Medical findings that explored the relationship between the Buddhist practice and how the brain operated found that Buddhist monks simultaneously use the brain's creative side and the brain's calculating side. They were, therefore, more open to creativity.

In a world where everything is always in motion, continually forcing us to move forward faster and more rapidly, many people feel the loss of their connection with nature.

Though nature is all around us, even in the major cities, what we have done to change Earth's pure form creates a disconnect from our minds. In Buddhism, you are connected to every natural thing in this world, and by practicing its teachings, you are brought back to that connection. It is an enormous draw for millions of people around the globe. You can think of it as connecting back to your roots.

If you are unsure of what this means, you only have to see what happens when you go somewhere you find inspiring. The feelings that you experience don't just come from external stimuli. They come from your inner self-recognizing the joy that lies in that ever-moving thing called nature.

This lack of an invisible deity often speaks to those that cannot find solace or belief in other religions where God is their governing body. Though there are many tales and teachings in Buddhism, there is no one holy book such as the Bible or Quran. Instead, the "bible" of Buddhism can be found in every natural effect on the planet, from the leaves on the trees to the worms in the ground. They are the past story, but you don't need to look to the past to find Enlightenment.

Moreover, the belief system of Buddhism can be described as "large-minded." It is not uncommon to find those of different religious backgrounds meditating together at various Buddhist centers, especially in the western world. Enlightenment, in Buddhism, is not based on who you believe created you, but rather by opening your mind enough to allow yourself to shine through. Once that is reached, all the answers you seek on creation will be known to you. Therefore, your title of faith is of no concern, though those who strive for Enlightenment usually find themselves identifying as Buddhist or other similar namesakes. Instead, they only explain if asked. The Life of the Buddha, the

Dharma is the doctrine and cornerstone of the philosophy of these religions. In the practical sense, it encompasses ethics, rituals, obligations, code of conduct, and virtually anything else that comes into a devout follower's life. The Sanskrit word "dharma" has proven difficult to translate directly, but its meaning is relatively concise in Buddhism. Dharma denotes "cosmic law and order," one of the most common translations of the word. The same term is also ascribed to all that the Buddha has taught to his followers – the Buddhist dharma. Therefore, it's not uncommon for "dharma" and "the Buddha's teaching" to be used interchangeably.

Interestingly, various Hindu scriptures and teachings have spoken of the Buddha and acknowledged his existence and life's work. Depending on the different Hindu traditions, the Buddha was more than just mentioned in passing. While followers of some traditions believe the Buddha to have simply been a holy man, others view him as one of Lord Vishnu's earthly incarnations, which would make him divine. However, as we proceed, you will find that this is the diametric opposite of how Buddhists perceive the Buddha because they tie no divinity concept to the Buddha.

The most significant overlap between Hindu's and Buddhists' beliefs is perhaps the concepts of Karma and rebirth. We will detail these later on, but the ideas are very similar between the two religions, with some key differences.

These are just some of the significant similarities, though, and the two major religions overlap even further in many other beliefs that are important to their philosophy. Meditation, for instance, is a crucial practice that Buddhists put great emphasis on, and the same holds for Hinduism. It illustrates that both religions' focus is primarily on the believer's inner state relates to the outside world. In that regard, both Hinduism and Buddhism also promote the virtue of detachment from all earthly things in a material as well as a mental sense.

Unlike Hinduism, however, Buddhism does not delve too deeply into the ceremonial or ritual practices found in most major religions. It might seem counterintuitive at first if you ascribe ritualistic connotations to meditation. That would be a very wrong way of looking at it because meditation has virtually nothing to do with rituals. Later on, as you will learn, meditation is a Buddhist's life's work in a sense, and it's a rather personal matter. A devout Buddhist works on his introspection and strives to perfect it from one day to the next, and you will see why as you read more.

The spread of Buddhist teachings was only gradual at first, though. But a great wind that would push the religion to new heights came when Buddhists received open support from Ashoka, the emperor. He held reign over the largest part of the Indian subcontinent in the 3rd century BCE as sovereign of the Maurya Empire. Ashoka was a great admirer of the Buddhist approach to spirituality, and he supported the faith with great enthusiasm. It is evident by inscriptions and carvings left behind him, which told his support and Buddhism's subsequent spread. This support continued through those who descended from Ashoka, and the extensive empire ultimately managed to successfully spread the Buddhist truth far and wide, beyond its borders to the north. These efforts also facilitated Buddhism's spread into Sri Lanka, where the Theravada tradition maintains a firm foothold today. Buddhism was also spreading westward over the subsequent centuries, and it may have gone much further had its spread not been halted in Persia in the 3rd century CE.

Looking at things from a certain angle, it could also be said that Buddhism came about as a product of its zeitgeist. It was a time when more and more intellectuals of varying prominence levels began questioning the traditional Vedic teachings and philosophies throughout Ancient India, giving way too many new ideas, one of which was undoubtedly the philosophy of Siddhartha Gautama. It was also the era that gave birth to Jainism, another Indian religion often compared to Buddhism. We'll look deeper into that comparison a bit later.

Chapter 3. Intelligence Beyond the Self, the Four Noble Truths

The Four Noble Truths are understood and accepted by the Buddhas as the actual reality. Buddhist teachings reveal that the Buddha began teaching the Four Noble Truths as soon as he had experienced Enlightenment.

According to these truths, all beings crave and cling to things and states that are not permanent. It leads to suffering, which in turn traps the beings who are stuck in the never-ending cycle of rebirth, suffering, and dying.

However, a path leads beyond this cycle. It is through the Fourth Noble Truth: The Middle Path. The Buddhas encourage those who wish to be awakened from the revolution, not just to understand but also to experience The Middle Path.

To understand and practice the Middle Path, it is a prerequisite first to understand all Four Noble Truths. Emeritus Professor Geoffrey Samuels, who played a crucial role in bringing Buddhism's teachings to the Western world, explained that the Four Noble Truths reveal what needs to be understood to begin the path that leads to Enlightenment.

Here are the Four Noble Truths:

Desire or Suffering (Dukkha)

The First Noble Truth teaches that one's desires are impossible to satisfy, and this causes pain or suffering.

Some liken the Four Noble Truths to be analogous to traditional Indian medicine, with the First Noble Truth being the diagnosis. In other words, it identifies and seeks to describe the disease in the form of Desire or Suffering. Some see this Noble Truth as a mere acknowledgment of the fact that people do suffer. If it's easier to understand in that way, by all means, adopt this stance while keeping your mind open to other interpretations.

Try the following exercise to consider how the First Noble Truth applies to your own life. Pause and reflect for a while on whether you have ever experienced feeling permanently satisfied. When you come to think of it, the concept of setting and attaining goals often leads to even more aspirations.

We, as humans, are in a constant cycle of yearning for a satisfying end to everything we do. However, this is impossible to do since achieving one goal, object, relationship, etc., opens doors to the next. In today's society of excess, it is even more challenging to find yourself satisfied. When we finally reach that financial goal for retirement, we strive to live other experiences that will satisfy us at the moment. Unfortunately, without realizing it, we spend our entire lives searching and wandering, attempting to fulfill a want that cannot be fulfilled. From the food we eat, the jobs we have, the money we make, and even the objects we desire, we are always searching for something we deem as "better."

Thirst or Craving (Samudaya)

The Second Noble Truth describes the primary source of Desire or Suffering, and it is one's "thirst" or craving for something in this world, which is impermanent. Your thirst or hunger creates Karma, which then causes a change in you that would only lead to a new desire. Thus, if you want this explained, it means that all suffering has a cause.

If you compare the Second Noble Truth with a medical diagnosis, you can describe it as the step to determine the root cause of the disease or the etiology.

To understand how the Second Noble Truth unfolds in your life, try to recall the last time you experienced pain and then reflect on what exactly caused it. Buddhists accept that when there is pain, there will always be a cause of that pain, no matter whether that is physical or mental pain. There are still reasons for this pain to happen.

Cessation of Desire or Suffering (Naroda)

The Third Noble Truth teaches that to end one's Thirst or Craving will lead to the end of suffering. It is only through this that Karma would no longer be created, and therefore one is awakened from the cycle.

Going back to the medical analogy concept, you could compare the Third Noble Truth with determining the cure for the disease or the prognosis.

The concept seems straightforward and straightforward, but its practice is what appears to cause us to continue in this self-absorbed cycle. Though you may think that you are kind, generous, and always helping, it is essential to realize that self-absorbed is not meant from a selfish standpoint, but in a way where your mind is creating these feelings to entice it to continue forward-looking to satisfy your next urge.

The Middle Path (Magga)

The Fourth Noble Truth explains that the only way to achieve Enlightenment is through the Noble Eightfold Path or the Middle Path's discernment and practice. The Middle Path symbol is the dharma wheel (dharma chakra), which has eight spokes representing its elements.

If you compare it with the medical diagnosis, the Fourth Noble Truth represents the part where the physician prescribes the right treatment for the disease that can help you cure it.

Buddhist teachers usually divide the Noble Eightfold Path into three core divisions: Wisdom, Moral virtue, and Meditation. Below is a comprehensive list of how each component of the Noble Eightfold Path fits into each category.

Meditation

Another word for meditation is Samadhi, and it is the final division of the Noble Eightfold Path. The whole concept centers on the conditioning of one's mind to install discernment into the Three Marks of Existence, let go of unhelpful states and reach Enlightenment. Full knowledge and dedication to practicing the final three of the Noble Eightfold Path – Right Effort, Right Mindfulness, and Right Samadhi – will fulfill these.

1.   Right Effort

Buddhist teachings describe Right Effort as your strength of will and mind as you choose to do good each day. It has the self-discipline to choose to think, feel, speak, and do what is right, even when challenging.

According to most Buddhist teachers, it requires more Right Effort to abstain from ill will and sensual desires. Ill-will includes anger, resentment, and hatred towards all other beings, while sensual desires are all sinful desires experienced through the five senses.

Your body is your temple, the avenue through which your true self can work to attempt to reach Enlightenment. Anything negative should be abstained from.

You may find this hard at first since your mind is accustomed to being distracted. However, when you learn to meditate and put the right amount of concentration into what you are doing, you will have fulfilled this requirement. You may find that you cannot let go of thoughts that are not relevant to the meditation process. However, everyone is guilty of this when they first try to meditate. If you can simply work your way through dismissing irrelevant thoughts, you will increase your effort.

Do not be harsh on yourself for this failure. It takes a while to be able to meditate. As long as you are making an effort, you understand what meditation is all about.

2.   Right Mindfulness

When being conscious of your body, you acknowledge and accept it for what it is. The same goes for one's emotions and thoughts. As you become aware of and recognize these states, you let go of worldly desires and all suffering attached to them.

One of the things that many Buddhists practice regularly is extreme mindfulness of thought. When you are stricken with emotion, especially the negative ones, you want to step back and take a pause. Realize that that emotion is created by your conscious mind and depends on your cultural understanding of the world around you. Once you understand the sentiment, you are feeling, gently remind yourself that it is not the truth. It does not merely come from your true self to explain it, and therefore it is not real.

Right mindfulness also covers letting go of those things that are of the past or perhaps worries that relate to the future. Mindfulness is indeed in this moment. If you look back in this book, you will be reminded of the Dalai Lama quotation, explaining mindfulness very eloquently. Mindful people are ever-present, and it is hard to reach Enlightenment unless you have that presence and understand its significance.

3.   Right Samadhi (or the state of intense concentration)

The final step in the Noble Eightfold Path, Right Samadhi, is about detaching yourself from desires related to the senses and from unwholesome states.

Then, you enter the first level of concentration called the first jhana. On this level, you maintain applied and sustained thinking, which will lead you to experience happiness gained from these detachments as you continue to concentrate.

Chapter 4. The Three Steps of the Way

A person who wants to enter Buddhism must first learn Buddhist morality and live accordingly. It is the first step, which is to cultivate character in one's behavior. Second, she should develop her mind with a wholesome attitude of thought. This step involves studying Buddhist scriptures and growing right views, free from ignorance and wrong ideas about life. The third step is to cultivate wisdom; this means seeing through the illusions of existence.

By following these steps, a person will gradually develop the ability to see things as they indeed are. Even if she learns many Buddhist doctrines and understands them, if at the same time she does not cultivate morality and mental development of wisdom, the result will be like that of a blind person who can explain in detail what an elephant looks like but cannot distinguish between one side and another.

Morality

A mind clouded by ignorance cannot know reality; it imagines everything as permanent, pleasant, and satisfying. Ignorance breeds desire, anger, fear, and greed. There are only suffering existences; all worldly existence is impermanent. Pleasures are not at all permanent; they always change into something else. The ultimate goal of life is happiness, but even the happiest moments will change into suffering because all things are impermanent. It is why we suffer.

Buddhism teaches us to transform this unsatisfactory and painful world into a pure land by practicing morality, cultivating wisdom, and developing our minds to obtain peace of mind so that our body and speech can express nobility.

Without this transformation, society cannot avoid the suffering it experiences daily. Therefore, morality is the first step on the path to free ourselves from wholesome or unwholesome actions; this is called self-control. Through the character, we can overcome our mental and spiritual weaknesses and realize the potential for the healthy development of mind, speech, and body. Once morality is developed, wisdom can be cultivated.

Wisdom

In Buddhism, wisdom is called prajna. It means understanding the true nature of reality through meditation. Some people say that Buddhism meditation does not exist; however, if someone goes to a Buddhist learning center for ten years without knowing about meditation or having any personal experience with it, that person will have learned nothing. Meditation is practiced to experience reality's true nature; this cannot be achieved without developing concentration and insight through a qualified teacher's technique.

When a person who desires to practice meditation learns the method from a qualified teacher, she begins by learning to sit properly. It helps to develop the power of concentration needed for the development of wisdom. It is why a practitioner must learn how to sit properly with her back straight and her head erect. She should also practice breathing exercises to help develop concentration, focusing on one subject uninterrupted for a long time. This kind of concentration develops in two different ways:

1. through physical means (as in breathing exercises), and

2. through mental means (as in mantra recitation).

The result of physical concentration is peace and stability. The effect of mental concentration is wisdom, which depends on one's ability to focus the mind on a single subject for long periods without being distracted.

From the beginning, one should practice focusing on a small detail, such as a pebble or leaf, or flower. After some time has passed, she can gradually expand her concentration to include more objects, such as branches of trees and then whole trees and so forth. The practitioner must continue to concentrate until the illusion created by her mind vanishes and actual reality is revealed. It is called "no self," meaning that she will see everything as empty because she will realize that there is no entity within phenomena. In this way, she will see the true nature of reality.

In the beginning, we should learn about the proper method from someone who has mastered it and then practices until we can do it without thinking about how we are doing it.

Mental Development

The concentration method should include stopping all thoughts by focusing on one object until there are no longer any obstacles for attaining higher concentration levels. If you reach the proper concentration stage, when you hear a sound or see a form, you will not be distracted by it. If you are distracted, it is because your concentration is weak. If you are not distracted even by loud sounds, it means that you have attained the first level of attention called "access concentration."

After attaining access concentration, no matter what thoughts or feelings arise from your mind, continue to focus on your object. It is called the second level of engagement, "absorption concentration." No matter what kind of thought arises during absorption concentration, continue to focus on your object without being disturbed. It is called the third level of attention, "momentary concentration."

This practice is the only way to reveal impermanence, suffering, and non-self. If you do not practice meditation, you will never understand the true nature of reality. All Buddhas and Bodhisattvas, those who possess perfect Enlightenment, attained it through meditation. Without it, they could not have achieved Enlightenment.

The Buddha said that when someone attains mindfulness or clear comprehension through meditation, she can see things as they are without any obstacles in her mind. People must develop concentration to understand impermanence as the Buddha taught us to do in his first sermon about impermanence: "All phenomena are impermanent; work happily for your liberation. All phenomena are painful; work happily for your liberation."

To work happily for happiness, we should first work to be liberated from mental and physical suffering by practicing meditation. We also need to understand that all things are impermanent and empty; therefore, they cannot bring us real or lasting happiness. It is why the Buddha said, "All phenomena are impermanent; work happily for your liberation." Working to be liberated from the sufferings of birth, old age, sickness, and death is the only way to achieve true happiness.

Every spiritual teaching begins with concentration because developing concentration is what leads us to insight or understanding. Therefore, without engagement, there can be no insight or wisdom.

We can also understand this from the teaching of the Four Noble Truths. The first truth, "All life is suffering," is a truth that can only be understood by those with concentrated minds, not distracted minds. People who are not concentrated cannot even see what is happening around them. Even if they saw it, they could not understand it because being distracted makes it impossible to see things as they are.

Just as we cannot understand what we experience in our daily lives when our minds are distracted, we cannot comprehend the first noble truth of suffering without developing concentration. It is why attention must come before insight; otherwise, understanding will be incomplete.

Sakyamuni Buddha taught that people are going through the cycle of birth, old age, and death because they do not know the Four Noble Truths. If we want to understand our experience, we need to be careful and try not to get distracted by things that cause suffering.

It is why meditating on suffering is the only correct way to contemplate it. When people practice this contemplation for a long time, they will develop insight into these truths. They will be able to give up all kinds of suffering and mental defilements such as sensual desire, ill-will, pride, and ignorance. When we have exhausted all of our mental defilements, we become liberated from them.

Chapter 5. Karma

What is Karma?

Strictly speaking, the meaning of Karma refers to any action, intent, and deed by a being. It summarizes the spiritual tenet of cause and effect, wherein the actions and intentions help shape the future of that being.

In a general sense, having good intentions and doing good deeds strengthen good Karma and promote the possibility of happiness in the future. On the other hand, having lousy intent and doing evil deeds can lead to bad Karma and, hence, the chance of experiencing pain and suffering.

In traditional Buddhism, Karma specifically refers to action based on the being's intentions. Such intentions would then determine the being's cycle of rebirth. The word used to describe the "effect" of Karma is Kampala. You can think of Karma as the seed and karmaphalas as the fruit of that seed.

For now, let us define it as the cycle of birth and death within the six realms of the mundane world, driven by ignorance, desire, and hatred.

Laws of Karma According to Buddhism

The literal meaning of Karma is to do, to make, or to cause. It comes from "kárma" in Sanskrit, to do. The common idea is that it's synonymous with cause and effect; you're doing something, and then you're reaping the consequences. It's translated in this way under Hinduism and other Eastern cultures. It's the catalyst that triggers the kind of life you have nowadays. If someone goes through struggles, it is because they are meant to purge past life actions.

Though initially is recording the sense of Karma was Hinduism, the religion, its root, is currently in Buddhism. Both agree that the natural laws of cause and effect are sufficient to explain how Karma works; if you do good deeds, you get the gain in this or the next life.

According to Hinduism's latest writings, Karma can be created in four ways: feelings, words, acts motivated by others, and oneself. Buddhism contemplates another theory of the nature of the cause and effect of Karma, which also aligns with this, only with five categories: impact of our behavior, seasonal changes, instincts of nature, rules of inheritance and will consist of mind.

Jainism is an exciting alternative to what Karma is. Karma is represented under this theory by particles that vibrate according to the mind, body, and speech. The present lives are the product of Karma and our present-day soul or consciousness. There is no higher outside entity that manages the concept of cause and effect.

Buddhism is a philosophy and religion made up of practical teachings, such as meditation, which aims to induce a transformation within those who practice it. To reach a state of Enlightenment encourages the creation of wisdom, knowledge, and kindness.

Existence is viewed in Buddhism as a constant state of transition. The prerequisite for us to take advantage of these changes is creating discipline in our minds. It would concentrate on favorable conditions, such as concentration and calmness.

The course aims to develop the emotions linked to understanding, happiness, and love. Therefore, all spiritual growth for Buddhism is materialized and complemented by social work, ethics, and philosophy research.

The Twelve Karma Rules

Similar to Buddhism, these are the 12 rules of Karma:

The great law: this law in the sentence "we reap what we sow" can be summed up. It is called the law of cause and effect: what we give to the world is what the world gives us back, but if it is anything negative, it will be multiplied by ten to return to us. If we give love, we receive love, but we get anger multiplied by ten if we give hate.

The rule of creation: we have to be part of life. We are part of the universe, and with it, we form a unity. Everything we see around us is a testament to our distant history. Create the lifelong options you want.

Humility law: that which we fail to recognize will continue to happen to us. If we can see only the negative aspects of others, we will be stopped at a lower level of existence. When, on the contrary, we humbly embrace what is happening to us, we will go up to a higher degree.

Growth law: wherever we go, here is where we are going to be. We have to continue and grow in our faith in the face of events, places, and men, and not what is around us. When we change our inside, we change our life.

Responsibility law: it is because there is something terrible about us that happens to us. Our reflex is about the surroundings. And we have to face our life circumstances responsibly.

The law of connection: all we do is connected to the world; however trivial it might seem. The first step leads to the last, and both are equally necessary as they are required to achieve our goals together. It interconnects current, future, and history.

Focus law: Two things cannot be thought about simultaneously. We went up slowly, one at a time. We cannot lose sight of our ambitions because fear and rage take hold of us at those moments.

Law of giving and hospitality: if you dream of anything that may be real, then the time will come when you will be able to prove it is. We must learn to offer and bring all that has been learned into action.

The rule of the here and now: being trapped in the past makes loving the present difficult. Repetitive thoughts, poor habits, and unfulfilled dreams make it difficult for us to move forward and renew our spirit.

Law of change: History must repeat itself until the lessons we need to learn are assimilated. When a troublesome circumstance presents itself many times, we must gain some information from it. We must map our course and follow it.

Patience and Reward Law: Rewards are the product of earlier actions. Hence more outstanding commitment, more significant effort leads to more gratifications. It is a patient and persevering work that bears fruit. We will learn to enjoy our role in the world; our efforts will be honored at the right moment.

Essential and motivating law: the importance of our triumphs and mistakes depends on the purpose and the time we expend to achieve the goal. We contribute to a universe personally, and so our acts cannot be mediocre: we have to bring all our hearts into what we do.

Karma as a Process

According to the Buddha, Karma is not an all-around determinant but rather a part of the factors that affect the future, with other factors being detailed and about the nature of the being. It moves in a fluid and dynamic way rather than in a mechanical, linear manner. Not all factors in the present can be attributed to Karma.

Be careful not to define Karma as "fate" or "foreordination." Karma is not some form of divine judgment imposed on beings that did good or bad things. Instead, it is the natural result of the process.

In other words, doing a good deed would not automatically entitle you to a future of happiness, and vice versa. After all, while specific experiences in your life are due to your past actions, how you respond to them is not yet determined. Of course, such responses to circumstances would then lead to their consequences in the future.

Karma as Energy

All beings continuously change due to Karma. For every thought, action, and word being produced, a kind of energy is released in different directions into the universe. These energies can influence and change all other beings, including the being that sends the power.

Think of the following scenario:

Janice and Carrie work in the same office with three other people. Janice notices that Carrie is continuously late and contributes low output to the team, if any at all. Because of this, Janice is irritated at Carrie. Each morning, whenever she sees Carrie at the office, she thinks Carrie is so annoying and incompetent. She should be fired. After weeks of entertaining such thoughts, she then decided to talk to her three co-workers regarding Carrie.

Chapter 6. Rebirth, The Effects of Karma on the Next Life

What is Rebirth?

Karma begets Karma - this is the essence of rebirth. Rebirth refers to the infinity of karmic tendencies. Thus, if you have good karmic tendencies, they will bring forth new good karmic tendencies. Unless you disrupt it by evil Karma, this process of good karmic tendencies will continue ad infinitum, and you will contribute to the better being of this world and yourself.

Understanding Rebirth

Death is but an impermanent end to an impermanent existence.

Through powerful meditation, one can recall one's past lives. If you possess this ability, you'll be able to put your present life into a meaningful perspective.

Karma and Reincarnation provide us with a plausible explanation for inequality. It shows why some men are born rich while others are born poor, why some babies are healthy while others are disabled. For some, this may be a pretty hard pill to swallow.

The belief in the cycle of rebirth is present in most of the major Indian religions, and it is most commonly called "samsara," which means "wandering." It is also one of Hinduism's core concepts, but Buddhism takes a somewhat different approach to this cycle's position. While Hinduism focuses much of its philosophy on the "atman," or soul, as the core of our being reincarnated repeatedly in samsara, Buddhism rejects the idea of soul or self altogether. The belief that we possess no soul and that self is an illusion of one of the Three Marks of Existence, which we will cover in more detail soon. All things considered, although Buddhist's view samsara as a painful cycle of suffering, it's important to note that each lifetime, no matter how difficult, isn't damnation.

The condition you have been born in reflects the lesson you need to learn in this lifetime. For instance, a person may be born rich because he needs to know the value of generosity. Alternatively, a person may be born poor because he needs to learn the value of hard work.

A common question asked by skeptics is this: If our souls never indeed die and if we are continually reborn in each lifetime, how does that explain that the world is more populated today than it was decades ago?

The human realm is but one of many other domains. When we pass on, we may end up in other realms. There are heavenly realms and lower realms. There are animal realms and ghostly realms. Likewise, beings from other domains may also be reborn into the human realm. Simply put, you could've been dwelling in another realm before you were reborn here in your present life. By understanding that we continuously come and go between these various realms, we gain more profound respect and empathy for other beings.

To be exact, most Buddhist teachings explain six realms of existence into which sentient beings are spawned. Those are the three higher realms of gods, demigods, humans, and three lower realms of animals, hungry ghosts, hell, or hell-beings. Sometimes, the kingdoms are viewed as only five, with the empires of gods and demigods being the same, which would make the human realm the second highest one.

Without reaching Nirvana or Buddhahood, being reborn into the realm of gods is the next best outcome one can hope for, resulting from the accumulation of perfect karma. There is one catch associated with this realm, though, which is precisely the fact that it is a heavenly environment. Namely, it is said that the joy, luxury, and ease of life in this realm pose a problem in that a person is prone to getting too attached, which constitutes terrible karma, of course. Therefore, if one who spawns into the godly realm is not careful and neglects their spirituality, it's quite likely that the next life will land him or her in a lower realm.

As for our human realm, even though it is primarily plagued by suffering and misfortune, it is still considered a reasonably fortunate outcome of one's karmic performance. Humans possess higher sentience and thus much freer will and independence of thought than other animals, which puts us in a position of ample opportunity to better our karma. It is said that animals suffer immensely due to them being ruled by raw instincts that they can't control.

Of course, the last two realms are the harshest. Those born into the realm of hungry ghosts will find themselves as creatures of great craving, hunger, and thirst. The fact that they are reduced to existing as subtle, invisible beings is also said to cause much suffering. That still doesn't compare to the hellish realm reserved for those that have accumulated significant evil karma. There are many descriptions of this realm across various traditions and texts, including multiple levels of scorching or freezing areas, realms of torture and great pain, and others.

You may be wondering how one gets out of these realms, mainly since there is a lack of awareness and free will to conduct good karma. In essence, the demerit that one acquires through terrible karma runs a specific course and eventually is depleted. According to one's degree of wrongdoing, particular lengths of time and punishment in hellish realms will be dished out to individuals. Remember, nothing in Buddhism is forever, and everyone can end their cycle of suffering.

Sooner or later, one will move up the bar ever so slightly and is presented with a chance to do better. Technically, one can be stuck in the lower realms indefinitely, but that will always be up to them personally. And while many of the rebirths into the human realm can be quite painful and tough on people, they should never forget that, unlike animals, they can commit to their karmic outcome truly and significantly accelerate the accumulation of good karma.

You might be wondering if that lack of free will in the lower realms means that karma can't get worse, in addition to there being no way to improve it. In general, this would be a correct assumption due to that fundamental issue of free will. To put it simply, there exist multiple realms that are below and are worse than the human one primarily to account for various levels of evil karma that people acquire, not because animals or hungry ghosts can do evil deeds and get themselves reborn into an even lower realm. Buddhists generally believe that animals and other inferior creatures are incapable of really doing any wrong, just as they are incapable of doing good. When animals kill, they do so out of necessity and a need for food or basic survival, not because they like it or following an ideology. Therefore, all there is for animals and other lower beings to do is live out their lives and wait for their bad karma to run out. It is life in one of the higher, conscious realms that determine how lowly you will be reborn, based on how evil your karma is. Animals generally can't find themselves reborn into the realms of hungry ghosts or hell. Instead, they can either remain in their domain or move up after they die.

About the Tibetan Book of the Dead

Those who have heard a few things about Buddhism in passing may have, at some point, also heard of something that is commonly referred to as the "Tibetan Book of the Dead." This piece of literature is intimately concerned with the concept of rebirth and death itself, but it's not quite as eerie as it first sounds. The Book of the Dead does not contain instructions on how to raise the dead or contact wandering spirits, but it is indeed a sort of manual.

The way that this book came to be in its current form in the West is quite a long story, but far more critical are its origins and subject matter. With all its gradual additions, reinterpretations, adaptations, and revisions, this "book" is rooted in the old literature of Bardo Thodol, meaning "The Great Liberation through Hearing in the Intermediate State." Various research efforts have uncovered that Bardo Thodol was most likely authored in the 8th century, after which it was buried at some point until being unearthed and revealed to the world by Karma Lingpa, a 14th-century man who is believed to have been a Nyingma teacher.

Chapter 7. Interdependent Origin

Buddhism began in northern India around 500 BC. The Buddhist tradition is named after a follower known as the Buddha or the Awakened. He was born in a region of north India, located today in southern Nepal. It was only a part of the large undifferentiated geographical unit that now refers to the Indian subcontinent.

The Buddha is the image of calm and contemplation. These are the experience of awakening, but the Buddha did not always sit in perfect reflection.

Upon awakening, he rose from his enlightened state and spoke to others on northern India's streets.

His life's main events occurred in the Ganges' so-called central region, which is still the Buddhist pilgrimage site.

In India itself, two major reform movements did not occur in the Buddhist community too long after the life of the Buddha:

• The Theravada: "The Teaching of the Elderly." These are a consciously conservative tradition. It starts in India and is practiced today in Southeast Asia: Thailand, Burma, and Sri Lanka. Try to reapply the practices of the first Buddhist community during the life of the Buddha.

• The Mahayana: "The big vehicle." It is a reform movement that has radically changed. Mahayana spread in different variants in China, Tibet, Japan, Korea, and Vietnam.

Before these movements grew in India, Buddhism was brought to Sri Lanka, just outside India's southern tip. Transported by Buddhist missionaries in the 3rd century BC From Sri Lanka, Buddhism brought to most Southeast Asia, including Indonesia.

Buddhism moved to India's northern part in China in the second century of the common era, transported north by monks. Merchants on the trade routes that stretched over India, Afghanistan, and then on the great trade routes called "silk "road" moved through central Asia and the main mercantile centers of northern China.

Here Buddhism encountered a sophisticated and ancient civilization. From China, Buddhism was eventually brought to Korea, Japan, and Vietnam. You could put together Korean, Japanese, and Vietnamese Buddhism as expressions of this significant East Asia strand.

Buddhism was transported across the Himalayas from India to Tibet. Today, the Dalai Lama, who is the head of the Tibetan Buddhist community, is one of the most visible Buddhist leaders and, in my opinion, one of the most active in the world.

Today Buddhism is widespread in much of the world, including Europe, Australia, and the Americas.

Buddha Can Date to 1800 BC

One of the most critical calculations in Indian history was based on the life of a certain Indian emperor named Ashoka. He was a Buddhist emperor responsible for spreading Buddhism to distant parts of India and neighboring countries and sending many Buddhist missionaries to these places. He built thousands of Buddhist stupas and created thousands of Buddhist monasteries throughout his empire, stretching from Iran to Bangladesh and Central Asia (Afghanistan) to southern India. Many stones and pillars, which existed throughout his kingdom, bore his edicts and proclamations on his subjects, written in Magadhi, Sanskrit, Greek, and Arabic. At first, he was a cruel king, killing many of his brothers to ascend to the throne. He inherited a vast empire and tried to expand it by fighting against the neighboring kingdom of Kalinga. He won the battle, but thousands of mutilated corpses' cruel sight during the war has completely changed his heart.

Several traditional historians are not aware of this controversy. They reject Megatheres as an unreliable writer and dismiss Indian scriptures as pure mythology. And almost all legal historians are blissfully unaware of the existence of two Ashoka's in Indian history. A handful of Indian historians know of this problem; they suggested that the Ashoka of Buddhist sources belong to the Gupta dynasty and ruled India around 300 BC. However, the Buddhist scriptures speak of Emperor Ashoka as belonging to the Mauryan dynasty, denying the arguments of the few Indian historians trying to get out of the riddle. It was the greatest enigma that has haunted Indian historical calculations for more than a century, almost like a mystery to Sherlock Holmes and Hercules Poirot.

Ashoka's rock edicts mention that Ashoka converted to Buddhism because of the remorse he felt for Kalinga's war. However, both Indian and Sri Lankan Buddhist scripts differ from this; these writings do not speak of Kalinga's war! They talk of Ashoka converted from the serene teachings of a certain Buddhist monk who is a novice Samudra/Nyagrodha15.

Why are Buddhist scriptures silent about Kalinga's war?

While the scriptures speak of 84,000 monasteries established by Ashoka, the proclamations are silent about this; they mention no activity related to Ashoka Buddhism. The Buddhist scriptures say of Ashokan missionary activities in Kashmir, Maharashtra, Sri Lanka, Burma, Thailand, Mysore, Himalaya, western India, and the Greek country. The Scriptures do not speak of officials called Dharma Mahapatra's in his kingdom, as the mandates profess. It was desperate to be known as the greatest of all the donors to the Buddha's faith. The Indian scriptures mention that it donated almost everything he had to Buddhist monasteries at the end of his life. He wanted to make sure that Buddhism spread throughout the world. In Bengal, a follower of Mahavira designed a photo showing the Buddha bowing at the feet of Mahavira. It decreed similarly on another occasion, promising gold to those who carried heads of killed non-Buddhists! And Ashoka has done everything to convert people to Buddhism, as some legends show. He wanted to turn his brother Veetashoka into Buddhism; to do this, he played a drama. One day invented his ministers to sit Vee Ashoka on the emperor's throne for a few minutes. Veetashoka told him that the death that hung in his head did not allow him to enjoy spiritual well-being. Ashoka then let him know, "On the off chance that you are absent to joys simply because of fast approaching passing.

The Ashoka of Rockedikte, however, gives an entirely different picture. In one decree, he confesses to the Buddha; but that's it. There is no evidence he has carried out missionary activities. None of his rock people mentions anything about the teachings of Buddha. The Ashoka of Rock Dedication speaks of the equality of all religions! One decree mentions:

The essentials can grow in different ways. Still, all of them have their restraint in the world. It is not without a good reason to praise one's religion or condemn the faith of others. If there is a cause for criticism, it should do mildly, but it is so. For this reason, it is better to have other religions. As a result, one's faith and other faiths benefit.

In contrast, one's religion and other religions are condemned differently; condemning others with the idea "Let me glorify my religion" only harms one's faith. Between the religions) Good to listen to and respect the teachings of others. Mistress of the Gods, King Payadas (Ashoka), wishes that all we should teach is other religions' ethical teachings. To those who are satisfied with their faith, the following should say: The lover of the gods, King Payadas (Ashoka), does not appreciate gifts and honors as much as he recognizes that the essence of all religions should grow. And for this purpose, many works - Dhamma Mahapatra's, Mahamatras, responsible for the women's quarters, officials responsible for remote areas, and other such officials. And the fruit of that is that your religion is growing, and the Dhamma is also becoming enlightened."

Some established historians could not explain these dichotomies and dismissed the Buddhist scriptures as unreliable. They focus exclusively on the rock arts to get an idea of the Ashokan's personality while relying on the Buddhist scriptures for historical purposes. We can see how selectively they treated the whole Ashokan episode - they dismissed Megatheres as a liar, rejected the Indian scriptures as pure mythology, shook off other Greek scriptures. They even turned away scriptures from the Buddhists! I think they have a lot to do when it comes to the Ashokan episode, though they believe currently their calculations are perfect.

He was a compulsive man, devout, and took steps to spread his religion far and wide by sending missionaries and buildings. The Buddhist scriptures speak of Ashoka, the Mauritian. The scriptures are mainly about India - Kashmir, Maharashtra, Mysore, Himalayas, West Indies. Buddhism was not widespread in India, so the scriptures speak of Buddhism's spread in India under the Moorish Emperor Ashoka.

The Ashoka of Edicts belongs to the Gupta dynasty of 300 BC. He was the one involved in the Kalinga War. It felt repentant and later converted to Buddhism. However, in his time, Buddhism was already widespread, and he did not have to send missionaries. Also, Buddhism experienced the surge of Shankaracharya in its day, and the Vedic religion made a comeback. Because of the theological attack of Shankaracharya, Buddhism was in a confused state regarding its ideology. Buddhism was in transition and offered little scope for missionary activity. So, Ashoka, the Gupta, was not in a bad mood about his religion but more tolerant of all faiths. And the places mentioned in its ordinances are mostly its neighboring kingdoms - the directives do not talk about India's locations.

The two Ashoka's are entirely different. If we think that the decrees have a place with one sovereign, while the stupas and religious communities have a home with another, the riddle is comprehended. Students of history combined the two Ashoka's into one.

So, if as per the Buddhist sacred writings, the date is 1500 BC. From the Buddhist Moorish Emperor Ashoka, we can rapidly get to the hour of the Buddha. Buddha goes before Ashoka by 200 and eighteen years. These would Buddha so somewhere close to 1700 BC. Chr. What's more, 1800 v. Chr. These relate roughly to the strict estimations, the Buddha's date to around 1800-1900 v. Chr. Dating.

Chapter 8. The Three Universal Characteristics

These three characteristics are always present or connected to the existence, and of which they speak to our nature of reality. They help us know what to do with this existence.

As it results of understanding these characteristics, we learn to develop the waiver or publication. When we realize that existence is universally characterized by impermanence, we give up the attachment to reality from suffering and not from the self. And once the attachment to existence is abandoned, we arrive at the threshold of Nibbana.

It is the purpose of understanding the three characteristics: it removes attachment, abandoning the illusion that leads us to think its wrong existence is permanent, pleasant, and connected to a self. It is the reason which the three characteristics are part of the content of wisdom

Buddhists believe that everything that exists in this world is subject to the following:

Anicca (Impermanence)

Everything in this universe has its limitation. Everything exists in its duration. When something appears, it will inevitably disappear just as surely as it had materialized.

It is where your Buddhist journey truly begins. Knowing what Anicca represents is the first step that every Buddhist takes, no matter if he or she ends up as a casual layperson practitioner, a researcher driven by curiosity, or a fully-fledged, ordained Buddhist monk devotes his entire life to the doctrine. More so than just knowing what it is and how it is defined, you must thoroughly consider impermanence. You have to ponder what it indeed implies for you, all your troubles or joy, and every single person you know and care about. Ultimately and preferably, it would help if you also meditated on the concept, as all genuinely devout Buddhists do.

You look around, and you see tangible objects. You derive comfort and safety from their solidity, from their permanence. Deep inside, you know that nothing in this world is permanent, and yet often, you choose to ignore that knowledge. That is where the problem lies. To successfully detach yourself from the material world, it is necessary to acknowledge Anicca. However, if you continue to nurture this kind of primordial ignorance, you will continue to fall prey to the poisons of hatred and envy.

In the usual spirit of the Buddha's teachings, this too is a concept that one can observe and draw their conclusion as to its validity. The way things work in nature as well as human history both tell the tale of impermanence. It is true of many great individuals and even empires, and although you could argue that at least their memory is permanent in the hearts and minds of others, it too will fade away given a long enough timeline. Please make no mistake; impermanence isn't law only in our realm either. Buddhism teaches that Anicca holds even in the realm of gods.

With that said, it is also a Buddhist belief that Nirvana is the one thing that is constant and permanent. Once a sentient being has achieved Nirvana, this state will never corrupt, come undone, or change in any way. Therefore, in the words of wisdom, Nirvana is "Nicca," meaning "constant" or "permanent."

Anicca or the Buddhist doctrine of impermanence is often referred to as one aspect of this faith that makes newcomers often misinterpret the religion as pessimistic or somehow inherently depressing. As you have indeed grasped by now, Buddhism is all about the contrary.

What I mean by this is that impermanence is, in many regards, excellent news for you. Incredibly comforting is that Anicca applies so broadly, both on the micro and macro levels of life. As long as you mind the concept of karma, knowing that nothing is permanent and that it ultimately does not matter can be a compelling motivator. This realization can push you to new lengths and help you achieve what you otherwise thought you never could. Even minor life's issues such as shyness, reluctance to take risks, and tiny, everyday frustrations can be done away with once you understand with all your heart that they are all transient. So, what if you embarrass yourself today while trying to achieve something you want, for instance

On the flip-side, you'd be right to wonder what the point of anything is when it's all impermanent and ultimately meaningless. Why even get out of bed and go about your daily duties and tasks if nothing is permanent? This kind of thinking almost always leads to destructive thoughts and actions, bound to gather bad karma over time and reflect poorly on the individual once his time in this life has come to an end. Buddhism still emphasizes our obligations and responsibilities because fulfilling them results in the accumulation of perfect karma. It's necessary to harbor the right thoughts and effect meaningful action if we improve our position in the cycle of rebirth, let alone if we strive to reach enlightenment.

The full embrace of Anicca is thus not meant to make us give up on life. Instead, it is intended to help you detach yourself and deal with the next, an all-important fact of life.

Dukkha (Suffering)

In essence, Buddhism teaches us that most of our Dukkha stem from Anicca. Unfortunately, the vast majority of humans have a strong urge to attach themselves to material possessions, moments, relationships, people, or ideas – things that are all transient. And because we are in a perpetual struggle to acquire these things and hold onto them, suffering is a fundamental fact of life.

However, this suffering doesn't merely pertain to our more noticeable forms of misery, such as outright depression, loss, anguish, or suicidal thoughts. Less intense but still unpleasant aspects of our lives, such as boredom, emptiness, or a lack of satisfaction, are part of this human condition. If life feels overly mundane and pointless, and this feeling puts weight on one's mind, then this is a manifestation of Dukkha. Many folks think that buying a new car or just acquiring more money will fill the void, and even though it may feel like that for a short while after getting what you want, the sensation never lasts. Instead, you will only crave more while the emptiness grows ever larger.

As one starts to contemplate these issues, it quickly becomes apparent that this form of suffering is rampant in modern, first-world societies. Material prosperity and luxury are not bad things in themselves, but it's obvious what we are looking at quite a few matters from a faulty perspective. Buddhism thus offers the Buddhist path as an alternate means of alleviating our Dukkha. As you have and will continue to learn, this means shifting focus inward as you go about your quest to find fulfillment and peace.

Nothing is ever meant to be satisfactory. Thus, you must learn to depend on nothing, whether it's a physical object, a person, or an emotion. A happy moment, no matter how beautiful, will not last. Success will eventually fade.

That said, it does not mean that you cannot enjoy success, happiness, or prosperity. You are encouraged to relish each wonderful moment in your life. Enjoy it but never cling to it.

On a fundamental level, you can see that Buddhist wisdom lets you have the best of both worlds and is all about shielding the follower of the path. The real beauty of the Middle Way is in that it does not prohibit or limit anything – it teaches you how to live with it in a way that makes you impervious to the trickery of Dukkha. That "it" is all that you own as well as everything and everyone you hold dear. The Buddha teaches you to live life to its fullest, go out there into the world and attain the good things in life, but at the same time, he teaches you to beware of letting your fulfillment, contentment, and happiness depend on those things.

As they are viewed in Buddhism, contentment and inner peace are not precisely what you think either. For instance, it's not about the peace that arises when you know that you have enough money not to worry about the scarcity of necessities for you and your family. That is merely the peace of material and existential security, and it refers to something very earthly and very human. The inner peace that Buddhism propagates is on the inside, and it is all-enveloping. Thanks to that knowledge of impermanence, it's the peace and stability of mind and spirit that endures through all tribulations.

That isn't to say that you will give up and sit back with your feet on the table when your family needs help –instincts will take care of that. However, it is to say that you will remain level-headed, pure in mind, and capable of thinking rationally and calmly, which allows practical problem solving and planning. Earthly life problems will need solving, but an enlightened Buddhist's state of mind and spirit remains unshakeable no matter the tribulations and hardships that come to pass. And that is the finest example of how a full acceptance of Anicca can help regular people keep Dukkha at bay.

Anatta (There is no "I")

Hence, you should also refrain from viewing other beings and things as separate entities. And since they are not separate entities, they can neither be owned nor controlled. Since "the self" is not real but merely an illusion, you cannot hold yourself. Thus, you cannot control yourself.

Nothing in this world is permanent. That includes your "self" as you perceive it. And that which is not permanent only serves to cause you pain. Why? Because you tend to hold on to it. And when you feel that it's gone, that is, when you can no longer perceive it through your physical senses, then you experience a sense of loss, a feeling of grief.

Would you willingly place your hand on a pile of burning coal, knowing that it will hurt you? Of course not! So why attempt to hold something knowing that it will only serve to hurt you in the long run? To try to save, own, or control anything will inevitably lead to suffering. Because you hold on to an illusion, but the moment you lose it, you experience pain as though the object of your mourning did exist.

Chapter 9. The Five Aggregates

Buddhism's main concepts are the five aggregates, or simpler terms, the physical and mental elements that make up each person. These are: form (rupa), sensation (vedana), perception (samjna), volition (sankhara) and consciousness (vijnana).

We will tackle the five aggregates in Buddhism, how they play a role in our spiritual journey to enlightenment, and why this concept is so crucial in Buddhist teachings on happiness. We will also examine how clinging to these aggregates can halt our progress and prevent them from causing us suffering. Finally, we will explore how emptiness (shunyata) could be considered the solution to misery and unhappiness.

Form

The form is regarded as the physical elements that make up a human being; it refers to concrete and tangible. In essence, form relates to body parts. It includes the five sensitive organs (the eyes, ears, nose, tongue, and body). The physical characteristics of our body have blood, bones, flesh, etc. It also includes our bodily fluids such as sweat, tears, etc. Form also includes anything else that belongs to our being – including our hair and nails (which are part of our body after all!). Forms can also refer to anything we consider to be out of our control, such as natural disasters, food, clothing, etc.

Form as the physical body carries a certain amount of emotional content; it is tied up with identity and self-issues to be painful. The pain of the condition lies in how we define ourselves. For example, if you hate yourself because you are overweight or have acne, this will result in suffering; some people may become anorexic because they hate their bodies, leading to pain and unhappiness. The reverse is also true; we can have a positive relationship with our bodies if we like them.

Our physical body can also be a source of pleasure. We can enjoy feeding ourselves, decorating our body and so forth. It is just as powerful as when we are suffering; it all depends on the mind and its relation to the body.

Sensation

The sensation is defined as the awareness of the pleasant or unpleasant qualities of things. It refers to feelings you have towards something or someone. If you like a sure thing, it gives you a pleasant feeling; if you don't like something, it gives you an unpleasant feeling. If there is no particular opinion towards something, then there is no feeling at all. It does not include physical pain or pleasure, such as liking ice cream or disliking broccoli (although this may be part of goza). It instead is referring to likes and dislikes of a mental nature.

Feeling or sensations refers to either pleasant or unpleasant feelings; it is tied up with desire and attachment to life. For example, when you like the taste of the food, it is pleasant; when you dislike the taste of something (like broccoli), it is unpleasant. We all want to enjoy pleasant feelings and avoid unpleasant ones; they become a source of pain or suffering. If we fail to understand this, we can spend our lives going after pleasant feelings and failing to recognize the suffering in life; why would we need Buddhism after all when life is good! Buddhist logic would suggest that we are not good enough to be happy permanently because the basis for happiness is not stable; if it were, why would anybody need Buddhism?

Perception

Perception refers to the awareness of sensory impressions. It also includes conceptualization, recognition, understanding, etc.; it relates to mental constructs such as views or ideas.

The third aggregate refers to perception. You can perceive a particular object in many ways. We could see it as a valuable item or something of little worth. We could also see it as useful or useless; maybe you would like to own a VW Polo, but you could just be looking at it out of curiosity and so on.

When we perceive things in the world, we also value them; things are good or bad, important or unimportant, etc. The emotional content here is pretty obvious.

Volition

Volition refers to our willpower – it is the mental effort we put into something. It does not mean physical exertion; rather an action of the mind (for example, wanting to do something). Such volition can lead us away from suffering or towards it depending on what we want. For instance, we can achieve great things; our lives may become frustrating by having lousy volition.

Recollection refers to memories, so when we remember something from the past, it brings pleasure or pain. We also remember things in the present but the past; for example, we could see a person and place them from a preceding time. This aggregate can be used to refer to things like positive memories from childhood or negative ones.

Consciousness

On the other hand, consciousness refers to the necessary awareness of being; it allows us to see, hear, smell, etc.

We all have impulses – thoughts or feelings that pop into our head for no particular reason; we may have some inclinations to act on them, but we may not act upon them because we choose not to. However, the way this is represented by Buddhist philosophy is an impulse that enters our mind unannounced and leads us to act.

We can see this happening all the time; things we see or hear influence us to do something. For example, if I say I want you to come here, you may decide not to because it is too far to come – your decision comes from your free will. It is an inclination based on a decision made by free will.

We also have inclinations that we make no decision about; for example, the thought of going out for a meal pop into our heads, and we go. Our impulse also leads us to act; there is no decision involved apart from whether we want to or not.

So, it is not our free will as some like to think, but the impulses that lead us to act. It is also true for the five sense desires; they are impulses that happen inside us, and then we work on them. These impulses (kama-raga) cause us suffering because they are subject to birth and death, just like everything else in this world.

It is what Buddha was suggesting. This illusion of free will reflects our ignorance and desire to be in control of our surroundings.

We make every choice influenced by many factors, including our culture, upbringing, habits, genetics, peer pressure, etc. This conditioning leads us to believe we have free will to choose what we want for breakfast.

As individual sentient beings, we have no free will. However, we have the illusion of free will because factors outside of ourselves influence every choice we make; this illusion leads us to believe in free will.

This illusion stops us from making spiritual progress because we spend all our time pursuing things within this world and aim to control everything. We do not let go of these things because they are ours, but they are not ours: they belong to the world of illusion and delusion. We need to let go of our desire to control everything; this is true happiness.

Five Aggregates and Happiness in Buddhism

In Buddhism, there are two types of happiness: worldly happiness and spiritual happiness. Spiritual happiness is sometimes also referred to as nirvana, but they are essentially the same. To understand what these two types of Buddhism happiness are, we first have to explain what unhappiness in general is, both in a worldly sense and spiritually.

The Buddhist view on unhappiness occurs when one has a negative outlook on the world or life in general. It is commonly thought that to be happy, and one has to have a positive outlook; this is the opposite of how Buddhism sees things. In Buddhism, happiness is not contingent upon having a positive outlook.

In the third century, BC Bodhidharma said the following: "If you want happiness, practice sorrow; if you want joy, practice zealousness," which implies that we need to experience suffering to achieve true happiness. In Buddhism, satisfaction is about letting go of the negative things that plague us in life. It is also about letting go of our desires and our greed. As long as we cling to such things, we will never experience true spiritual happiness – this clinging on to negative things causes us suffering.

If you look at each aggregate's meaning, you will notice that they all have emotional content; each total is tied up with certain emotions, both pleasurable and painful (but mainly painful).

The Five Aggregates and Goza

Briefly, we shall now show how the five aggregates relate to goza in Buddhism. The five aggregates are also referred to as our body, mind, and speech, which are the external aspects of our existence, while vedana, sañña and sankhara are our inner feelings which is what we have been looking at so far. Goza refers to that which stands on its own and is not tied up with anything – it is called dukkha-samuccheda-Durham (the cessation of the suffering that comes from despair). So, we can see that the five aggregates are tied up with grief and are a source of pain; they are also the basis for craving, leading us to experience more suffering. They are also what binds us to this world – they are our attachments. As long as we have these attachments, we cannot achieve spiritual happiness, which is what Buddhism is all about – it is meant to liberate us from such things.

Chapter 10. Mahayana - The Great Vehicle

Mahayana Buddhism

The Dharma wheel turns for the second time. Buddha teaches the Sutras of Perfection of Wisdom and the Sutra of Discernment of Intention. In addition to personal enlightenment, the Buddhist is concerned with the redemption of all sentient beings. Since the endeavor transcends personal goals and involves all of humanity, Mahayana Buddhism is also called the "great vehicle" or the "great way."

The monastic ideal gives way to secular orientation. Although the Sanskrit Tipitaka is also considered the core of the traditional scriptures in Mahayana Buddhism, other sutras are also used. Also, the Bodhisattvas in Mahayana Buddhism play a fundamental role as helpers of humanity on the standard path to enlightenment.

Mahayana Buddhism spread mainly in the north, to Nepal, China, Mongolia, and Japan. Mahayana Buddhism began to develop around 100 AC. The term Mahayana means something like a "large vehicle." The aim was to emphasize that it was suitable for many, while the Hinayana ("small vehicle") was only good for a few. The term Hinayana was initially intended to be slightly derogatory.

Mahayana

In Mahayana, the notion is that one's spiritual path is not enough for achieving full enlightenment. Thus, the focus should be on gain for all sentient beings. Monks are encouraged to prioritize sharing their insight, and lay practitioners should meditate towards developing a state of mind in which they distance themselves from the notion of self.

In Mahayana, the Buddha is seen as a deity of sorts which consists of three parts. Meditation is practiced by visualizing the Buddha, seeing oneself as the Buddha, or repeating the Buddha's name.

The teachings of Mahayana consist of texts that can have different interpretations, which can all be true at the same time. The goal of Mahayana is attaining bodhicitta and Buddha-hood as soon as possible. It is since an enlightened being other beings the most.

The Six Perfections of Mahayana Buddhism

In the Mahayana path of Buddhism, it is said that the Buddha spoke of 6 training bases for total and complete enlightenment. These training bases became known as the 6 Perfections. The 6 Perfections are as follows: Generosity, Morality, Patience, Energy, Meditation, and Wisdom. A closer look at each perfection will help you understand its particular importance in the path to Nirvana. However, there is a significance to the given order of the 6 Perfections. The first three perfections are virtuous, while the last three are spiritual.

1. The perfection of Generosity – Generosity is believed to be the gateway to dharma. Think of it as your very first step in Buddhism. Generosity in Buddhism is not as simple as being generous in your life right now. Sure, you might donate to a charity once in a while, but what are your intentions behind that donation? A tax deduction? Bragging rights? Generosity in Buddhism is giving to others without expecting anything in return. It is selfless and pure. You want no recognition; you shy away from it. You want only to give to others because it is the right thing to do,

not because it makes you feel proud. You grant to others because it makes you feel good to help people, to bring joy and compassion into their lives.
The perfection of generosity can be divided even further than just general giving and helping. Generosity is divided into four categories: giving of property, giving Dharma, giving refuge, and giving active love.

The giving of active love refers to wishing happiness and joy to all creatures. You want to spread the love, spread the joy, everywhere that you go. Sure, you can want to someone a joyful day, and their day might not be pleasant at all. But if you're going to them a festive day every single day, perhaps they will start noticing the joy in their lives more often – all because you put the seed of joy in their minds.

2. Perfection of Morality – Morality in Buddhism does not mean blindly following rules, lists, and sets. All of those lists are guiding tools that you should use to achieve your path to Nirvana. No two courses are ever the same. When you are enlightened, you will know how to react to any situation without reminding yourself of any lists. Morality is the Buddhist way of developing compassion. There are three categories of character: protecting body, speech, and mind from unskillful deeds, protecting others as we defend ourselves, and performing skillful acts protects us from unskillful deeds.

Performing skillful deeds ensures that we are protected from performing unskillful stunts is self-explanatory. By doing only skillful deeds, you are not able to perform unskillful acts. How can you do something unskillful when all of your time is taken up by skillful deeds?

3. Perfection of Patience – Patience in Buddhism means being patient, tolerant, and enduring. You can withstand so much more than you even know. There are three categories of patience: patience when someone harms you, patience when you are suffering, and tolerance of keeping concentration.
4.
Patience when someone harms you simply means not getting angry with someone when they physically or mentally bring harm to you. It also means that you cannot seek revenge on the person by trying to harm them back. Think of this patience as a coat of armor that protects you always from harm.

5. Perfection of Energy – Energy is about being courageous in your path to enlightenment. You must develop and nurture your character, you must have spiritual training, and you must dedicate yourself fearlessly to helping others around you. You approach all aspects of Buddhism with energy, courage, and with integrity. There are three kinds of power in this perfection: the strength of the mind that halts desire for ordinary things, the energy that shields us from growing tired and weary in our pursuit of Nirvana, and the energy of confidence in ourselves to attain enlightenment.
6.
The energy of the mind keeps you focused on the dharma. Your love of everyday things in life should never be greater than your love of the dharma. You actively pursue the dharma at all times of your life. You do not lay in bed for hours, thinking of nothing – you get up early and continue on the path to Nirvana. You never waste any time in your pursuit of enlightenment.

7. Perfection of Meditation – Meditation refers to the intense concentration that nurtures your mind and brings you awareness and clarity. You must be able to calm and still your mind, as mentioned earlier when talking about knowing your mind. You should be able to clear your mind and practice mindfulness meditation without distraction from your mind. Meditation takes time to learn – you must practice, practice, practice.

8. Perfection of Wisdom – Wisdom is the realization and understanding of emptiness, that all things are without a "self," that all items are empty. It is an unequaled type of wisdom because it is the truth of Buddhism. Through the practice of the other perfections, you will attain this wisdom. Understanding emptiness in all things will help you to rid yourself of ignorance.

Chapter 11. How to Find Enlightenment

When a human being has satisfied his basic needs – food, water, shelter, security, and so on – he begins to wonder about the purpose of existence or the essence of life. The Buddha himself had reflected on this, especially as he may have been a noble whose basic needs were fully satisfied.

Helping Others

Buddhism teaches compassion because it enables one to value life in general. The Buddha himself chose to help guide others towards the path of Enlightenment because of mercy.

To find the essence in life in this aspect, you may begin taking on a sense of responsibility for other beings, especially those who are in a more difficult position than you are. Perhaps you can volunteer for a local charity organization or use your skills for the welfare of others.

Cultivating the Four Divine Abodes

Meditation is the recommended way to cultivate the Four Divine Abodes, namely:

- *Loving-kindness,*
- *Compassion,*
- *Sympathetic bliss, and*
- *Equanimity*

1. In a quiet and peaceful place, spend some time reflecting on any of the Four Divine Abodes.

For instance, if you will meditate on Loving-kindness, reflect on how to describe this feeling. Try to embrace this as part of who you are, and by meditating on them, you will find that your meditation has real purpose and that you come closer to understanding what enlightenment is.

2. Visualize a person in your life who can easily make you genuinely feel this quality. If you meditate on loving-kindness, you might think of a loved one you care for with all your heart. Often, these are the people who bring out the best in us. Through their actions and belief in you, you can see what it's like to incorporate these qualities into your life.

3. As you invoke the feeling of the quality, let it reverberate from within you to your surroundings.

In the case of loving-kindness, you can visualize your loved ones and other people you do not usually care for in real life. Through practice, you could even direct it towards those whom you do not particularly like. The point of this is that you overcome your prejudices and make yourself capable of shutting off prejudice and seeing beyond it.

4. Continue to extend the feeling of the quality towards all beings in the world. Visualize it pouring from your heart towards them.

You can continuously practice this form of meditation so that the Four Divine Abodes will eventually become more natural to you. Embracing these qualities will then enable you to see the true essence of life. It helps you to become more optimistic. It allows you to

---

increase your mindfulness and energy levels so that the energy you give off is positive and helps those around you see joy and happiness in their own lives.

Generosity

To be excellent means to be open to helping others without expecting anything in return. There are several ways to become more generous to others, but in traditional Buddhist teachings, there are four ways:

1. To share the teachings of the Buddha

Leading others towards a path that frees them from suffering is a great thing to do. It enables others to think and act for themselves and gain the right motivation to live a meaningful life. When you experience the positivity of your belief in Buddhism's philosophy, you can impart that to others and share with them the joy that this brings to your life. Each person must choose their route through life. You cannot select it for them. However, you can influence those you care about to learn the generosity of spirit from knowing you. Give without expectation of thanks or return. When you do, you feel nearer to the spiritual awakening than when you add strings to the things you give.

2. To protect other beings

Other living beings, humans and animals alike, have to live through life-threatening conditions every day. The only way for them to be saved is by helping those in better positions than they are. In day-to-day life, this could mean giving to the poor or being generous with your time when people are sick and in need of company. There are many ways that you can give your protection to others, and it's entirely possible that you already do this with your family. Extend your protection to people around you who are less well off than you.

3. To inspire and motivate others

You can also practice what you teach through meditation and follow the teachings of the Buddha. When others see that you are capable of it, they might be inspired to do the same. Inspiration does not involve any expectations. You can share what you know about Buddhism's teachings, but you cannot influence people to follow the way simply because you say so. They need to see your example and to be inspired by it, rather than being expected to follow a way that does not seem natural to them.

4. Offering material goods

Living beings need food, shelter, clothing, and other materials to improve their quality of life. Your generosity in the form of such gifts can tremendously benefit them. This way is easily most associated with the concept of altruism. In the Protestant and Catholic religions, people give alms. These are collections of money that are used for the benefit of the church or of other people. When you have things that you no longer need, there are always those who have less than you. Offering them the things you know will make their lives more comfortable should become a natural way forward for those who believe in Buddhist philosophy.

Moral Behavior

Moral behavior in exercising self-discipline so that you do not cause harm to other beings. The effort placed into choosing the more difficult but morally upright path instead of the easy but wrong one is one way to uphold this Perfection. Another is to cultivate genuine compassion for others through prayer, meditation, and good work.

Through constant practice, moral behavior will become more natural and spontaneous to you.

Patience

The more you practice the teachings of the Buddha, the more naturally patient you will be. Being patient protects yourself and others because it restrains you from allowing feelings such as ill will and anger to transform into destructive actions. As your patience continues to grow, you will notice that such negative emotions become weaker until you can no longer feel them.

To help you develop patience, here are traditional Buddhist practices to try:

1. Acknowledge and Accept Suffering

However, by accepting this reality, you develop the patience to go through these negative experiences. Through this, you do not become overwhelmed by feelings of regret, resentment, or anger associated with these events in your life. The acceptance of the Four Noble Truths will help you with this. The very first Noble Truth tells you that suffering is something that happens in life. However, when you strengthen your ability to accept suffering, you are more potent when such an event causes suffering.

2. Stay calm

Staying calm despite frustrating or dangerous events leads to good karmic results. At first, it might be a challenge to remain calm when someone is attacking you. However, by taking a step back, you can analyze the best steps you can take based on the situation before you react.

3. Develop patience in pursuit

As you continue to practice the Buddha's teachings, there will be times when your old habits resurface and tempt you to steer from the path. However, you must remain patient in your efforts even if you do not always see immediate results. To do that, simply draw yourself back by reminding yourself of the teachings that have led you to start your journey in the first place.

Effort

The effort, in this sense, refers to one's commitment and perseverance in choosing to do what is right. It also means doing things with enthusiasm instead of feeling as if you are abstaining and resisting something. Some Buddhist teachers even emphasize that effort is the foundation of the other Perfections because, with it, the rest would naturally fall into place.

To practice Effort, you must understand and acknowledge the presence of the three obstacles that impede it. These are defeatism, trivial pursuits, and laziness.

Concentration

Meditation is the key to improving your concentration, so take the time to practice it each day. Start with simple meditation exercises, such as sitting and breathing meditations. Once you become accustomed to them, you can move on to deeper levels, such as those that enable you to reduce physical pain and emotional trauma. To sit and meditate, you can choose to use a seated stance on a cushion on the floor where your legs are bent at the knees and crossed at the ankles. It is hard for people who are new to meditation to take up the more traditional lotus position at first, and this position, provided your back is straight, is a good position for meditation. Your hands can be cupped with your palms facing upward and your thumbs touching. If you use a cushion for meditation, it's an excellent idea to sway from left to right and back again to ensure that your body is grounded and comfortable before starting the breathing exercises. When you begin to meditate, make sure that you are not busy or free from distractions.

Practices of Buddhism

Buddhism's primary emphasis is on overcoming our shortcomings and fully enhancing our positive potential. Limitations include a lack of clarity and an emotional imbalance that confuses us about life. Consequently, we conduct ourselves compulsively, motivated by troubling emotions like frustration, greed, and naivety. Our positive potentials include our ability to communicate, understand reality, empathize with others, and better ourselves.

The Fourteenth Dalai Lama

We all care about our physical hygiene, but taking care of our mental state is just as critical. We need to remember the antidotes to our upsetting state of mind, remember to apply them when necessary, and remember to retain them.

To remember all the antidotes, you must:

Learn what they are.

Contemplate them until we understand them correctly, knowing how to apply them, and being convinced that they will work.

Practice applying them in meditation to become familiar with them.

Buddhist Practice, Preliminaries, and Rites
Medicine Buddha

The mantra and the medicine Buddha image are perfect for your health and that of others, for your mind in short. Meditate on the Medicine Buddha idea, and if you accompany it with a bowl, the result is perfect.

The Third Ray, Active Intelligence, connects with the fifth Center. It is recited by visualizing the Blue Medicine Buddha, or instead, a sphere of blue light, which in essence represents the Medicine Buddha.

They can be visualized on the forehead or crown. In reciting the mantra, the reciter visualizes rays of light and nectar emanating from the sphere of light, penetrating the head's peak and clearing all diseases, tensions, and blockages.

With the same procedure, healing water can be obtained, increasing the power of medications and medical treatments. It helps recite the mantra while visualizing the Medicine Buddha pouring over the medicine we are taking, imagining that the prescription is filled with the mixture of Buddha's light energy.

Gong Bath

When we listen to the Gong's sound, deep relaxation is created—freeing us from the torrent of thoughts that our mind generates.

During a Gong Bath, you will experience sensations inside and outside the body. The sound caresses you as if it were a wave. At the cellular level, vibration also works by harmonizing all body cells by the physical principle of sound resonance. A Gong Bath is an experience that will never leave you indifferent. Let yourself go, flow like water, and let the sound guide you.

Dalai Lama Guru Yoga

Through the practice of Guru Yoga, we are inspired by the example of the spiritual master. By placing ourselves under his guidance, we progressively reveal our mind's essential nature, developing and training its positive qualities.

Guru Yoga is essential in Vajrayana Buddhism because, on this path, achievements depend on the purity of commitment (Samaya) and how we perceive and relate to the teacher.

The Dalai Lama himself wrote the Dalai Lama's Inseparability Guru Yoga Practice with Avalokitesvara (Compassionate Buddha). It contained a meditation on Avalokitesvara and a complete meditation on the gradual path to enlightenment.

Shabab Duchen

Shabab Düchen is one of the four most crucial Buddhist tradition celebrations: prayer and virtuous actions. Shabab Düchen is the celebration of the Buddha's descent from the paradise of Tushita to give Dharma teachings to his mother, Queen Mayadevi. It is part of the Tibetan Buddhist tradition to dedicate this day to prayer and virtuous actions. In this celebration, it is believed that the or merits of all right actions are multiplied by 10 million times, and adverse actions also give this same multiplier effect.

Lama Chöpa

This Buddhist ceremony is observed during the "days of Tsog" in the Tibetan calendar. It is an indispensable practice for Vajrayana practitioners. Guru Yoga is the root of the spiritual path and the basis for reaching all spiritual realizations. Compiled by the First Panchen Lama, the fundamental pillar of this practice is devotion to the teacher. Still, it also contains all the essential instructions of the stages of the path and those related to the locations of generation consummation of the Supreme Tantra.

Offering the Tsog is very important to keep commitments and avoid obstacles, as we place ourselves under the care of dakas and dakinis, who grant us realizations. Furthermore, our health, merits, and joy increase by doing this practice. As it is an offering ritual, you must attend it with offerings of flowers, food, or drink.

Initiations

A tantric initiation is a power transmission ceremony that activates our Buddha-nature's evolutionary factors, stimulating them further. Receiving initiation requires a fully trained tantric master and prepared and receptive, and that our participation is active in the process.

The initiations are allusive to a specific tantric entity: Vajra sattva, Chenrezig, Tara, Manjushri. They are usually accompanied by teachings related to said entities' qualities, and receiving them implies the teacher's authorization and blessing to perform them independently. Many of them indicate a firm commitment on our part, both philosophical and daily practice.

Vajra Sattva Practice

ONE FRIDAY A MONTH AT 6:30 P.M.

Doing the Vajra Sattva practice and reciting the 100-syllable mantra 100,000 times purifies negativities, provided it is done correctly, with all factors complete. If the recitation is done without the four elements, we cannot filter the negativities in their entirety. However, if the meditation and recitation of Vajra Sattva are appropriately done, with the four opposing powers, and we recite the mantra 100,000 times, all negativities are purified. Repeating the mantra 21 times every day prevents negativity from increasing.

Chod Practice

ONE FRIDAY A MONTH AT 7:00 P.M.

The practice of Chöd is part of the cultural heritage of Tibetan Buddhism. The traditional approach of Chöd cuts self-esteem, and clinging to a real existence of the "I" creates the conditions under which the conventional bodhicitta mind can develop, which holds others as dearer than oneself, and the Ultimate Bodhicitta mind, which sees reality as it is.

By cutting out our habitual selfish patterns of thought and behavior, we allow the natural openness, clarity, and sensitivity of the mind to manifest. Strong and spontaneous compassion arises when we experience our union with the universe and with all sentient beings that inhabit it.

With this practice, we simultaneously train the body, speech, and mind through meditation, visualization, sound, and rhythm. Like all tantric practices, Chöd can only be performed after receiving the lineage's initiation and instructions by a fully qualified master. The family to which the Chöd practice that we follow in our center belongs to the Wensa Tradition's Gelugpa lineage.

It is also known as the Chöd practice of Padampa Sangye and belongs to the Manjushri collection. Chöd was a private practice of Lama Tsongkhapa. The great master Gyelwa Ensapa Losang Dondrup, the first Panchen Rinpoche, received the Lama Tsongkhapa lineage initiation, which had been transmitted continuously until it reached him.

Praises at 21 Taras

WEDNESDAYS AT 7:00 P.M.

Tara is a Buddha with a feminine aspect, who, out of great compassion, promised to lead to Enlightenment in a single lifetime, all the beings who entrusted themselves to her. As long as we remain in samsara, we will suffer various kinds of sufferings and setbacks, so we will often need help. Tara acts with us as a mother would with her child; she protects and cares for us, ready at all times to come to our aid.

She is known as the mother of all Buddhas since entrusting herself to her with honesty and determination leads to the state of Buddhahood. The praise of the twenty-one forms of Tara was composed by the Buddha himself and is a widespread practice in all Tibetan Buddhism schools. Its recitation brings great because being a Sutra, the very words of Buddha,

This practice is very suitable to eliminate obstacles, fears, diseases, achieve prosperity, well-being, abundance, and happiness. Given the current circumstances, it is necessary to create the causes for temporary and ultimate well-being, both for ourselves and our environment: family, friends, colleagues, fellow citizens, compatriots, and all sentient beings in general. To alleviate hunger and disease, wars, injustice, and to ensure that all beings enjoy the qualities of enlightenment. It is delicious to recite the Praise at 21 Taras as often as possible.

Prostrations

TUESDAYS AT 7:00 P.M.

The prostrations are a vital act of respect towards the Buddha, the Dharma, and the Sangha, which constitute the Three Jewels. They are also an antidote to pride, and it is a form of accumulation of merit and purification of negativities. There are two types of physical prostrations, short (5 points) and long. The prostrations performed in this practice are the long ones.

For most Buddhists, there are at least three situations in which we must prostrate ourselves unless we go on a pilgrimage trip or do certain specific practices:

When entering a gompa: It is a sign of respect for performing three prostrations before the main altar. Also, when you are going to leave until another day.

In the presence of the teacher: When you wait for the lama to enter to offer to teach or lead a puja, you have to wait for him to sit on his throne. Then three short prostrations are done before sitting down, and they are repeated when the lama gets up to leave.

When placing and removing the altar: Immediately after setting up the altar and just before beginning to remove it, three prostrations should be made at a time.

The mantra that is usually recited when doing prostrations is Om Namo Manjushriye, Namo Sushriye, Namo Utama Shriye Soha. What it means: I pay homage to the impeccable Buddha Mind, I pay tribute to the noble and glorious Dharma, and I pay homage to the Glorious Order (Sangha).

The prostrations to the Thirty-Five Buddhas of Confession are a powerful method if carried out as the first activity in the morning, to purify any negativity created during the night, and as the last thing in the day, to purify negativities. In which we may have incurred during the day. Through this practice, the mind, speech, and body participate in the purification process.

How to practice Buddhism

Unlike any other spiritual philosophy, Buddhism, neither better nor worse, but unique, teaching less about the value of divine deities and rules and more about a way of life that can change our inner world and, ultimately, the world around us. This practice reverts to what is now known as Nepal and started 2600 years ago. While there are many schools within Buddhism today, there is a common understanding that all Buddhists share.

Yet why is it that people practice Buddhism? While there are several explanations, one of the core concepts is in his belief that all beings are experiencing the essential wear and tear of birth, maturity, illness, and death, so we must go beyond this normal wear and tear, life, and death.

Chapter 13. Guidelines for Practicing Buddhism

Throughout the centuries, Buddhism practices have been transforming based on the people who continue to uphold them. How the methods are adopted is based on the culture of different societies.

Yet, one thing remains the same, and it is that the core values of Buddhism are preserved. Such virtues are being strong-willed, generous, kind, and selfless are universally accepted and timeless.

You will learn how they can help you to become stress- and anxiety-free at the least, and how they can help you stay motivated as you follow the Noble Eightfold Path.

Mindfulness Meditation

When you talk about Buddhism, you cannot avoid mentioning the concept of meditation. It is the core of the practice. Additionally, scientific studies can attest to its mental and physical gain. Meditation is a generally accepted and widely recommended way to reduce stress in everyday life, improve cognitive and emotional intelligence, and increase positive thinking.

Theravada Buddhism Meditation:

- Anapanasati
- Satipatthana
- Metta
- Kammatthana
- Samatha
- Vipassana
- Mahasati
- Dhammakaya

Vajrayana and Tibetan Buddhism Meditation

- Ngondro
- Tonglen
- Phowa
- Chod
- Mahamudra
- Dzogchen
- The Four Immeasurables
- Tantra

Zen Buddhism Meditation

- Shikantaza (sitting meditation)
- Zazen
- Koan
- Suizen

Chanting and Mantras

Another common practice in Buddhism is chanting. Buddhist monks in different parts of East and Southeast Asia practice regularly chanting to improve their concentration and reflect deeply on Buddhist concepts.

Buddhist's modernists use phrases in their spoken language to create mantras that help them sink deeper into their meditative state as well.

You may be familiar with the "Om," a sacred mantra that Buddhists chant at the start of all mantras. According to ancient Hindu texts, Om is the eternal sound in the past, present, and future. It embodies birth, life, and death, and it is used and heard every day. Interestingly, it is said that by chanting "Om," the vibrations it causes helps relax the body and mind.

There are also centers whose gurus give individual chants to students based upon the year, time, and place of birth, and these are personal to the student.

Chanting is found useful in many ways because it allows the student to concentrate on a given thing rather than allowing the mind to wander. Although this was not the specific purpose of mantras, it helps to cut out unnecessary thought processes that help the student meditate more successfully. It also allows the student to breathe since some mantras are used in rhythm with the breathing and help the student breathe and chant the mantra on the outward breath.

Vegetarian or Vegan Lifestyle

While it must be noted that the First Buddha himself never mentioned anything against the consumption of meat, many Buddhists choose to live the vegetarian or vegan lifestyle.

Therefore, by harming another being, one is breaking the self as well.

Some Buddhists who choose to eat meat do so only out of necessity. For instance, those living in cold climates can only survive on a diet rich in fat and protein. In such cases, the Buddhists would then choose only the meat of ethically raised animals. In other words, the animals lived a full and relatively happy and free life and were slaughtered most humanely and painlessly for their meat.

Ultimately, the decision to choose your diet rests in your hands, as the Buddha himself explained. Of course, no one is exempted from eating meat's karmic results, mostly if the living being was slaughtered specifically for you. It is worthy of note since Buddhist monks are often given food, and there is a story about a Buddhist monk who was extremely hungry. He was given a chicken plate and looked forward to eating it until he was told that the chicken had been slaughtered specifically for him. In this case, he was not permitted to eat it since this goes against Buddhist belief, and he was considered the cause of the killing.

As you can see, many – if not all – of Buddhism practices can easily be incorporated into the modern lifestyle. It is up to you how you perceive and practice these rituals each day. After all, it is only through experience that you can truly witness the gain of these practices.

Would it surprise you to know that Buddhism is not a religion? At least, not in a sense wherein it is an institution that dictates how one should believe in divine power. Many people make that mistake and avoid Buddhism because they think it contrary to their church's teachings. However, you can practice Buddhism in conjunction with your personal belief and religion or complement it.

Your real self is what can be understood to travel from life to life during reincarnation. In different belief systems, these are given names, such as the soul, though what name you give it isn't vital. It is merely crucial that you recognize that these two parts of you exist and that, if you are unhappy in your life, the harmony or balance is missing, and that's where Buddhism helps you to align these values so that both parts of you are in connection with each other.

Each living being has the opportunity to become enlightened in each life they live. There is no set course or prewritten script for your life.

However, things get interesting here because when you follow Buddhism's path, you do not have an "end goal." It is a paradox for one to declare that they are going to practice Buddhism to reach enlightenment.

Who is The Buddha?

The word "Buddha" translates to "the enlightened one" or "the awakened being." It refers to any being who has achieved this state. However, you might be curious to know about the first Buddha.

According to legend, the first Buddha was named Siddhartha Gautama. Many believe that he was born around 563 B.C. in a land that is now found in Nepal. It is said that The Buddha was born a royal, shielded from the suffering of the kingdom of his father, who built a grand palace around him void of religion or human suffering. The King created an entire world inside those castle walls and, as his son grew, led him to believe that the world was one of happiness, empathy, and joy. The King was told by seers when the prince was born to either be a great warrior or a spiritual leader.

Later in his life, after he had married and was raised, he ventured out into the world and saw humanity's truth. He met an older adult and found that all people age and eventually die.

At the age of twenty-nine, he found that neither his power nor fortune brought him true happiness, and he wanted to understand the world outside of the palace walls.

Therefore, what he did was he set out to explore as many religions across the world as he could to find the answer to the question that we all ask ourselves, "Where can one find happiness?" He tried many ways, including fasting, and when he found that fasting was not helping him in the way that he thought it might, he decided to meditate on the problems he faced. While others still practiced going without food and had believed that Siddhartha had given up the practice, he had taken himself on another route – one that would lead him to enlightenment.

Several years into his spiritual pilgrimage, the Buddha discovered "The Middle Path" while meditating under the Bodhi tree. This path is a way of balance, not extremism, which he found only through trial and error. He sat for days under that Bodhi tree seeking the answers he had initially set out to find. During this meditation, Siddhartha had to face the evil demon known as Mara, who threatened to stand in the way of his Buddha status. He looked to the earth for guidance and the land answered by banishing Mara and allowing Siddhartha to reach full enlightenment. Such discernment led him to achieve the perfect state of culture. After this life-changing experience, the Buddha lived the rest of his days sharing what he had discovered. The followers of the Buddha's teachings called his principles the Dharma, or "Truth."

It is thought that Buddha or anyone who reaches the state of perfect enlightenment in their life no longer continues on the circle of rebirth. Instead, the Buddha is believed to sit outside of constant reincarnation and sends teachings and guidance to those searching for their freedom of self. They no longer have to sit through what Buddhists believe to be an endless cycle of suffering known as life.

Though Buddhism as a practice can bend and move on a scale depending on your dedication to the teachings and heritage, anyone can practice the Buddhist way of living. There is always extreme importance put on the word empathy throughout the teachings of Buddhas through the generations. Compassion is not just reserved for humans but every living creature of this world.

At this point, you must be eager to learn the different teachings of the Buddha. Keep in mind that the Buddha's teachings are vast to such an extent that they grew into many Buddhism kinds. These teachings can bring wisdom to anyone, whether seeking to find their real self through enlightenment or those that wish to understand the world around them a little bit better. These teachings are for the young and old alike, regardless of religion, status, gender, or heritage.

You have to discern the truth for yourself because your truth will not be everyone else's. With the constant changes that happen throughout life, the Buddhist belief encourages that you embrace the moment and are ever-present in it. For westerners, this is always a little difficult since we are always striving to better ourselves, although sometimes the betterment that we seek is detrimental. If you were to talk to Tibetans, they do not find merit in people trying to prove that they are better than others. Boasting is not part of the Buddhist way of life, which contrasts with life in a modern society that encourages competition and heroics with very little to do with betterment from a Buddhist perspective.

Siddhartha Gautama's idea was to encourage people to understand that their actions dictate the outcome of different life stages. It is always something that westerners find hard to understand. However, when you see how Buddhist philosophy includes other elements, you will see that the whole picture of your life has been covered and that there are actions you can take to increase your awareness and sense of happiness. Our current Dalai Lama was once asked what surprised him the most about humankind, and his answer will give you something to think about, which relates to modern times and which you can probably identify with.

Chapter 14. The Roots of Evil

The Roots of Evil

The following are the Three Poisons that every Buddhist must strive to avoid. They are regarded as the primary source of evil manifested through our actions, speech, and thoughts. They are considered as blocks to positive karma.

Greed

It includes an insatiable desire for:

- Riches
- Fame
- Sex
- Sleep
- Overcome greed by performing simple acts of generosity.

Anger

Practice calmness and patience. Do not allow anger to dictate your actions. Once you do, you will enable it to dictate your karma and dictate your future life quality.

Ignorance

As a Buddhist, you are urged to embrace the truth. Let go of prejudices. Stop clinging to delusions. Use your intellect and your senses to carry out observations in an objective manner.

Think of life as a wheel that turns round and round. Depending on your past life deeds, you may be born on top or at the bottom. And so, this goes on and on until you are finally able to experience the awakening. The purpose of reincarnation is to give you a chance to escape the ever-turning wheel of life eventually. It is done by achieving enlightenment. Accordingly, to do this means you must first successfully become free of the Three Poisons.

Remember to also apply the wheel metaphor to this very life and not just the excellent rebirth cycle. The suffering, temptation, and hardship that, as you have learned, come into every life are things that oscillate a great deal. Since both sorrow and happiness are subject to the doctrine of impermanence, the very life that you are traversing now is certainly also reminiscent of a great wheel, although not as great as the one of Samsara. Nonetheless, Anicca will always have you alternating between the top and bottom of the revolution, between the good times and bad, health and sickness. Luckily, you now know how to deal with these cold facts of life, and all you have to do as a Buddhist is to strive toward enlightenment. As long as you do, you will always end up better than you started, no matter how far you manage to get.

Radical Teachings

Some of Zen's traditional stories describe masters using unorthodox education methods, and many practitioners today tend to interpret these stories overly literally.

For example, many are outraged when they hear stories like that of Master Linji, the founder of the Rinzai school, who said, "If you find the Buddha, kill the Buddha. If you find a Patriarch, kill the Patriarch." A contemporary master, Seung Sahn, also teaches his students that we all need to kill three things: kill our parents, kill the Buddha, and kill our teacher (in this case, Seung Shan himself). However, neither Linji nor Seung Sahn was speaking literally. They wanted to say that we need to "kill" our attachment to outside teachers and things.

When visiting temples or Zen practice centers, beginners who have read many of these stories and expect to find iconoclastic teachers are often surprised by the conservative and formal nature of practices.

Zen and Other Religions

Since the mid-twentieth century, Zen has been open to interreligious dialogue, having appeared in countless meetings and conferences worldwide.

In Zen temples and centers of practice worldwide, it is common for many non-Buddhists to attend activities and practice zazen. This practice is generally well accepted by teachers since Buddhism is a religion of tolerance that sees other religions as valid spiritual paths and is open to anyone who only wants to meditate without any religious affiliation.

In some schools, Sanbo Kyodan, the acceptance of practitioners of other religions is so high that a practitioner can receive the Dharma transmission and become a teacher without needing to leave their faith.

Statements like that of the former Pope, who called the Dalai Lama "godless," naturally had a considerable and (of course) adverse effect on the population's masses.

Therefore, most people are unaware that the Buddha did not regard himself as either God or a messenger of God. He merely explains that the teachings Dhamma (Pali) or Dharma (Sanskrit) can be experienced through his meditative vision (of contemplation). Furthermore, Buddha refers to the individual's self-reliance in learning this technique and urges against a dogmatic adherence to his teaching. Self-responsibility is the highest here.

The Illumination

In Zen, enlightenment is generally called satori or kensho. The kensho is the initial glimpse, so to speak, of the true nature of reality and of itself. It's a shallow form of enlightenment. On the other hand, Satori is a more profound and more lasting experience in which the practitioner has an intense experience of Buddha's Nature and sees his "original face."

But it is not a visionary experience. Although some people suppose that enlightenment experience should lead those who experience it to universes of intense light or something worth it, the testimony of Zen masters contradicts this hypothesis. When asked about how his life was before and how he stayed after satori, a modern Zen master replied, "Now my garden looks more colorful."

In enlightenment, the practitioner is not distracted.

Another common assumption is that when being enlightened, the flow of thoughts stops. The practitioner stands as a polished mirror, reflecting the actual reality without ideas that will hinder it. On the contrary, dreams do not stay - what happens is that the practitioner gives them up, lets them go, forgets them, and forgets himself. When the Fifth Patriarch, Hongren (in Japanese, Daiman Konin, 601-647), decided to choose who would succeed him, he proposed to his disciples that they try to capture Zen's essence a poem; the author of the best poem would be his successor. When they received the news, the monks knew who the winner was: Shenxiu, Hongren's oldest student. No one bothered to compete with him. They just waited, and Shexiu wrote his poem and hung it on the wall:

"This body is the Bodhi tree.

The soul is like a bright mirror.

Take care that it is always clean,

leaving no dust accumulates on it."

All the monks liked it. Surely Hongren would enjoy it too. However, the next day there was another poem hanging by the side, which someone had preached during the night:

"Bodhi is not like a tree.

The bright mirror shines nowhere:

If there is nothing from the beginning,

Where does dust accumulate?"

The monks were amazed. Who would have written that? After a while, they discovered: the author of the poem was Huineng, the monastery cooks. And realizing his achievement, it was to him that Hongren extended his cloak and his bowl, making Huineng the Sixth Patriarch.

Like all Buddhist schools, Zen sends its roots back to Indian Buddhism. The word Zen comes from the Sanskrit term dhyana, which denotes the typical meditative practice state. In China, this term was transliterated as channa and soon reduced to its shorter form. From there, it translated to Korean and finally to Japanese as Zen.

According to traditional accounts, the Zen practice style was taken from India to China by the Indian monk Bodhidharma (in Japanese, Daruma), circa AD 520. Although modern scholars have questioned this account's origin and authenticity, Bodhidharma's story (or legend) is the fundamental metaphor of Zen on the core of its practice.

In Second Counts Registration Lamp Transmission, one of Zen's oldest texts, Bodhidharma, went to China. Due to his wise fame, the Liang Dynasty's territory was immediately summoned to the famous Emperor Wu-ti court. The emperor, who had broadly supported Buddhism in China, asked Bodhidharma about the merit he had gained by supporting Buddhism, hoping that this merit would ensure him a good life in his next incarnation. Bodhidharma replied, "No merit." The emperor, enraged, then asked, "Who is this that is before me?" (in present-day language, something like "Who do you think you are?") Bodhidharma replied, "I do not know." Dazed, the emperor concluded that Bodhidharma must be mad and expelled him from the court. One of the ministers then asked the emperor: "Your Imperial Majesty knows who this person is?" The emperor said he did not know. The Minister said, "He is the Bodhisattva of Compassion, bearer of the Seal of the Buddha's Heart." "Full of regret, the emperor wanted to call Bodhidharma back, but the minister warned that he would not come back even if all the Chinese went to pick him up. Other people, however, were intrigued by his response and followed him to the cave where he had gone to live. They became his disciples and discovered that Bodhidharma was the spiritual heir of Mahakashyapa, one of Buddha's great disciples.

According to traditional teachings, Bodhidharma could not answer because his true nature and the true nature of all things were beyond discursive knowledge, definition, and words. It is to this direct experience of reality that Zen aspires.

Mahakashyapa, of whom Bodhidharma was a spiritual heir and successor, had himself this experience and was enlightened. According to the sutras, Mahakashyapa was Buddha's only disciple to understand his Lotus Speech, in which Buddha, without saying anything, simply raised a flower. It was an immediate reality, beyond words.

After training his disciples for many years, Bodhidharma died, leaving his student Huike (Japanese, Daiso Eka). Huike was the second Patriarch of Zen and went through a succession line of which little is known until arriving at Huineng (in Japanese, DaikanEno, 638-713), the sixth and last Patriarch. Huineng, one of the greatest masters of Zen history, participated in a famous dispute when his master succeeded: a group of monks refused to accept him as patriarch and proposed another practitioner, Shenxiu, in his place. Huineng was forced to flee to a temple in southern China under threat, but in the end, supported by most of the monks, she was recognized as a patriarch.

A few decades later, however, the feud was resurrected. A group of monks, claiming to be Shenxiu's successor, faced another group, the Southern School, which presented itself as Huineng's successor. After heated debates, the Southern School eventually prevailed, and its rivals disappeared. The records of this dispute are the earliest historical records of the Zen school we have today.

Later, Korean monks went to China to study the practices of the Bodhidharma school. When they arrived, what they found was a school that had already developed its own identity with strong Taoism influences, formerly known by Chan's name. Over time, Chan eventually settled in Korea, where he received the name Seon.

Similarly, monks came from other Asian countries to study Chan, and the school spread to neighboring countries. In Vietnam, it was called Thien, and in Japan, it became known as Zen. These schools have grown independently throughout history, having developed their own identities and characteristics entirely different from one another.

Zazen

For Zen, experiencing reality is experiencing nirvana. To experience reality directly, one must detach oneself from words, concepts, and discourses. And to separate yourself from this, one must meditate. Therefore, zazen ("sitting meditation") is the actual application of Zen.

Chapter 15. The Four Stages of Enlightenment

The Four Stages of Enlightenment:

- Arhats are Buddhists who seek to enlighten themselves.
- A Pratyekabuddha is someone who retreats from the modern world to find enlightenment.
- A Bodhisattva is an aspiring Buddha who seeks to inspire not just himself but for others as well.
- A Buddha refers to someone who has reached the stage of perfect enlightenment.

It is up to you to determine your degree of involvement in Buddhism. The best way to conduct your journey is to proceed at your own pace. Remember, you are free to incorporate whatever teachings work for you. Likewise, you are free to leave the ones that don't.

Keep in mind that reaching Nirvana or Buddhahood is not necessary for Buddhism to improve your life. It's also worth mentioning that some traditions, such as Theravada, maintain that monks can only attain nirvana. On the other hand, Mahayana traditions believe that everyone can achieve this supreme enlightenment without being ordained. Either way, Nirvana is the apex of spiritual growth in Buddhism, and individuals who are recognized as having reached this point are not very common. However, millions of people practice Buddhism with only a vague aspiration towards Nirvana while gaining much fulfillment from the lifestyle regardless.

Is being Buddhist that easy?

Yes! These are other steps that will help you live life the accurate Buddhist way:

Be Responsible for Your Own Life.

There is no supreme being who will be watching over you every second of your life, ready to reward or punish you as he sees fit. Unlike other religious teachers in history, the Buddha did not require his disciples to be close to him at all times. He encouraged them to wander, to meditate on their own, and to preach in different places. Then, the followers would gather once a year to listen to the Buddha's new teachings.

As mentioned at the beginning of this book, Buddhism is meant to be a way of life. As an aspiring Buddhist, you are encouraged to live life and experience for yourself the truth in the Buddha's teachings.

Receive the Teachings

You don't have to be Buddhist to practice the teachings of the Buddha. As mentioned, your degree of involvement depends on you. Often, Buddhist groups and teacher's Buddhism offer classes and meditation instructions for free. They welcome anyone who is self-motivated enough to seek them out actively.

Gain a Deeper Knowledge of the Teachings

Read more books on Buddhism. Find a teacher if you wish. However, understand that receiving someone as a teacher involves a commitment on both sides. There are different traditions of Buddhism. Before you decide to receive formal initiation, make sure that the ceremony you choose is right for you. Alternatively, you may opt to remain a layperson while observing the basic precepts of the Buddhist tradition of your choice.

Choose a Tradition

Theravada

Theravada is considered one of the main branches or traditions of Buddhism and the most historic. Its teachings revolve around the most well-known Buddhist concepts, such as Nirvana, the Noble Eightfold Path, and escape from Samsara.

Teachers of this tradition do not claim to have any spiritual authority. Think of a fellow traveler who happens to know more about the area. He occasionally nudges you towards the right path when you lose your way. Put merely, Theravada teachers are more like mentors.

Mahayana

It is the second major branch of Buddhism, and it includes many other traditions, such as the famous Zen school. Mahayana is the more adaptable form of Buddhism, and it has included numerous additional rituals and teachings over time.

An exciting difference between Mahayana and Theravada teachings is how Mahayana Buddhists contemplate the idea of higher enlightenment at the end of the journey. Namely, this tradition doesn't believe that a follower will necessarily escape the rebirth cycle but will instead remain in this state to facilitate and assist others' awakening. Therefore, instead of reaching Nirvana, a follower of the Mahayana teaching aspires to attain Buddhahood by traversing the bodhisattva path, which we mentioned above.

Vajrayana

Teachers of this tradition have substantial authority over their followers. He initiates trainees, and they follow his rules dutifully.

Vajrayana is the only school of thought that is sometimes considered the third branch, but many views it as a part of the Mahayana tradition. All the other rules may fall under any one of the ones we mentioned thus far.

Tibetan Traditions

Instructors of Meditation may be monks or lay practitioners who assist you in developing your practice.

Lamas are teachers that are usually monks, although not in all cases. They possess advanced meditation training and have disciples who revere them.

Geshes refer to teachers who possess advanced academic training. Their expertise is in interpreting and clarifying the scriptures.

Zen

Teachers of this tradition are often called "teacher" or "master." It is to signify that they possess substantial spiritual authority. Close personal training with a Zen master is an essential part of Zen practice. Besides masters, the Zen tradition also has meditation instructors and teachers who all function under the master.

Chapter 16. Zen

Zen Buddhism is the Japanese name of a school that originated in China in the 5th century and is related to the Great Way (Mahayana). It, too, relies on explanations given by the Buddha himself to his disciples. Many Zen schools regard knowledge and conventions as useless ballast. Enlightenment should breakthrough in a flash through self-arising insight.

Particularly well-known in the West are Zen meditations. The participants sit still for hours or ponder a paradoxical question (Japanese: Koan) to exhaust the constant flow of inner ideas. Zen Buddhism was mainly passed on in Japan.

What is Zen Buddhism?

Zen Buddhism, like any other form of Buddhism, originated from Buddha.

After his enlightenment, he developed countless ways to teach his disciples to reach the experience of awakening. It was reported that on one occasion, a large number of his disciples assembled, and Buddha approached them, as he usually did when he wanted to give a teaching. This time instead of talking, he raised a lotus flower with one of his hands without saying a word and just sketched a soft smile. All the disciples gathered there could see the gesture but did not realize what he wanted to convey. However, one of his chief disciples, Mahakashyapa, could understand and grasp the message that the Buddha sent beyond any word. This particular event, in which the Buddha could silently communicate something of the spirit of awakening, is considered the beginning of Zen's great tradition.

Without depending on words or letters, Zen tries to bring the practice and teaching of awakening beyond any doctrine, scripture, or conventional communication method. Zen Buddhism is a concrete and immediate way of emitting the essence of Enlightenment experience and seeing things as they are. It is pointing directly to the mind.

Zen Buddhism is a branch of late Indian Buddhism called Mahayana. The Mahayana has several philosophical backgrounds. One of the schools called Madhyamika, which emphasizes the empty nature of things from the Shunyata doctrine - Zen Buddhism likewise stresses that the mind or consciousness is identical to what he perceives, emphasizing the Mahayana philosophical school called Yogachara. According to this doctrine, to reach the full experience of awakening, one must directly contact the nature of Mind or consciousness in its most profound sense. In this way, Zen Buddhism considers the Mind to be identical with reality, and this means that if we want to reach full awakening, we have to approach that which allows us to perceive it directly. We have to contact our mind directly - this is carried out through meditation.

History of Zen Buddhism

Zen or Zen-Buddhism is the Japanese name of the Ch'an tradition, originated in China, and associated with Buddhism's origins is the Mahayana branch, Sanskrit, "Great Vehicle," doctrinal synthesis of the Buddha's teachings Gautama Buddha, performed by various Buddhist schools around the second century. Cultivated mainly in China, Japan, Vietnam, and Korea. Zen's essential practice in the Japanese and monastic version is Zazen, a type of contemplative meditation that aims to bring the practitioner to the "direct experience of reality."

In Japanese monastic Zen, there are two main strands: Soto and Rinzai. While the Soto school places greater emphasis on silent meditation, the Rinzai school makes extensive use of koans, riddles, or charades. Zen is currently one of the most well-known and expanding Buddhist schools in the West.

According to Allan Watts, an Englishman who became famous for Zen's spread in the West from the third decade of the twentieth century, Zen's original form is no longer in China. What is closer to this original version is found in traditional Japanese art forms that have been cultivated and transmitted according to this tradition.

There are several legends within the Zen tradition, transmitted and renewed by the oral tradition and parts of Chinese and Japanese folklore that intertwine with history. Narratives of oral tradition, many of which are compiled into literary anthologies, maybe, according to different views of theorists, considered legends, folklore, and mythology literature.

Zen-Buddhism's origins have pointed to the Flower Sermon (mentioned earlier), whose earliest source comes from the 14th century. Gautama Buddha joined his disciples to a Dharma speech. When they entered, the Buddha remained utterly silent, and some thought he was tired or sick. The Buddha raised a flower silently, and several disciples tried to interpret what this meant, though none of them did adequately. One of the disciples, Mahakashyapa, silently looked at the flower and obtained a unique understanding beyond the words - prajna, or "wisdom," directly from the mind of the Buddha. Mahakashyapa somehow understood the true inexpressible meaning of the flower, and the Buddha smiled at him, acknowledging his knowledge and said:

"I possess the pure eye of the Dharma, the wonderful mind of Nirvana, the original form of the report, the delicate Dharma portal which does not depend on words or writings but it's a special communication outside the scriptures, this I pass to Mahakashyapa."

Mahakashyapa is, by this rare gift of understanding, considered the founding patriarch by Chinese Zen, or (Ch'an).

In this way, through Zen, a path was developed that focused on direct experience rather than on rational beliefs or revealed scriptures. Wisdom was passed not through words but the lineage of the direct transmission of mind to the mind or a teacher's thought to a disciple. It is commonly believed that this lineage has continued uninterrupted from the Buddha's time to the present day. Historically this belief is debatable because of the lack of evidence to support it. According to DT Suzuki, the idea of a line of descent from Gautama Buddha is a distinctive Zen institution. He believes scholars invented it through hagiography to give legitimacy and prestige to Zen.

Philosophy and Practice of Zen Buddhism

Zen is a branch of the Mahayana Buddhist tradition and is fundamentally based on Siddhartha Gautama's teachings, the historical Buddha, and the founder of Buddhism. However, through its history, Zen also received influences from the countries' diverse cultures it has passed through.

Its formative period in China, in particular, determined much of its identity. Taoist teachings and practices exerted considerable influence on Chinese Chan. Concepts such as Huawei, the fluid nature of reality, and the " non-carved stone" can still be identified in Japanese Zen and related schools." Even the Zen tradition of "mad masters" is a continuation of the rule of Taoist masters. Another influence though minor, came from Confucianism.

Such peculiarities have led some scholars to argue that Zen is an "independent" school outside the Mahayana tradition - or even Buddhism. These positions, however, are a minority. The vast majority of scholars regard Zen as a Buddhist school within the Mahayana tradition.

All Zen schools are well-versed in Buddhist philosophy and doctrine, including the Four Noble Truths, the Noble Eightfold Path, and the parasites. However, Zen's emphasis on experiencing reality directly, in addition to ideas and words, always keeps it within the limits of tradition.

This openness enabled (and allowed) non-Buddhists to practice Zen, such as the Jesuit priest Hugo Enomiya-Lassalle, to receive the Dharma transmission and many other non-Buddhists.

Zen Practices and Teachings

In general, Zen's teachings criticize the study of texts and the desire for worldly achievements and focus on a dedication to meditation (zazen) to directly experience the mind and reality. However, Zen does not become a quietist doctrine - the Chinese Chan Baizhang (in Japanese, Hyakujo, 720-814), for example, devoted himself to manual work in his monastery and had as his motto a saying that remained famous among Zen practitioners: "A day without work is a day without food."

Zen has a long tradition of meditative work, from manual to refined activities such as calligraphy, ikebana, and the famous tea ceremony - in addition to martial arts. Zen has always been connected.

However, these practices are well-grounded in the Buddhist scriptures, especially in the Mahayana sutras composed in India and China, particularly the Huineng Platform Sutra, Heart Diamond Lankavatara Sutra, and Samantamukha Parivarta, a part of the Lotus Sutra. The significant influence of the Lankavatara Sutra, in particular, led to the formation of Zen's "mind-only" philosophy, in which consciousness itself is the only reality.

Zen is not a style of intellectual or solitary practice. Of course, temples and centers always assemble a group of practitioners (a sangha) and conduct daily activities and monthly retreats (sessions). Also, Zen is seen as a way of life, not just as a set of practices or a state of consciousness.

Zen and Meditation

Likewise, Zen is the school of Buddhism that takes reflection as a direct way to reach awakening. All schools of Buddhism also take meditation as a practice and try to achieve full awareness. However, Zen is among the different traditional schools that take meditation as the primary tool to reach this achievement.

The word Zen is of Japanese origin and is derived from Chan's Chinese name, which Mahayana Buddhism practiced in China from which Zen arose. In turn, the story Chan is a transliteration of the Sanskrit word Dhyana. The term Dhyana describes the experience of meditative absorption that occurs after an effective concentration. In the ancient discourses of the Buddha, up to eight different levels of this absorption are detailed.

They were observing our nature and awakening to Buddhahood. Buddhahood happens when you reach your ultimate enlightenment. Zen considers that any person has the potential for Enlightenment and Buddhahood in his experience; this is a very particular feature of Zen Buddhism. When practitioners become involved with any aspect of their practice, be it conscious attention, compassion, or whatever they assume, that quality is already inherent in their experience. Consequently, the method consists of opening up and discovering what already exists in its condition; this makes Zen practice very positive, affirmative and allows its practitioners to progress naturally and directly. In essence, Zen affirms that we are all Buddhas, and training helps discover this fact more deeply.

A peculiarity of Buddhist ethics can be found in Zen Buddhism. Here, the prohibition of intoxicating means is emphasized. It is related to the fact that in Zen Buddhism, the right mindfulness has a significant role. Moreover, intoxicants prevent a clear and always alert mind. Another peculiarity that only occurs in Zen Buddhism is the great importance of goodness and compassion. In Zen Buddhism, the idea of universal love is emphasized as much as the concept of charity in Christianity. That is why nonviolence, peacefulness, and love of one's enemies are sought.

The Three Jewels of Refuge

Also known as the 3 Refuges or the Triple Gem, the 3 Jewels are where Buddhists can take refuge. Taking refuge in Buddhism means seeking shelter and security, a sense of safety and well-being, by taking a vow, a vow on each of the 3 Jewels. It is an intellectual and spiritual commitment to the path of Buddhism. The 3 Jewels are different levels of an awakened mind. The 3 Jewels are the Buddha, the Dharma, and the Sangha.

With this Jewel, you are acknowledging the Buddha as an enlightened man, not a god, who followed a specific path to Nirvana – an approach that you, too, can follow. You acknowledge that the Buddha held supreme wisdom and compassion, that he was entirely pure, and that he can show you the way to enlightenment. You are also acknowledging the teachings of the Buddha. Since the actual Buddha is no longer in this world, you embrace all of the other Buddhist teachers who continue to spread his supreme knowledge worldwide. You seek refuge in enlightenment, knowing that there is a path to enlightenment, and you can follow that path to Nirvana.

You must trust and accept the Dharma to practice Buddhism; you must also trust in yourself that you are mindful of the moment in practicing Buddhism. You are embracing the way to Nirvana by embracing the lessons of Dharma. The Dharma is your guide; therefore, you seek refuge in the Dharma to protect you and show you how to Nirvana.

You cannot achieve enlightenment alone – you need other Buddhists' help to help you find your way to Nirvana. You can compare it to belonging to a church. When you are a member of a church, you attend that church faithfully. You actively participate in the church and its functions. You do not participate in other churches of other religions because the church you attend is your church – it is your chosen religion. The Sangha is the community with which you surround yourself. Your fellow Buddhists will help you see your truth, and you will help them see their validity, as well. There are no demands in the Sangha, no expectations – it is a community of like-minded people who seek enlightenment, just like you. Fulfillment comes from the Sangha because you are accepted and welcomed without question and judgment.

The Three Higher Training

The 3 Higher Training are some of the most critical aspects of the teachings of the Buddha. These pieces of training are essential on the path to liberation and enlightenment. Regardless of which Buddhist way you are on, which instructions you follow (Mahayana, Theravada, and Vajrayana), these three pieces of training do not change – they are essential to all the Buddhist paths. These higher training all work together to help you reach a state of enlightenment. The 3 Higher Training are ethical discipline, concentration, and wisdom.

Ethical discipline gets your mind ready for meditation. It would help if you had an exact reason to meditate. You cannot have any negativity in your mind, or you will not correctly meditate. It would help if you were disciplined to simplify your life, and simple life is the Buddhist way. You have to make an environment around you to maintain a peaceful, happy state of mind.

Concentration is that actual act of meditation. It is when you transform your mind. Your mind becomes a clear space through meditation levels, free of negativity, pure, and ready for enlightenment. After reflection, when your mind reaches the most hygienic level, wisdom follows. With understanding, you can find even more ways to simplify your life, to be disciplined. The more you discipline yourself and your life, the more you can open your mind to higher meditation levels, creating even more wisdom. A simple, disciplined life leaves you more time and energy to devote to meditation, leading to more knowledge and awareness, leading to more discipline.

It is easy to see that the 3 Higher Training are a circle of individuals and, yet, dependent on each other. Each training takes you to another level of the next, and then the process starts over. With each time you simplify, meditate, and gain wisdom, you are that much closer to reaching enlightenment – to reaching Nirvana.

The path of enlightenment has a few principles that are the foundation of Buddha's teachings. These principles are divided into three categories, which are prajna, sila, and samadhi.

Prajna

One of the first principles of the Buddhist path is prajna, also known as wisdom. Prajna is regarded as enlightenment, which is the main focus of Buddhism. When it comes to prajna, understanding is a lot different than knowledge. Knowledge is what you know, a collection of facts. Wisdom comes out when you are most calm and pure. It's obtained through meditation and cultivation and comes at the end of your path.

Sila

The word sila translates to moral values and is essential in the path's progress as it's the foundation of qualities. There are two principles that sila is based on, and these are the principles of reciprocity and equality. When Buddhists talk about the direction of equality, they are speaking about the equality of all living things, including the equality of security and happiness.

Samadhi

Samadhi translates to mediation. As a Buddhist, you want to obtain pure freedom, which you can do through mental development. You need to purify the mind, and the only way to do this is through meditation or samadhi.

All three of these practices work together to purify the mind so that you can obtain complete freedom. You can't have one without the other.

Chapter 18. The Three Poisons – Diseased Roots

Moha or Delusion

The Buddhist concept of moha can be translated to delusion, dullness, or confusion. A being's ignorance can be traced to this root. According to traditional Mahayanists, it is the reason for a being's destructive thoughts and actions. In the Wheel of Life, moha is represented by the boar.

The cure for Moha lies in Wisdom or prajna.

Raga or Greed

The Sanskrit word raga translates to "color" or "hue," but it represents the qualities of greed, lust, desire, and sensual attachment. All forms of craving, significantly those sensual and sexual, fall under this poison. Any being who seeks and finds excitement over worldly pleasures that the senses can feel is afflicted by it. The rooster is the symbol for raga in the Wheel of life.

The cure for Raga can be found in Generosity or dana.

Dvesha or Ill Will

The term dveshais Sanskrit and means "hate" or "aversion." It is represented by the snake in the Wheel of Life. Harboring dvesha towards anything, including other beings and yourself, leads to suffering.

One can be cured of Dvesha through Loving-kindness or metta.

If you take a look at an image of the Wheel of Life, you will see at the center the Three Poisons as their animal representations. Specifically, you will notice that the snake and the rooster are coming out from the mouth of the boar. It means that the first poison – delusion – is the source of the latter two toxins – greed and ill will.

However, what is a delusion? It is the mindset attached to a false sense of self and reality. To help you recognize the presence of the first poison, here is a famous Buddhist story:

The moon is hidden in the clouds, but the stars are out and are enough to guide you as you follow the path that is familiar to you. Then, ahead of you, you see something.

It is long and winding, and it appears as if it is ready to strike out at you. You feel a sense of panic as your body is suddenly frozen with fear. Then, the clouds moved, allowing the moonlight to shine on this coil, and you realized it is merely a piece of rope.

After doing so, you realize that there was no snake in the area in the first place. It was just the idea of the possibility that struck you. Your mind relaxes, and your heart drops back to its average rate as you continue to follow the path.

After reading this analogy, what do you think the "snake" represents? If you believe that it means your false sense of self, then you are right. But as long as you hold on to the idea that that piece of rope was a snake, then you will continue to feel fear, stress, sadness, disappointment – suffering. However, through wisdom as symbolized by the moonlight, and if you make an effort to look around, you will discover that this false sense of self does not exist.

Therefore, the Three Poisons cure acknowledges that your concept of who you are or should be is false. Once you let go of this, you can move towards cultivating wisdom, generosity, and loving-kindness.

Be open to relearning and letting go of certain things in your life. However, if you do stumble, just pick yourself up, brush yourself off, and move on. There is no deadline or competition towards Enlightenment. Remember that the Buddha himself said that all beings are equally capable of reaching it.

The Buddhist philosophy will help you come to terms with whatever you perceive as your weaknesses and strengthen your resolve against the things that give you problems. You are more capable of embracing life to its fullest.

The way that this variation of Mindfulness Meditation works is that it combines focus and detachment. This meditation can be performed anywhere, including at home, at work, or anywhere in between. Since this form of meditation will require the most practice before you can do it effectively, it is probably best that you start practicing it at home. It will allow you to focus more efficiently while also providing a calmer environment to meditate in. The trick to mindfulness meditation is to focus on a single activity and then take the same mental step back you did in Open Awareness Meditation. By doing this, you can be focused while also being detached. The huge advantage of this meditation is that it will allow you to develop the Buddha Mind while living your day-to-day life. You won't have to find a quiet time or a quiet place to perform this meditation. Instead, this is a form of meditation that you can achieve no matter where you are and what else you are doing.

The ideal way to begin practicing this meditation is to perform it while you are doing household chores. Any household chore will give you the focus point you need for the concentrative element, provided that it is a chore that will take at least 10 minutes to perform. That said, washing dishes is a perfect chore for Mindfulness Meditation. While you might feel that you pay attention to washing dishes typically, this will require greater focus. The point of focusing on the words now isn't to ensure that you are doing a good job; instead, it is to make sure that your mind is clear of all thoughts and feelings not associated with washing dishes.

Once you have achieved total focus on washing the dishes, you go to the second phase of the meditation—the open awareness phase. At this point, you should shift your attention from washing dishes to the other things going on around you. Again, it is essential to take in a few details while focusing on a person before moving on to the next focus. Now you are an active observer, both participating and observing. At this point, you should perform a feeling of being present yet detached from the environment you are in.

Additionally, the opportunity to lose focus is increased in this scenario as you are actively performing a task while not necessarily being alone. Even so, that is the whole point of this method. This form of meditation is designed to help you take your learned skills of concentration and detachment and to be able to apply them in the regular world. The necessary steps of this meditation are as follows:

- While washing dishes was used as the example above, it is not the only chore available. Folding clothes, sweeping a floor, vacuuming, washing a car, or any other such activity will do as well. Any task that involves machinery should be avoided, such as mowing a lawn, as any lapse in concentration could increase the risk of serious injury. Could you keep it simple and keep it safe?

- Begin to perform your chore as you usually would.
- Stay focused on your breathing until your breathing becomes natural and relaxed. Additionally, stay focused on your breathing until your body and mind reach a more relaxed state.
- Next, begin to focus on the chore you are performing. Focus on the task the way you would on a candle or other object using the Concentrative Meditation techniques.
- Stay focused on the object until all unrelated thoughts and feelings in your mind fade away.
- Once you have achieved a clear mind, begin to shift your attention to other things using Open Awareness Meditation techniques.
- Focus on each object or person for no more than 5-10 seconds, being sure to take in details of each thing you pay attention to.
- Keep doing this until you feel detached from your environment. You want to feel like an observer with no attachments to anything or anyone around you.
- Maintain this practice for at least 10 minutes. As you get better at the technique, you can increase your time as much as you want.

The one thing that separates the Mindfulness Meditation technique from the Concentrative and Open Awareness techniques is that you will perform it even when you are actively involved in life. The more that you practice Mindfulness Meditation while doing everyday things is the better you will become. Eventually, you will find that the meditation will evolve into an actual way of life. Instead of intentionally performing Mindfulness Meditation, you will begin to practice it out of habit. After a while, it will change your whole way of life as it will redefine your state of mind. With this, a severe reduction of stress, anxiety, anger, and any other detrimental mindset will follow. Before long, you will begin to live a life of focus and detachment which will lead you ever closer to the state of Nirvana that frees you from all human suffering.

Chapter 19. Combating Stress, Anxiety, and Depression with Buddhism

Suffering is an inevitable part of life and, until you have reached the state of Enlightenment, it helps to know how to cope with each challenge you face. Stressful situations can stir feelings of pain and anxiety, more so if they have to do with the things that you are most attached to. The good news is, Buddhist teachings can show you ways to cope with such emotions and events. The most effective of these is Mindfulness Meditation.

Mindfulness is the trait of paying close attention to the present moment. It allows you to see the reality for what it is, unclouded by assumptions and expectations. Studies show how effective mindfulness meditation is in reducing stress both instantaneously and over the long term.

It triggers you to either face the problem or flees from it. In both cases, the body and mind react in the same way.

Consider the Best Ways to Respond to Stress and Anxiety

The body responds to how the mind perceives a stressful situation, so the best way to feel less stress is by calming the mind first. Therefore, the stronger your reason is, the more resistant your body would be towards stressful situations. Begin by recognizing your power to choose.

For instance, you can use your journal to reflect on how you usually responded to these situations. There are plenty of healthy options. Here are some that are in line with the principles of Buddhism:

- Practice breathing meditation to regularize heart rate and breathing. You will find that this is covered in detail within the pages of this book.
- Go on walking mindfulness meditation to temporarily step away from the stressful situation and allow your mind to think deeply.
- Stay away from intoxicating substances that will only impede your judgment (particularly alcohol).
- Exercise with mindfulness to train the body to be more resistant.
- Detach yourself from the situation as if you are a mere spectator.
- Chant a mantra that helps strengthen your mind, such as "everything is going to be alright," or "I am calm and collected."

Once you have positive responses to stress and anxiety, you can then practice them regularly through meditation.

Breathing Meditation

Mindful breathing in and of itself merely is aware of your breath without changing it. Practicing it is a great way to acknowledge and express gratitude for the ability to breathe and help you regulate it during stressful situations.

Breathing meditation, on the other hand, can be done using a variety of techniques. One is deep breathing meditation, which is incredibly effective at reducing stress and anxiety. Here are the steps to do it:

1. Sit or lie down comfortably. Keep your back straight and shoulders relaxed. You can choose whether to use a hard chair and keep your feet planted flat on the floor or whether you want to use a cushion, bend your knees and cross your ankles. Your hands need to be posed, one cupped by the other with the palms facing upward and your thumbs touching each other.
2. Focus on your natural breath, noticing each movement of the body as the air passes through from your nostrils to the upper abdomen.
3. It will help you feel the air entering your body and create a pivot motion that will tell you that you live sufficiently profoundly.
4. Begin breathing deeply. As you inhale, notice how your belly rises, but not your chest. As you exhale, see how your stomach falls while the trunk remains relatively still. As you breathe, this movement should form a rhythm.
5. Another breathing meditation to try for stress and anxiety relief is by counting your breaths. It helps you to relax and calm the mind as well as the body. Here are the steps. After a while of meditating in this manner, you may not need to count but will know the length of your breaths instinctively by the rhythm they form in the movement of your stomach.

Mindfulness in Walking Meditation

I have included this aspect of meditation because it is useful when you are away from home and face stressful situations. You may find yourself having to meet with people who cause you stress or face a meeting that worries you. Walking meditation will help you overcome the fear and strengthen your mind to be clear-headed and meet whatever anxiety is calm.

1. Loosen any clothing that may be restrictive.
2. Stand with your back straight and start to take steps, with your head slightly lowered, watching each movement of your feet.
3. Breathe in, move the foot forward, and be aware of all the foot muscles' movement.
4. Feel your other foot lift off the ground, move forward, be conscious of the muscles' movement in the leg, the knee, and the calf.
5. Be conscious of the foot touching the ground and continue to breathe in and out using your nostrils for the inhalation and feeling the air go through to your lower chest area.
6. When you breathe out, move your leg in time with the breath so that you are always in rhythm with your breathing.
7. Think of nothing else at all. If thoughts happen, let them slide away into the background and go back to your concentration on walking and meditating.

This kind of meditation helps you alleviate the types of stressors brought about by events in life. Interviews, meeting new people, or going to a meeting can all be precursors to this kind of stress, and this type of meditation can help you keep your composure and control what you are feeling inside of yourself. Be in the moment. Be in the steps that you take. Breathe.

Be Mindful of Your Thought Patterns

Modern-day stressors are not the leading cause of your stress and anxiety. It has more to do with your perspectives. The teachings of the Buddha offer plenty of ways to transform your thought patterns for the better.

However, anyone can get distracted from these because of the demands of daily life. See Things from a Different Angle.

Imagine yourself in someone else's shoes, such as someone you admire (perhaps the Buddha himself?). How do you think this person would perceive the situation? How would he respond to the source of stress? Sometimes this exercise can change how you see things yourself. You may have already done this in your everyday day-to-day life. I am thinking as a child thinking that I was a concert pianist when I had piano practice, and it's almost the same thing, except that you are using that other person as your focal point and looking at the situation from the angle that person would see it, rather than seeing it as yourself. It helps you to avoid distraction and to use inspiration to guide you.

Identify the Individual Parts of the Stressor.

Seeing a big issue as a whole can be taxing, emotionally and mentally. Therefore, it would be a good idea to break the subject down into smaller, more manageable parts so that you can stop procrastinating and start solving it. It may hurt you to think about the things that stress you initially, but when you can identify them and dissect the problem into smaller portions, it is easier to cope with. We put off dealing with stressors because, in themselves, they cause us stress, and we believe in avoidance. However, if you dissect the problems, they become smaller and more manageable, and you can gradually expose yourself to these stressors so that they don't cause the same psychological damage. Let me give you an instance. If you have problems with relationships, write down the issues in a list format and work on one of them at a time until they become less of a problem. If you are stressed by going into a public place, try entering an area where you are more aware of who is likely to be there and gradually spread your wings a little and include new people into your circle so that you are not so anxious with strangers.

Consult an Expert.

If you acknowledge that you alone are incapable of solving your stress and anxiety problem, do not be afraid to approach an expert. Receiving guidance from someone who has already gained the wisdom to solve such problems will benefit you greatly and enable you to solve the problem for yourself later on in life. The subconscious mind works when you have stressors because it responds to how your mind has taught it to respond. You can change this programming by mild exposure to the trigger and gradually realize that you can react positively to whatever that trigger is. Professionals help people to do this if they are afraid of doing it on their own.

CHRISTIANITY

Christianity refers to many religious traditions that have grown from a single source. These include Catholicism, Protestantism (which has many divisions), Copts, Eastern Orthodox Christianity, and countless small sects. All of them have in common the teachings of Jesus Christ as they have evolved over the past 2,000 years. Christianity has had an incalculable effect on the world, both on its culture and language and its political and social development. Western governments have established national holidays around Christian rituals, and we live by a calendar that measures time according to "Before Christ" and "Anno Domini" (in the year of Our Lord).

Chapter 20. Mudras to Combat Stress

We live in an age of anxiety. When we are stressed, we acknowledge it yet still refuse to address our stressors like they're the plague. This fallacy leads us on a continual cycle: experiencing more stress and more tension, leading to fatigue, physical illness, or worse. It's time for you to take charge!

What Does Mundras Mean?

Mudras are a type of symbolic hand gesture in Hinduism and Buddhism. While there are many different mudras, each one represents something about the religion.

In Hinduism, people often use mudras to show spiritual powers or blessings and represent aspects of the god or goddess they worship. Buddhists may use a mudra to represent Buddha's teaching and serve as an offering during meditation. In yoga, mudras are used to help balance the body.

Mudra means "seal" or "sign." A mudra can be made with any part of the body, but most commonly, it is made with the hands or fingers. Often a mudra is incorporated into a yantra, which symbolizes a sacred diagram and has a specific set of hand postures. Yantras represent cosmic principles that create and sustain the world; they are used for meditative purposes by Hindus and Buddhists.

It is said that through the use of mudras and yantras, the body can be purified and aligned with the universe. By using mudras, people are believed to increase their energy and creativity.

By incorporating specific mudras into your daily routine (they can be practiced anywhere!), you will learn how to manage your stressful lifestyle while simultaneously improving your physical and mental well-being.

If you're feeling stressed, have a hard time sleeping, or need some help increasing your self-confidence, try these mudras! Mudras are hand gestures that can help with physical and emotional ailments. They can also provide more peace of mind if you're worried about an upcoming event.

Different Mudras to Help Physical and Emotional Stress

1. Gyan mudra: Place your right thumb and middle finger on your forehead and press the tip of your ring finger against the advice of your thumb to form a circle. Hold it for as long as possible for the best effect.

2. Ashwini mudra: Alternately press your ring finger and thumb tips against each other while you keep the rest of your fingers extended. Inhale deeply and hold for five to ten seconds.

3. Gyan mudra with Anahata chakra mudra: Place your right hand in the Gyan mudra, but instead of touching your forehead, connect the middle of your chest with it. Make an Anahata chakra mudra with the rest of your fingers (see below), and hold it for as long as possible.

4. Bhand Mudra: The Bhand Mudra is similar to holding a ball under your hand or cupping it from underneath.

5. Anahata chakra mudra: Interlock all of your fingers except for your index and pinky fingers. Straighten them out while you keep them touching. The pinky finger should extend straight out, while the rest should be bent at a 90-degree angle.

6. Gyan mudra with Sushumna Anahata Chakra mudra: Use both hands to make each mudra as described above, then hold them together (as if in prayer) against your chest with the fingertips touching or overlapping slightly.

7. Bharam: Place your hands, palms facing upwards, and fingers slightly separated on the sides of your face.

8. Antakshari mudra: Point your middle finger at someone else, then wiggle it at them while you make that hand gesture with your other hand right after. Do it repeatedly quickly for best effect!

9. Gyan mudra with closed eyes: As in Gyan mudra, this time with closed eyes and **one** hand closed around the other fist when tonguing through the lips.

10. Gyan mudra with Anahata chakra mudra: As in the description above, use a Gyan mudra instead of touching your chest.

11. Gyan mudra with Sushumna Anahata Chakra mudra: As in the description above, but use both hands to make each mudra as described above, then hold them together (as if in prayer) against your chest with the fingertips touching or overlapping slightly.

12. Bharam: Place your hand's palms down on either side of your head and press hard enough so that you feel some pressure while keeping the two palms facing each other and fingers apart.

13. Gyan mudra with closed eyes: As in Gyan mudra, this time with closed eyes and one hand closed around the other fist when tonguing through the lips.

14. Gyan mudra with Sushumna Anahata Chakra mudra: As in the description above, but use both hands to make each mudra as described above, then hold them together (as if in prayer) against your chest with the fingertips touching or overlapping slightly.

15. Gyan mudra with Anahata chakra mudra: As in the description above, use a Gyan mudra instead of touching your chest.

16. Bharam: Place your hand's palms down on either side of your head and press hard enough so that you feel some pressure while keeping the two palms facing each other and fingers apart.

17. Gyan mudra with closed eyes: As in Gyan mudra, this time with closed eyes and one hand closed around the other fist when tonguing through the lips.

18. Gyan mudra with Sushumna Anahata Chakra mudra: As in the description above, but use both hands to make each mudra as described above, then hold them together (as if in prayer) against your chest with the fingertips touching or overlapping slightly.

19. Gyan mudra with Anahata chakra mudra: As in the description above, use a Gyan mudra instead of touching your chest.

20. Bharam: Place your hand's palms down on either side of your head and press hard enough so that you feel some pressure while keeping the two palms facing each other and fingers apart.

21. Antakshari mudra: Point your middle finger at someone else, then wiggle it at them while you make that hand gesture with your other hand right after. Do it repeatedly quickly for best effect!

22. Gyan mudra with closed eyes: As in Gyan mudra, this time with closed eyes and one hand closed around the other fist when tonguing through the lips.

23. Gyan mudra with Sushumna Anahata Chakra mudra: As in the description above, but use both hands to make each mudra as described above, then hold them together (as if in prayer) against your chest with the fingertips touching or overlapping slightly.

24. Bharam: Place your hand's palms down on either side of your head and press hard enough so that you feel some pressure while keeping the two palms facing each other and fingers apart.

25. Gyan mudra with Anahata chakra mudra: As in the description above, use a Gyan mudra instead of touching your chest.

26. Gyan mudra with closed eyes: As in Gyan mudra, this time with closed eyes and one hand closed around the other fist when tonguing through the lips.

27. Gyan mudra with Sushumna Anahata Chakra mudra: As in the description above, but use both hands to make each mudra as described above, then hold them together (as if in prayer) against your chest with the fingertips touching or overlapping slightly.

28. Bharam: Place your hand's palms down on either side of your head and press hard enough so that you feel some pressure while keeping the two palms facing each other and fingers apart.

29. Gyan mudra with Anahata chakra mudra: As in the description above, use a Gyan mudra instead of touching your chest.

30. Bharam: Place your hand's palms down on either side of your head and press hard enough so that you feel some pressure while keeping the two palms facing each other and fingers apart.

31. Gyan mudra with Anahata chakra mudra: As in the description above, use a Gyan mudra instead of touching your chest.

32. Bharam: Place your hand's palms down on either side of your head and press hard enough so that you feel some pressure while keeping the two palms facing each other and fingers apart.

33. Gyan mudra with Anahata chakra mudra: As in the description above, use a Gyan mudra instead to touch your chest.

34. Bharam: Place your hand's palms down on either side of your head and press hard enough so that you feel some pressure while keeping the two palms facing each other and fingers apart.

35. Gyan mudra with Anahata chakra mudra: As in the description above, use a Gyan mudra instead of touching your chest.

36. Bharam: Place your hand's palms down on either side of your head and press hard enough so that you feel some pressure while keeping the two palms facing each other and fingers apart.

37. Gyan mudra with Anahata chakra mudra: As in the description above, use a Gyan mudra instead of touching your chest.

38-53 Repeat steps 13-37 three more times, always starting with 13 and 53.

54. Shambhavi mudra: This is the same as Gyan Mudra, except that you use your right hand to form the Gyan mudra and your left hand to form shambhavi mudra.

55-57 Repeat steps 13-37 three more times, always starting with 13 and ending with 57.

58. Utkanthi mudra: Keep both hands open and upturned.

59-61 Repeat steps 13-37 three more times, always starting with 13 and ending with 61. The "C" is the center. Each of the 13 numbers is assigned a letter. The numbers from 1 to 9 are designated A, B, C, D, E, F; the numbers 10 to 90 are assigned G, H, I, J, K; and the numbers 100 to 999 are assigned L. For example, 4225 is 5 (J) and 23 (L).

Purpose of the Mudras

The purpose of a mudra in Hinduism is to prevent evil influences from entering the body through the hands and encourage good energy from holy figures to enter the body. The hands are believed to link to one's heart directly, so they are seen as an avenue for sending love and receiving love. As part of prayers or rituals, mudras have been used since ancient times in Hinduism.

Different types of mudras involve different finger positions. Some might use a single fist position, while others may include the thumb or entire fist to create an almost meditative state. The mudra is supposed to bring about divine energy, healing, and blessing, all with one simple gesture of the hands.

A mudra can be performed with a hands-on lap while sitting. A mudra can also be performed during a conversation or even when holding a pen or pencil.

Ancient yogis studied how the mind responds when one uses mudras and recited mantras using specific hand gestures, such as "Gyan Mudra" (the motion used when chanting the mantra "Om Gum Ganapataye Namaha," meaning Glory Be to Lord Ganesh).

Mudras are still commonly used in Hinduism to bring about positive life changes and to deliver a message that a person wants to communicate to the world.

Chapter 21. Start Your Day with Positive Motivations and Thoughts

How to Develop Positive Core Beliefs and Balanced Life

This famous quote by Buddha signifies the importance of living each day mindfully. It is imperative to incorporate values and principles into our daily lives. It ensures peace and tranquility in the world. Living each day mindfully will not be comfortable in the beginning. You may feel the need to give up. However, living mindfully is the only way to solve issues we face in our daily lives. Man must learn to be at peace because everything in this world keeps changing with time. He must understand that expecting something to last forever will only bring forth distress.

Pursuit of Happiness

Life is often seen as the pursuit of happiness. The yearning for pleasure is an instinct. Nobody wants to be unhappy. When a person is happy, he wants the feeling to last forever. He does everything within his capacity to maintain it. When a person is unhappy, he tries to push the feeling away. He either broods about it or thinks of ways to forget the factor that's making him sick. Every other desire of a human being is incidental and ancillary to the desire for happiness. Man seeks money, wealth, company, and other aspects to attain happiness. However, Buddha said, "there is no path to happiness. Happiness is the path itself".

Letting Go of Clinging

When we are happy or have something, we like, we tend to make it last forever. We do not want to accept that the world is dynamic. We do not want to get change. Similarly, when we are facing something negative, we are scared that it will last forever. A real Buddhist would know otherwise.

Don't Take It Personally

"Why did this happen to me?" We ask ourselves and the people around us when things do not go our way. We are demanding explanations for why something negative has happened to us. The only practical answer is that negativity and misfortune may be bestowed on anybody. There is no need to take this personally. Instead, realize that the suffering is only temporary and move on in life.

Opening to Love

Buddha, in his sermons, emphasized the importance of love. He said that the best and most important kind of love is one's love for oneself. Only when one loves oneself will one be able to love another. It is genuine. It is not possible to share something you do not possess. If a man does not love himself, then there is no love inside him. He will not be able to love others. We are often distressed and upset about "not being loved." Sometimes people are sad because the person from whom they crave love does not love them back enough. It causes suffering. The sting of love can be the worst and most unbearable pain in the world. It is why people are often scared to open up to love or to expect love. If love can hurt us so much, why does Buddha ask us to be open to love? Perhaps the reason is that Buddha's definition of love is different from ours, or maybe because he understands this emotion's depth far more than we do. When you love someone and expect them to love you back the same way, such love can no longer be called selfless. If love isn't selfless, it isn't loved at all. It is merely attachment. It is the attachment that causes pain and not loves. The Bible says that love is patient, kind, selfless, and all-forgiving. Being able to love that way is putting an end to a lot of suffering that we endure.

Buddha advocated the Love Kindness meditation to help people develop this ability. This meditation focuses on nourishing the feelings of love and compassion in your heart. The Buddha asked his disciples to meditate on someone they love. However, he asked them to ensure that their focus must be on the emotion of love and not on the person they are thinking of. Men must strive to foster the feeling of compassion within them. They must feel for other fellow beings. Man must realize that the whole world is his family and that every other deserves to be loved.

Buddha said that hate is not an answer to anything. Hatred, greed, and ignorance are the main reasons for suffering in this world. Man must develop the ability to love and take care of another as much as he loves himself. It will ensure peaceful co-existence between beings. It can change the reason for one's existence, to redefine every aspect of him once and for all. Only the rays of love can warm a cold soul or heal a broken heart.

Love has the power to open the inner eye and to fill one with bliss and peace. However, one must have the insight to differentiate between love and attachment. It was able to make this distinction that will change one's life forever.

Anger Management

One day a young boy fought with his mother. He said things that he didn't mean because of his anger. It left his mother deeply wounded. The young boy's father, who had listened to the mother and son's conversation, called the boy aside and walked him to the wooden fence guarding their home. He asked the boy not to speak when he is angry. The son did as he was told. After a few days, the boy ran out of pins. When the young boy confronted his father, the father asked the boy to remove the nails one by one from the fence whenever he was angry. Once again, the boy took his father's advice.

Freedom from Fear

We live in fear every day. Fear of death, fear of losing someone we love, fear of being poor, fear of being unsuccessful, etc. – these are only some of the fears we face every day. Living in fear is as good as being half alive.

When we are in a good state, we are scared of losing it. When we are in a bad state, we fear it will last forever. The most profound reason for this is desire. It is our desire to be happy always and our desire never to be sad. However, this is an impossible goal to achieve. Further, there is no way to put an end to suffering. Old age and death are also unavoidable in life; there is absolutely no point in dreading them.

Compassionate Life

Compassion is the highest level of love and kindness. Buddhism stresses the importance of developing love and service in one's life. Understanding also means 'empathy to other beings.' Man must feel sympathetic to other fellow beings. He must pay special attention to increase positive feelings like love and kindness within him.

Similarly, man must make a conscious effort to ensure that negative feelings are discarded from the mind. Man must have to ability to move beyond self-centeredness. It is easier to be compassionate when one realizes that his fellow beings also have wants and needs. They also want happiness and companionship.

Chapter 22. How Do I Begin to Practice Buddhism?

The Five Precepts of Buddhism are the fundamental ethical guidelines for Buddhists. However, they are not regarded as a rigid set of rules and gentle suggestions on living a life free from suffering. After all, the Buddha always emphasizes the being's power of choice.

Below is a description of the Five Precepts as well as suggestions on how to put each of them into practice:

The First Precept: Do Not Intentionally Kill Any Living Being.

The followers of Buddha should not entertain the idea of causing harm or, worse, killing any other living beings, whether human or animal. Instead, they cultivate genuine concern for and loving-kindness towards the welfare of others.

You can bring the First Precept to mind each time you are tempted to hurt a living being, be it an insect or another person. The least you can do is avoid having anything to do with the senseless killing of animals, such as for sport or overconsumption. It is this First Precept that has inspired many Buddhists to become vegan.

The Second Precept: Take Only What Is Given to You.

This precept greatly discourages stealing and "borrowing" items from others without returning them. By following this precept, Buddhists seek equality in the distribution of resources, and, at the same time, they wish to instill the value of generosity in themselves.

To put the Second Precept into practice in the modern world, you can work towards living within your means and paying off debts that you owe. Many Buddhists have turned to the minimalist lifestyle because it guides people to let go of consumerism and live meaningful lives. In this day and age, this is also a common practice because the simplicity of this precept is that it gives so much back. The common saying that "less is more" really comes into its own when examining how it applies to modern-day living.

The Third Precept: Do Not Misuse the Senses.

In the traditional sense, the third precept advises against letting one's sexual drive dominate one's life, as it is understood that it leads to suffering. Instead, Buddhists are encouraged to live a contented life with thoughts and actions that serve a meaningful purpose.

However, you may interpret the Third Precept as something that encompasses all abuse of the senses. For instance, it can be taken as advice against overeating, which leads to many sufferings, such as obesity. Instead, the Buddhist is guided towards doing things (including food consumption) in moderation and useful purposes.

Misuse of the senses can include an excess of anything that causes suffering. Excess drug consumption, excess smoking, or any quantity that touches the senses is considered to be against this precept.

The Fourth Precept: Do Not Speak of Falsehood.

The Buddha teaches that one should not lie, slander, and engage in malicious gossip. Instead, one should only speak words of truth and kindness and be motivated by positive intentions when engaging in a conversation with others.

It can be tempting at times to talk negatively about something. However, now that you have learned of this Precept, perhaps you can practice mindfulness in the way you speak. If you find it hard to hold yourself back from saying things that could hurt others, you might want to consider writing in a diary. It is a great way to begin acknowledging and monitoring your thoughts before turning them into spoken words. It is hard for people to accept that hurtful thing you say to people comes back to you and hurts you as much as those to whom the words were directed. By being true to yourself and kind to others, you suffer less, and you can feel better about who you are. Your journal is simply a means to record your negativity so that you don't make the same mistake again.

The Fifth Precept: Avoid Intoxicants.

The Fifth Precept emphasizes the harm caused by drinking alcohol and taking unnecessary stimulants and drugs. Buddhists are on the path towards improving their concentration and cultivating rational thought. Therefore, this precept is a gentle reminder of what causes the opposite of these.

However, following them rests solely on your own volition, especially since the Buddha encourages everyone to think and experience things for themselves rather than to follow through blind faith. The Five Precepts are reasonably straightforward and logical for people to follow and help put mindfulness in your life. Note them down in short form to be reminded of them and correct your behavior when you see yourself being taken away from them by life in general. Your awareness of these Precepts makes you more responsible for your actions. By accepting these seriously, you lessen your suffering and control how your mind can perceive mindfulness.

Chapter 23. The Five Impediments

The Five Hindrances

The Buddha's teachings taught us that five hindrances exist that stop us from reaching Enlightenment. These mental states are known as hindrances because they help bind us to our suffering and ignorance. Realizing our Enlightenment means freeing ourselves of these hindrances.

Hindrances can't be ignored or pushed under the rug. They will only go away once we've realized they are states we've created for ourselves. Once we can perceive this, we can begin the path towards Enlightenment.

For hindrances, one must practice and meditate. The initial step is recognizing the block, then acknowledging it, and finally understanding you're the one who's making it real.

Sensual Desire

It refers to anything from the desire for sex to desiring certain foods. When these feelings arise, the first thing to do is recognize your feeling, acknowledge it, and then try and observe the desire and not give in to it or chase the feeling.

Ill Will

Feeling anger and rage is often an easy to spot hindrance. The cure for this is to try and cultivate Metta or loving-kindness. Metta is a virtue that Buddha taught should be used in times of ill will and anger.

We often get angry because someone has bruised our ego. One needs to practice letting go of anger, acknowledging its presence, and admitting that anger is born from pride and ignorance.

Sloth, Drowsiness, or Torpor

Many people find they have trouble keeping up their energy or staying awake during meditation. The Buddha taught that we should always pay attention to the thoughts we are chasing when getting tired and then shift the mind elsewhere. If that doesn't work, try switching to walking meditation, pinching yourself, or splashing water on your face.

If this type of drowsiness occurs regularly, as you continuously feel low on energy, you need to find out if there's some psychological or physical cause. Any health issues should always be resolved in a timely fashion.

Worry and Restlessness

This particular hindrance comes in many different forms. Some of these forms include remorse, anxiety, and feeling rushed. Trying to meditate when in this state of mind is not a comfortable proposition.

If you're in an anxious state of mind, don't try and force the anxiety away. Instead, try to imagine your body as if it were a container. Observe the anxiousness moving around freely, don't attempt to separate or control it.

People who have PTSD or chronic anxiety disorders may find meditating to be incredibly intense. Skepticism or Uncertainty

Doubt and skepticism aren't good or bad. In reality, it's something you can start working with. Never ignore doubt or tell yourself to avoid feeling doubt. Instead, keep yourself open to what your skepticism and doubt are trying to warn you about.

Throughout life, we often get discouraged when our experience practicing meditation doesn't quite live up to what we expected. It is why it's important to remain unattached to any expectation. The effectiveness of our meditation sessions will differ over time. Some meditation sessions could get deep, while others could be filled with frustration.

Don't let those challenging periods get you down. Frequently, in the end, they bear the most beautiful fruit. That's why it's important not to label our meditation sessions as being good or bad. Avoid attaching any expectations.

In between these services, the monks might be assigned to work in the garden, clean or repair the monastic buildings, accommodate visitors (monasteries were often treated as inns by travelers), or copy manuscripts in the monastery's scriptorium.

Medieval Copyists

Monks in the Middle Ages spent a great deal of time copying manuscripts. Before the invention of the printing press, this was the only way of preserving texts, and the monks regarded it as a sacred charge to copy the gospels and other religious writings. They also copied many manuscripts containing works by ancient authors from Rome and Greece (though countless others were lost). The monks not only copied these works; they illustrated or illuminated them. Many illuminations were extremely rich in detail and skill and represented one of the major art forms of the Middle Ages. One of the greatest examples of monastic illumination is the Irish Book of Kells.

Although many monasteries were the targets of raids by the Northmen beginning in the ninth century, the institution survived, revived, and flourished in the High Middle Ages during the tenth through fourteenth centuries. Thanks to them, Western Europe inherited the rich religious traditions of early Christianity and much of the literature, philosophy, and other ancient Greece and Rome learning.

THE REFORMATION

Christendom Transformed

The Reformation is the name given to a dramatic upheaval within the Catholic Church between 1500 and 1625. These are only approximate dates since various church reformers before 1500 and continued reform and conflict after 1625.

Martin Luther (1483–1546) was the most influential reformer, with which the Reformation is most associated. Luther attended the university at Erfurt, aspiring to become a lawyer. However, in 1505 he had a terrifying experience. While traveling from Mansfield to Erfurt, Luther was struck by lightning. As he lay in the road, he prayed to St. Anna, promising that he would become a monk if she helped him survive. He did stay, and true to his word, he entered an Augustinian monastery in Erfurt.

Struggle and Disillusionment

Luther's time at the monastery was unhappy. He began to question the God of the scriptures as well as his relationship to God. He sought to purge himself from sin through fasting, meditation, and self-flagellation. By 1507, when he was ordained a priest, he wondered if he was really up to such a task. In 1510 he traveled to Rome. He was happy when he got there, but his happiness was short-lived. Rome was a city of corruption and materialism with a religiously indifferent population.

To Be or Not to Be?

Decades after Luther defies the papacy, Wittenberg was still highly symbolic of change and turmoil. In Hamlet, Shakespeare makes the young prince of Denmark, tortured by indecision and by unaccustomed thoughts, a former student at Wittenberg.

Luther found the core of his answer in St. Paul's letter to the Romans. From this, he derived the essential element of his philosophy: People achieve salvation by faith alone. If they believe in God through Christ's sacrifice on the cross, they are absolved of sin and will receive God's grace. It has nothing to do with doing good deeds — donating money to rebuild St. Peter's cathedral in Rome, for example.

In this, Luther attacked a prevalent practice of the church: indulgences. The church raised money for its vast projects by soliciting donations from Christians. In return for these donations, the church granted an indulgence from sin. Luther was offended by this idea, mostly as it was practiced by Johann Tetzel (1465–1519). In 1517 Tetzel was on a mission from Rome to raise funds for the rebuilding of St. Peter's basilica. In his preaching, Tetzel promised that the Christians who donated their money to this venture would be given an indulgence, which consisted of granting the pardon for past sins without penance, the release from the purgatory loved ones, and the clearing of sins that have not yet been committed.

Chapter 24. Symbols of Buddhism

Six symbols were used to represent Buddha in the early years of Buddhism. There was never an image of Buddha himself used until the Buddha statue, which wasn't created until after Buddha's death. Buddha's vision was never used in early art as it was said that he did not like to be revered as a person and was reluctant to accept images of himself. The six symbols used most often in early art were the Eight Spoked Wheel, the Bodhi Tree, an Empty Throne, Buddha's Footprints, The Lion, Deer, and Stupas.

The Eight-Spoked Wheel

The Buddha is known as the Wheel-Turner. It was he who set a new cycle of teachings into motion and changed the course of destiny. The eight spokes in the Eight-Spoked Wheel symbolize the Eightfold Noble Path. There are often three swirling segments illustrated in the hub of the wheel that represent the Triple Gem.

The wheel is often looked at in three parts, the hub, the spokes, and the rim. Many people consider each piece to relate to the Buddha practice aspect, with the seat representing discipline, the spokes representing wisdom, and the rim representing concentration.

The Bodhi Tree

It is the tree that Prince Siddhartha sat beneath when he reached enlightenment and became the Buddha. Tree worship had been a part of India's culture before Buddha came into existence, so the Bodhi tree's development to become a holy symbol was natural and isn't surprising.

An Empty Throne

The symbol of the throne is a reference to two distinct parts of who the Buddha was. First, it is a reference to Prince Siddhartha's royal ancestry. It is also a reference to the idea of Enlightenment being a spiritual kingship.

Buddha's Footprints

Traditionally, the footprints symbolize the physical presence of the Enlightened One. It is said that before his death, the Buddha left an imprint of his foot on a stone as a reminder of his presence on earth.

The Lion

Traditionally, the lion is a symbol of strength, regality, and power. Since the Buddha was a prince, it became a fitting symbol. Buddha's teachings are occasionally referred to as Lion's Roar to indicate his teachings' power and strength.

Deer

This symbol also has two origins. Buddha's first teaching was in the Deer Park, Sarnath. It was also said that Buddha's appearances were so wondrous and his presence so peaceful that even the animals came to listen to what he had to say.

Stupas

Stupas are a symbolic grave monument used to represent the enlightened mind of the Buddha. They have been being constructed since the early days of Buddhism. A stupa is a square base, a round dome, and a cone shape with a canopy. These monuments have been made in all shapes and sizes.

The Buddha Statue

The most commonly recognized Buddha symbol today is the Buddha statue. The first Buddha statue was created during 500-550 B.E. Before this time, there was no image of Buddha used as a symbol. Buddhists use the figure because they find that the image gives them a transparent role model on their paths towards their Enlightenment.

Buddha statues can be found in a variety of poses. He was sitting, standing, smiling, or laughing. His hands are also found in a variety of gestures, called mudras. Each of these postures and gestures carries a different symbolism and relates to varying qualities of the Buddha. These qualities include balance, compassion, grace, and wisdom, courage, and determination. A couple of examples of common mudras that are found on Buddhist statues are:

-The Gesture of Meditation: Both hands are resting on the lap with palms facing upwards;

-The Gesture of Fearlessness: The right hand is slightly elevated with the palm turned outwards; And

-The Gesture of Debate: Explaining the Buddha's teachings, with the hands raised and tips of the thumbs and forefingers touching each other.

Non-Buddhists often use the Buddhist statue in their home or business to encourage an atmosphere of well-being and calm. It is especially true of psychotherapists and alternative healers.

Offerings

While some people believe that Buddhists worship the Buddha statues, this is not the case. Buddhists bow and make offerings in reverence to the Buddha himself, not to the image. They are reflecting on the virtues of the Buddha and inspire to become like him. The Buddha images are not necessary for this reverence. They are used by many Buddhists who find them helpful in keeping their focus. There are five traditional offerings used to show respect to the Buddha, flowers, light from lamps or candles, incense, water, and food. Each of these offerings represents something different.

Flowers: Flowers are offered to the Buddha to signify the practice of generosity. They are also used as a reminder of how quickly things change and that nothing lasts forever.

Light from Lamps or Candles: Light is offered to signify wisdom. The beauty of the light is said to dispel ignorance. By providing light to the Buddha, one is reminded to lead their mind to wisdom and question all things around them.

Incense: Buddhists offer incense to the Buddha to signify moral ethics and discipline. It is meant to remind one to be peaceful towards all things.

Water: Water is used to signify purity. Since water is used to cleanse, by providing water to wash the Buddha, one also cleans their minds.

Food

Food is used to remind us to give our best to the Buddha. Since food has many tastes, it is used to signify "Samadhi," which is ambrosia to feed the mind.

Other Reformers

By this time, the dispute had spread across Europe, where it had social and theological impacts. In Germany, peasants wanted to participate in newfound religious freedom, and they also demanded social, political, and economic reform. They formulated twelve demands:

1. Each parish should choose its pastor.
2. Some forms of tithing (that is, church taxes) should be abolished.
3. Serfdom, the tying of peasants to the land, should be done away with.
4. Peasants should have the right to hunt and fish freely.
5. Peasants should be able to collect building materials and firewood voluntarily from forests.
6. Lords should stop imposing oppressive workloads.
7. Peasants should only work according to what is "just and proper" according to an agreement between lord and peasant.
8. Rents should be affordable.
9. There should be equal justice for lord and peasant.
10. Unfair division of land should be done away with.
11. The death tax should be abolished.
12. If any of these demands did not adhere to the word of God, they would be scrapped.

Chapter 25. Why is Buddhism True?

Buddhism is the oldest religion globally, and it is the belief that all living beings possess Buddha-nature. It's a philosophy concerning liberation from pain and what causes pain in the first place.

Buddhist teachings currently emphasize morality and widen our circle of concern to include all beings. If you are looking for meaning or truth in your life, if you want to live humanely or be less selfish, if you wish for greater happiness and contentment -- then Buddhism is for you.

Buddhism is Unique in Several Ways

One: It is the only religion without a God, our creator. Two: It is the only one that denies a soul exists. Three: It is the only one that prohibits a person has free will over his/her actions (this is not a flaw, but rather, it emphasizes how our environment shapes our actions). Four: It does not require faith or belief in anything except for Buddha's teachings (although such faith may develop over time). Five: It does not believe in everlasting life after death or reincarnation, but rather, it considers liberation from pain can be attained during one's lifetime. Six: It is the only religion that makes no distinction between priests and ordinary practitioners, and it allows everyone to reach enlightenment.

Buddhism is not concerned with matters of faith nor beliefs. Instead, it's concerned with wisdom and reason. Buddhism asks you to examine what you believe in and why you believe in them. Although there are several myths about Buddhism's origins (most of which were created by non-Buddhists), the teachings themselves do not provide any answers as to why they exist. The Buddha himself said he did not create his education, but instead, they were discovered through the careful investigation into our human nature and the reality we live in. They are simply insights that are universally true (when correctly understood).

When people ask why Buddhism is true, the best answer is: it works. That's the bottom line. If you believe in Buddha's teachings and put them into practice in your life, they will help you to reduce suffering and attain greater happiness. The methods that Buddha taught (called dharma) have been used for over 2,500 years by millions of people worldwide to help them lead better lives. It may not be perfect, but so far, it is the most successful method we have discovered.

Understanding Buddhism

In recent years, Buddhism has experienced increased interest from those who want to have the tools to deal with their minds. Perhaps this is due to our modern world's instability and chaos, or maybe it is because people seek a more compassionate religion. These points are both valid, but they don't give us a clear picture of what Buddhism is all about. Here are the basics of what Buddhists believe and how they understand Buddhism to answer your question.

What exactly does an adherent of Buddhism believe? Buddhists believe that we suffer from a fundamental misunderstanding: that our existence revolves around our self-interests. In our daily lives, we frequently face challenges to our happiness. We are beset by fears, desires, and other impulses that cause us to behave in ways that are detrimental to ourselves and those around us. It is because we are so focused on the idea of our "self" that we don't see or understand anything else. We don't recognize that there is a larger reality, one in which many life forms are interconnected in many ways. Buddhism teaches us that this perspective is rooted in ignorance and self-centeredness.

But Buddhism isn't necessarily pessimistic about human nature; it only says that we do not understand it very well yet. Instead, Buddhism focuses on changing our perspective of life to bring peace into the world. To know how it works, we have to trace the source of all suffering back to something called "ignorance." Ignorance is not a lack of information or knowledge; instead, it is delusion or a misguided understanding that prevents us from seeing things as they are. The Buddhist doctrine states that ignorance causes our suffering. Most of us suffer because we are always plagued by negative thoughts and emotions that cause us to behave in ways that make us unhappy and those around us painful.

Another way to think about this concept is to imagine a fish swimming around in an aquarium. It wouldn't know anything else existed, so it could only perceive its environment based on what it could sense from inside the tank. When a fish crashes into the side of the aquarium, it doesn't know that there is nothing to fear. It thinks that there is an obstruction in its way and changes direction to go around it. The fish doesn't know that there is nothing there. The same thing happens with us; we only have the senses we were born with, so when we are faced with a threat (like pain), we cannot easily discern what or why we should avoid it.

Buddhism teaches us that this kind of ignorance is caused by a fundamental misperception of reality: our own identity. This understanding came from Buddha himself, and he explained that our suffering is caused by a fundamental misunderstanding of what we think we are. We are not separate individuals; instead, we exist within a web of interconnectedness. We are all part of the same reality that has the same goal: to be happy and avoid suffering.

As humans, however, we have never had the opportunity to experience life in this way because we always see things from a self-centered point of view. Only when you understand your fundamental nature will you begin to see yourself as part of everything else in existence. At this point, you become enlightened and understand everything relating to your life instead of just yourself.

Five Senses in Buddhism
- Manas (the faculty that receives input from the mind).
- Mahan (the faculty that receives input from other sense faculties and throughout one's body).
- Ahan (the faculty that works on a person's feelings and emotions but can only be experienced by oneself).
- Jung (the faculty that works on an organism's internal activities but can only be experienced by oneself).
- Beau (the faculty that works on an organism's unconscious mind but can only be experienced by oneself).

By only using our five senses, we are deceived into believing that things exist when they don't or that they are what they are not. Things don't exist as we perceive them to be. They only live in the way reality makes them behave. If you drop a pebble off a tall building, it will appear to fall slower than an apple. The speed of things depends on how we perceive them to be. What seems real is often not real; what doesn't seem real is often real.

It is why the Buddha emphasized engaging in the careful investigation when investigating reality. Detailed analysis means taking time to observe things carefully and deeply, rather than rushing through them quickly. All the knowledge we have today is a result of such careful investigations into reality. Even science has confirmed that our five senses do not give us an accurate picture of reality (try doing simple experiments with mirrors or lenses to experience this yourself).

What is "Buddha nature"? It is the potential for attaining enlightenment that all living beings possess. What does "enlightenment" mean? Culture means to be liberated from suffering. What is liberation from suffering? It means no longer being controlled by delusions, such as the idea of a separate self or the concept of a permanent soul. It means no longer being maintained by selfish desires but rather acting according to what we feel is right instead. All living beings can be liberated from suffering. Still, not all will achieve this goal in their lifetime because they fail to practice Buddha's teachings accordingly (the instructions are straightforward and easy to understand). What is "delusion"?

Delusions are beliefs in things that do not exist or which are not right. For example, believing that you're a separate person from others is a delusion that causes you suffering. Misconceptions cause us to act differently than we would if we were free of them. What is the "Middle Way"? It refers to following a path between the extremes of self-indulgence and self-mortification (or self-harm). It means to avoid thinking that material wealth is the most crucial thing in life because it doesn't provide happiness.

Suffering from internal causes (e.g., being dissatisfied with what we have). To overcome suffering, we need to learn how to deal with its internal and external causes. What is "emptiness"? It means the absence of inherent existence (or "self-nature") in anything (e.g., in me, in you, in a tree, in the grass). It's merely un-true that things exist separately from each other (like the idea that I'm a separate person from others). When one understands this concept, one does not strive to hold on to things or cling to things anymore. What is "dependant arising"? It refers to the fact that all phenomena and situations arise dependently on other conditions. For example, my computer is composed of many parts. If each piece were changed slightly (or removed), it would no longer be my computer. The computer depends on all its features to existing.

In the same way, all things in the world depend on other things to come into existence. What are "the three poisons"? They are the three primary delusions that bring suffering into our lives: hatred, ignorance, and self-grasping (or selfishness). Why do we mistake ourselves for being a separate self from everything else? It happens because we cling to impermanent phenomena and situations as permanent. The Buddha taught us about "all-pervading space." What is this? It means being free of any concepts of "inside" or "outside," which are just ideas that we make up. Everything is equally everywhere (it is spacelike). For example, I am around, within me, and outside me. I am not only inside my body; just as much, I am not only outside my body. Wherever there is a thought "I" or thought of "mine," there I am. When studies are not present anymore in our minds, then the concept of "inside" disappears. The same can be said about the ideas of "outside" and "others." Then one realizes that everyone and everything is together within a spacelike-mind of equanimity: one sees the world as it is – without any separation between self and other.

For example, we might have the concept of "others" by thinking of rich or poor people with different skin colors or different religions. It will make us feel "separate" from them. That would make it hard for us to contact that person because he/she is not like us. But if we see the world as it is, we can see the world as one without any separation between self and other than just mere thought constructions. There is no such separation anymore and thinking in terms of "us" versus "them" would be incomprehensible. Then one realizes that everyone and everything is together within a spacelike-mind of equanimity: one sees the world as it is – without any separation between self and other.

Chapter 26. Why is Buddhism so Popular?

There are many reasons why Buddhism has become so popular, including its popularity in different countries and its similarities to Christianity.

Buddhism has many similarities to Christianity, including the following: both are based on a book; both religions have monks and nuns who follow stringent rules, and both religions have many followers around the world.

In Buddhism, there is no Bible like Christians follow. Instead, Buddhists follow a book called The Tripitaka. It is a collection of scriptures they believe were passed down from Buddha. Like Christians, Buddhists have rules they must follow to be good followers of the religion. Monks and nuns are required to live in temples and take part in daily activities such as meditating. They wear robes and shave their heads, which is the opposite of what most people do in the United States.

Buddhism has become very popular with many people around the world because of its similarity with Christianity. Players from the Boston Celtics, Los Angeles Lakers, Chicago Bulls, New York Knicks and several other NBA teams all follow Buddhism. Buddhism is not exclusive to a single race, country, or group of people. Over the centuries, a generous portion of the Western population has benefitted from Buddha's teachings.

Buddhism is on the rise nowadays in many countries. Cultural perception of religion in different parts of the world is an essential factor in this regard. Suppose you were living in East or Southeast Asia. In that case, you'd find that being a committed Buddhist is a thing of tradition and heritage, making it a relatively conservative way of life. In most Western countries, though, that is not the case, especially in America. Buddhism has a shroud of exoticism and mystery around it, as it comes from foreign parts in the Far East. It makes the philosophy very attractive to young, progressive people who are open to new ideas and experiences, thus helping Buddhism spread. Apart from this aesthetic appeal, Buddhist teachings' actual substance is undoubtedly what makes it attractive, if you will. It is a religion with a straightforward philosophy to relate to anywhere globally, maybe even more so in the West than in developing countries. Today, there are more than eight million Buddhists in the United States alone.

Siddhartha Gautama, known as Buddha, founded Buddhism. As a young boy, Buddha's father protected him from the outside world to keep his son away from anything wrong that might happen to him and prevent him from ever leaving home. Buddha grew up believing the earth was filled with evil people who would try to hurt him and his family or steal their things if he ever left home. At the age of 29, Buddha left home to see what the outside world was like. He learned how good people indeed are and saw how much pain people were going through. He also knew that life is full of suffering.

But as Siddhartha Gautama found out 2,500 years ago, self-deprivation is not the path towards enlightenment. Take a look at the face of the 14th Dalai Lama. He's always smiling, brimming with energy, and radiating with the beauty of life. It is the real face of Buddhism. Buddhists are encouraged to laugh, to love, and to enjoy life. The whole purpose of the awakening is not just to end suffering but also to achieve indescribable joy.

The bottom line is that those monks burned themselves not because they wished to embrace death more than life. How much suffering and pain was alleviated from the many people who found themselves oppressed is a thing of history.

The political change that Thich Quang Duc managed to effect is documented. Whether or not this was a worthy sacrifice that acceptably transcended the core Buddhist precepts is up to the beholder to decide.

Buddha realized he could help other people overcome their pain and suffering by teaching them about his life views. After becoming a teacher, he taught thousands of followers about how they should live their lives to avoid suffering. These teachings became what we now know as Buddhism.

The name "Buddha" comes from two words in Sanskrit, "Budhu" and "dha." Together they mean "awakened one. Buddha taught that everyone should learn to meditate and achieve enlightenment. He also taught his followers the importance of attaining selfless acts, speaking with kindness, and ignoring all harmful things around them.

In each Buddha's teachings, he said people should believe in karma, a spiritual force that rewards good deeds and punishes terrible acts. While Buddha never wrote down these teachings, monks took notes on what he was teaching to preserve it thousands of years later. The Tripitaka is a collection of his teachings passed down from monk to monk over many years until they were written in Sanskrit. In the 700s, they were translated into Chinese and later into other languages like Tibetan and Japanese.

Buddhism is a religion that teaches peace, calmness, and reliance on discipline. It also introduces the importance of meditation and can be considered an eastern form of thought. Buddhism is so popular because it's a way for people to find happiness through self-power and control.

In many ways, Buddhism is similar to other religions. Probably the most common faith in the United States is Christianity. There are more than 300 million Christians in America today. This religion is based on the Bible and teaches people to be good followers by following a book called The Bible, which tells them how Jesus Christ will save them from their sins and help them go to Heaven when they die. Christians believe any person who follows God's rules will go to Heaven afterlife. In Buddhism, followers must follow Buddha's teachings and live a good life without sin before entering Nirvana or paradise after death. With Christianity, followers are forgiven for their sins by asking God for forgiveness. With Buddhism, followers must take care of their karma.

In another 20 years, it is estimated that 3 percent to 5 percent of the United States will be Buddhist. In other countries like Thailand and Japan, 40 percent of citizens follow Buddhism, and many people in Taiwan and China. The main reason why Buddhism is growing so popular is that it is being exposed to more people around the world.

You May Ask Why Buddhism is So Popular?

Well, one reason is because of its similarity with Christianity. It's becoming more popular because of the connections it has with other religions in this country, such as Hinduism and Jainism. With more people following the faith, there might be more spread of misinformation about Buddhism's history.

Buddhism is increasingly the world's most popular religion. With some 6.2 billion people, it accounts for about half of the world's population. At one time, Buddhism was mainly a product of India; now, it's practiced in more than 110 countries worldwide and accounted for as many as two-fifths of all active followers of non-Christian faiths. It is estimated that there are between 235 million to 600 million Buddhists in China alone, but the country does not officially recognize any religion other than Christianity, Islam, and Taoism. (Wikipedia)

The rapid growth of the number of Buddhists in the world is due to several reasons, such as.

In other words, unlike many different religions, Buddhism presents no supernatural claims; it has no theology and does not ask its followers to accept anything on faith. It is entirely based on observation and reason. It makes Buddhism very easy to understand and follow.

Buddhism is a rational religion that appeals to people who are accustomed to a scientific way of thinking. The Buddha explained his findings in simple terms without using any supernatural concepts.

Buddhism emphasizes following the middle path. It discourages overindulgence in sensual pleasures as well as excess in self-denial. The Buddha showed a practical and balanced way of achieving real happiness.

The Four Noble Truths and The Eight-Fold Path summarize Buddhism's essence most practically so that one can practice and achieve inner peace even in this very life.

The Buddha's message applies to all people, irrespective of their birth, gender, color or caste, etc. He has not given any special privilege to any particular group of people.

The eightfold path is a universal guide that applies to people of all races and nations. It shows a practical way leading to the ultimate happiness.

Buddhism offers excellent hope because it teaches that everyone can achieve enlightenment in this very life. After death, one merges back into the infinite consciousness and achieves Nirvana. Hence the real essence of "self" never dies, and there is no fear of death or any other worries regarding it.

It asks them to observe and verify its claims on their own and come to a rational conclusion based upon this observation. Thus, it appeals to people who like to think for themselves without blindly following any authority figure or dogma.

When you enter a Buddhist temple, you'll see numerous statues, incense being burned, flowers being offered, and monks prostrating themselves in front of the altar. Buddhists do not worship Buddhas in the same way as followers of other faiths worship their gods. Prostration in Buddhism is performed as a conscientious deed as opposed to being a mindless ritualistic act.

As we know these things in a few other significant religions, worshiping and idolization would be somewhat contradictory to Buddhism's core principles. Whereas Islam, Christianity, and the like worship Gods that are perceived as eternal, omnipresent, omnipotent, and unchanging, Buddhism perceives everything in this universe, except Nirvana, to be impermanent and essentially meaningless, as you will learn in detail later on. Therefore, it could be more accurate to consider Buddhism as a form of utmost dedication and devotion to the truth instead of an idol or divine ruler and creator.

More so than worship, the Buddha himself is simply respected and admired for his achievements. You can think of Buddhism as a large club of devout followers dedicated to carrying on the torch and preserving what they believe in, and It has been the most enlightened way of comprehending the world and life itself. The Buddha set an example that is followed voluntarily, but much more important than the man himself is each journey that those who seek awakening will travel. The whole of Buddhist commitment is a very earthly attitude toward a worldly achievement attributed to a born man and has died like everyone else. What sets the Buddha apart is how he lived that entirely natural life and passed on knowledge to those who cared to listen, and that is what Buddhism is all about.

Chapter 27. Why are Buddhist Nations Poor?

Buddhist nations are the poorest in the world. The question is why.

I am going to start this article with a cliff note. The reason for Buddhist nations being poor is that they are inherently more spiritual than materially minded.

It can be a turn-off to commercial purposes, and it is not their natural way of thinking which leaves them in poverty. Not only that, but we can also say that Buddhists have a philosophy of what we call "parallel living," meaning that they do not believe in scarcity and plenty, but instead believe in equality for all, thus no need to preach about how many gold bars one person has compared to another person since you cannot increase your happiness by having more material possessions.

If a person is spiritual and wants to have more wealth and material things, he cannot call himself spiritual. That is like me saying that I want to marry the most beautiful girl globally, but I will only have sex once a year with her since, for Buddhists, the most significant aspect of life is family and social relations.

If one is to be spiritually rich, then he/she needs to be materially rich since his/her desires will not be sated by just being in constant spiritual bliss.

Speaking of which, the reason why India is not imperfect is not that it was never Buddhist. Still, instead, it was because they milked their spiritual ideals and harmonized them with materialism. It had made India one of the richest and strongest pre-colonial countries. But when India started its liberation struggle, they never allowed themselves to make money since it insulted the Indian idea that they would fight for freedom with their empty coffers. To my mind, this has made India into a third-world nation today.

I need to start at the beginning. What is the purpose of life? Some would say that it is to procreate and spread your genes, while others would say that it is to be happy in all aspects of life. I say that there are multiple purposes in life for different people and different nations at different periods. Some want to procreate and spread genes while others desire power, for others money, for others spiritual harmony. All these are valid, but only if it is the natural way of thinking for one's people.

India was never concerned about power and materialism because they had a spiritual leader. The same goes for the Chinese, Koreans, Vietnamese, Cambodians, etc. I am not saying that all Buddhists are inadequate or that all non-Buddhists are rich. Instead, I am pointing out history that these Asian nations have become impoverished in ancient times because they started to value other things in their lives. Thus, their economies went into the gutter.

Let us take the example of the Japanese after WWII. They focused their energy on rebuilding their economy. Again, I did not wish this to happen to Myanmar or other Buddhist nations, but I just pointed out how Japan became rich and prosperous.

For centuries India was known for its spiritual leaders who preached about spiritual harmony in their lives, while China was materialistic.

Buddhist countries are among the world's lowest since their economic rise began over 50 years ago. Their geography partially explains it; they're both landlocked and near volatile regions of political tension. And various studies have shown that Buddhist cultures have a different relationship to money than Western cultures, leading to less emphasis on economic growth as progress for their people and more focus on social stability and happiness within a community.

But there's a more fundamental reason for the disappointingly poor economic outcomes of Buddhist nations, and it lies in the teachings themselves. Buddhism's core precepts have a worldview that stands in direct opposition to capitalism, and this clash has had its consequences.

The Core Values of Buddhism Opposed Capitalism

Buddhist economics' core value is non-attachment; one should not become too attached to material goods or money but rather see them as brief and ultimately meaningless. It is a perfect setup for a stagnant economy; people can start new ventures taught that all material goods are ultimately useless? What attempts at innovation are made by individuals who don't believe they have anything to gain materially from their work? The answer is obvious.

The next core value of Buddhism is non-violence. It leads to pacifism and ultimately subjugation when confronted with stronger nations. Non-violence also implies that people who enjoy violence are wrong. So, Buddhist societies are often very liberal in their attitudes towards tolerance of homosexuals, transgender people, and other sexual minorities who engage in non-reproductive sex. They're also illiberal in their attitude toward murderers or aggressors since, according to Buddhist precepts, both violence and sexuality are inherently selfish and harmful for society.

The third core value of Buddhism is non-competition. It leads to a caste system, where people are taught that they should not try to rise above their station in life and that faking the appearance of "productivity" through heightened economic growth statistics is wrong. These values reinforce each other in a slow fatalistic cycle; homogenous cultures discouraged from competition lead to economic stagnation and higher levels of violence within their societies.

It's no surprise, then, that the modern "beige Buddhist" countries are some of the world's poorest. Lacking entrepreneurialism or motivation, they stagnate economically and have high levels of societal violence. They're also some of the most liberal places on Earth, which is often a sign of moral decadence in a society that's been around for too long.

The problem of what to do about Buddhist cultures is a difficult one. There are certainly downsides to Westernization in terms of cultural and economic homogenization. Still, there's no reason not to expect improvement from Buddhism as it becomes more integrated into the global community. It has happened many times before; Christianity was once very hostile towards capitalism and was opposed by thinkers like Adam Smith but eventually embraced capitalist ideals and became one of its greatest champions.

Buddhism teaches you how to be in harmony with your spiritual self, while the West teaches you how to connect with your material desires, thus helping you make money and spread your genes. And it worked in India for centuries since they were never poor when they were harmonizing their spiritual nature and worldly desires.

Also, this is why Buddhism is more individualistic than other religions, and the same goes for India who is even more individualistic than China or the Islamic nations.

Now we can see why Buddhism is in decline. It has lost its natural followers (Japan, Korea, China). Instead, it has gained a nation of people interested in being rich such as Myanmar (Burma), but the ruler is very poor. It again will create a gap between the rich and the poor since the rich will not want to share their wealth with an individualist society that

doesn't respect them or Buddhism itself. Thus, this creates a self-destructive cycle that needs to be broken.

I am writing this because my dislike for Buddhism would be wrong since spiritual practices are essential if you want your ideal life. And I also do not have a problem with people who want to be rich since all my life I have been materialistic (as most other people who live in the West). However, because I have realized after all of my material desires are sated, I still can't call myself being happy in life.

I am just pointing out how much the world is changing and how these changes will affect Buddhism. In Thailand, their Buddhist monks leave their monasteries to become businessmen, while Myanmar (Burma) balances spiritual harmony with materialism.

According to Buddhism, one of the critical reasons for poverty is greed. By reducing one's attachment to material possessions and living a simple life, Buddhist nations can better protect their natural resources and reduce pollution. Furthermore, Buddhist nations are characterized by higher savings rates and infrastructure investments than many other countries.

In economically troubled Asian countries like Thailand, Japan, India, or China (which feature the largest number of Buddhists), people who practice Buddhism don't spend money on luxury items like expensive cars or designer clothes that might have been purchased in more affluent times. They don't spend money on gambling because it's considered a sin within Buddhism. The practice of Buddhism also doesn't encourage people to accumulate wealth for the sake of showing status - it's discouraged.

Critics point out that Buddhist nations are still impoverished and much lower than their Muslim neighbors. According to World Bank, India's GDP in 2010 was $1.8 trillion and is predicted to pass China in 2012.

On the other hand, Muslims are forbidden by Islam from practicing usury (the lending of money for interest). However, most of the banks in Islamic nations are owned by non-Muslims. Because the Quran forbids lending money for a part at all, from an ethical perspective, it makes no difference whether a bank is owned or managed by a Muslim or not. It has caused much controversy amongst some Muslims concerning debt.

The Arabian nations are some of the world's most imperfect, and their governments have been unable to provide adequate services for their citizens. Many poor people live below the poverty line and can barely afford food, clothes, etc., in their homeland. The Arabian nations are heavily dependent on foreign remittances, mostly from the Middle East and Europe. Arabian countries also have some of the highest birth rates (one of the reasons for poverty) globally, with about 50% of their populations being below 15 years old.

Several predominantly Muslim countries are among the richest in the world. They include Saudi Arabia, Kuwait, U.A.E., Oman, Qatar, Bahrain, and Turkey. Oman is ranked as the third-wealthiest country in the world (as of 2004). However, a study by Harvard economist Alberto Alesina found that Muslim countries were more likely to suffer from civil wars than other countries with similar income levels.

Chapter 28. Is Buddhism a Science?

Buddhism and Science

Over the past few decades, Buddhism and science have started to work with each other. Scientists look more closely at Buddhism to understand and explain the universe, as Buddhists are beginning to use more scientific tools. One of the biggest reasons this has come to be is that science studies the mind, and Buddhism focuses heavily on the mind. Of course, one of the most significant studies of the reason lies within psychology when it comes to science.

Buddhism and Psychology

Buddhism and psychology go together because Buddhism teaches that you need to remain positive, be compassionate, and remain calm to reach your enlightenment. While it's stated differently in the science of psychology, it holds the same beliefs. In psychology, there is a lot of talk about how people will have better self-esteem and feel overall better about themselves and their tasks at hand if they have a positive self-image and thoughts about themselves. Of course, like Buddhism, there is a fine line between having positive thoughts about yourself and becoming arrogant.

Dependent Origination

In Buddhism, dependent origination means that everything is connected. It means that something else is caused if something happens, and this keeps going as one thing will always cause another thing. When it comes to science, this can often be compared to evolution. Through evolution, not only does human life continue to exist, but we have changed over time because of our surroundings—or as Buddhism would put it because something happened to make us change.

Other Similarities

There are a few other similarities between science and Buddhism. One of these is that both studies believe that there isn't one creator of the universe that exists. Just like science, Buddhism likes to focus on logic and reasoning.

The Chinese Challenge

Xavier died before making it to China, and another Jesuit, Matteo Ricci, undertook his missionary work in that nation.

Finding that Confucianism was ensconced in Chinese culture and represented a serious challenge to Christian doctrine, Ricci taught that Christianity was not new in China. Instead, it was a unique expression of existing religious beliefs. Instead of bombarding his way with force and wrath, he learned the culture and the language of the region and made attempts to talk to the Chinese leaders, honoring them with gifts and friendship. When Ricci died in 1610, there were 2,000 Christians in China.

The Clocks

Among the gifts, Ricci gave the emperor during his stay in Beijing were two clocks. The emperor loved them, but at some point, they stopped working.

After Ricci's death, Johann Adam Schall von Bell took over missionary work in China. By the time of his death in 1666, there were more than 300,000 converts in the kingdom. In 1692, to reward years of Jesuit effort, China passed an edict of toleration. Although it seemed that things were ripe for the conversion of the entire nation, the Jesuits, Dominicans, and Franciscans quarreled over the correct practice of Christianity in China, and things collapsed.

SCHOLASTICISM

The Marriage of Aristotle and Christianity

During the twelfth century, there came a revival of learning within the Christian Church. Universities were opening all over Europe, and people began to study, think, and question. Art, literature, music, and science quickly came to the forefront of education.

Cathedral schools were established to promote the understanding of Christianity. These schools were open to all, and their object was to study the faith within the fixed bounds of church law. A cathedral school education consisted of the seven liberal arts:

1. Grammar
2. Rhetoric
3. Logic
4. Arithmetic
5. Geometry
6. Astronomy
7. Music

The growth of education stemmed from enthusiastic schoolteachers; often monastic scholars eager to spread their wealth of knowledge. This enthusiasm would take many educators away from medieval thinking's restrictive bonds into a mysterious world of questions just dying to be asked.

Gerbert of Rheims

Gerbert of Rheims (later Pope Sylvester II) was a brilliant monastic scholar influenced by Christian bishops and Muslim culture. Gerbert discovered the inquisitive thinking of Muslim learning and decided to incorporate it into his teaching methods.

The Value of the Question

He gave his inheritance to his brothers and traversed all of France to learn from great thinkers. He became a lecturer (professor) at the University of Paris and wrote Sic et Non (Latin for Yes and No), in which he posted 158 questions with answers drawn from Christian scripture, pagan writings, and church leaders.

Abelard took the ancient Greek method of consistent questioning and applied it to medieval study—something many church leaders did not welcome. At the Council of Soissons in

1121, Abelard was condemned for his writings on Trinity's nature and was soon living in seclusion in a monastery.

Abelard and Héloïse

While teaching in Paris, he became fascinated with Héloïse, niece of the canon of Notre Dame. Abelard seduced her; he made a secret marriage with her, but when Héloïse publicly denied they were married, her uncle confronted Abelard and had him castrated. Héloïse spent the rest of her life in a convent, and the two lovers are today buried together in Paris's Père Lachaise cemetery.

A New Age

Once interest in questioning had begun, there was no way to stop it. Schools opened all over Europe. They developed a teaching method that incorporated Abelard's format of posed questions and answers. The technique was called "Scholasticism," which gradually became a means of arriving at difficult conclusions through questions and debate. By arranging information and questioning the details, students would come to a logical conclusion.

Less than 100 years after Abelard's death, schools opened in Paris, Oxford, Cambridge, and Bologna (among many other cities). The Europeans called these schools Universitas, a Latin word that in the Middle Ages meant any corporate group.

Many had been translated from Arabic since Islamic scholars revered the ancient Greek thinkers and preserved many of their works. The writings of the Jewish philosopher Maimonides and the Muslim thinker Averroes were widely circulated.

St. Thomas Aquinas, a Dominican monk, and scholar were called to examine Maimonides and Averroes' texts. While he refuted some of their propositions, he reconciled others with Christian thinking in a massive work titled Summa Theologica. The book was never finished, but many scholars regard it as the Scholastic movement's intellectual high point.

PAUL OF TARSUS

Paul's Travels

According to the scriptures, Paul made three significant trips during his life:

1. Palestine and Antioch (ancient Syria, now Turkey)
2. Thessalonica (the city in ancient Macedonia)
3. Philippi (the city in ancient Macedonia) and then on to Corinth and Turkey

Chapter 29. God in Buddhism

Place of God in Buddhism

Westerners are often curious about the place of God in Buddhism. There is no "God" figure in Buddhism, and that's a good thing because it means that Buddhists don't require any kind of outside sustenance for personal or spiritual growth.

Buddhist meditators are encouraged to cultivate an attitude of "non-attachment" from the things around them (including material goods, success in life, and even their personality). This freedom from attachment frees up the mind and body to pursue enlightenment.

Buddhists don't believe in God because they don't think that God is necessary for them to fulfill their spiritual path or destiny.

Buddhists don't believe in God because they understand that the universe is self-sufficient and can work perfectly well without a godlike figure interfering with its workings.

Buddhists don't believe in God because they understand that there is nothing outside of themselves that can save them from their suffering. It's up to each person to liberate themselves from suffering through personal effort and the cultivation of wisdom.

In this way, Buddhists believe that they are on a journey of self-redemption. They don't need God to do it for them.

The "God" figure is commonly misunderstood by people who are unfamiliar with Buddhism. In most religious traditions, including Judaism, Christianity, and Islam, the idea is that God created the universe and then turned his attention to other matters. In contrast, the universe takes care of itself. Early Buddhist scholars were aware of this idea and wrote about it in comparison with Buddhist beliefs. The Buddha himself said:

"Loving-kindness has no limits; loving-kindness knows no boundaries. Whether we are rich or poor, all human beings are the owners of their actions. Nobody else is the owner of their actions, just as nobody else is their wealth. One who doesn't own wealth can't give it away; one who doesn't own actions can't either."

In this way, Buddhists believe that the self-created universe doesn't need God to run it; it runs itself. They also believe in karma and rebirth and that karma is carried forward from one lifetime to another by individuals. If one "lives wisely" in this lifetime, they will live well in future lifetimes. In this way, Buddhists can be said to have some belief in life after death, but it's still an individual journey and not one that requires the intervention of any "God" figure.

Buddhists don't believe in God because they understand that there is no need for God to create the universe or run it. They think that it establishes itself and runs itself, and so, as a result, they don't need to "worship" anything or anyone. That's why Buddhists often refer to themselves as being "unbelievers.

However, this does not mean that Buddhists do not respect or revere their teachers in the same way that Christians respect and revere Jesus and Mohammad. Buddha himself was a teacher who lived his life in ways that were worthy of being studied. He acted with good intentions towards others, he cultivated wisdom in the same way as anyone else would, and he encouraged others to do the same. Buddhists believe that these are necessary actions to follow, whether one is a Buddhist or not. They believe that all human beings should act well towards one another without regard for personal reward or gain.

However, Buddhists do not worship Buddha in the same way that Christian worship Jesus. Buddhists have a great deal of respect for other religions and religious people because they see it as a personal journey that is unique to each individual. They believe that it's better to encourage others to be useful rather than telling them how to live, and thus they would not want to tell someone else how to live or how to interpret their sacred texts.

Buddhists also tend not to believe in "prophets" of any kind. They don't believe in prophets because they understand that any person can act as a prophet and speak for God. They also understand that people can be self-delusional to interpret their inner desires as God's will.

There is another reason Buddhists do not believe in prophets: They know that many so-called prophets have spoken words of hatred and violence towards other human beings. The Buddha himself said kindly towards others, never spoke with anger or hate, and always treated others as valuable individuals to be respected. That's why Buddhists have respect for their teachers but no "prophet" or "God" figure.

Buddhists don't pray because they don't see prayer as a necessary part of their spiritual journey. They often say that prayer is harmful because it requires people to believe that things outside of themselves can save them from their suffering. They understand that everything results from the individual choices they have made in the past, and thus they strive to cultivate wisdom and compassion in their hearts.

In summary, Buddhists do not worship God or pray to God because they believe in karma and rebirth. They also do not need to rely on divine intervention because there is no separate entity that needs to save them from suffering. They believe in acting with wisdom and compassion towards others and that these actions themselves are worthy.

It is not to say that Buddhists do not believe in kindness or goodwill towards their fellow human beings. They certainly do, but the Buddha did not teach that a person needs to believe in God or a "higher power" to be kind or good-hearted. That's why some people call themselves Buddhist unbelievers because they understand that it's possible to arise from suffering without believing in something outside of oneself.

Buddhists may have different opinions on this question than Christians do, but they neither worship God nor worship the Buddha himself. They see God, Jesus, and the Buddha as human beings who were great teachers. They believe that these individuals were wise and compassionate people, and they try to follow in their footsteps. It's important to note that Buddhists don't think that a person needs to be religious to be good or wise.

Buddhist beliefs focus on compassion for one another rather than believing in divine intervention. It is not to say that Buddhists do not have a strong belief in karma or fate; instead, Buddhism is very much about being self-reliant and taking responsibility for your own decisions.

The Buddha taught that everyone could help others, and if everyone used their talents for this purpose, then the world would be a better place. It is this attitude that Buddhists appreciate rather than any specific religious practices. It is also why Buddhist teachings are seen by many as compatible with Western philosophy and religion because they are consistent with other beliefs regarding humanism, social justice, and peaceful coexistence.

The main reason why Buddhists do not worship Buddha or God is that they understand that all forms of self-deception stem from believing something about yourself without evidence to support it. They do not see any good in worshipping a god or a Buddha or even yourself. The Buddha taught that it's essential to treat everyone with honor and respect, regardless of their beliefs or background, and that is why Buddhists do not worship God.

"I believe in working out my salvation. If I were under the impression that I could only be saved by making myself acceptable to the Almighty, I would be reduced to despair - if God does not love me, why should I love myself? But if we work for each other's goodwill and love, it is the greatest glory we can give to God. I believe that those who live the good life do not need a father's conception in heaven to make them good. I believe in working for the secular goodwill and love of my fellow men, and respect to God is not necessary to promote that."

The history of Buddhism is profoundly intricate and multifaceted. For the sake of this post, allow me to give you a glimpse into the religion's conception.

Buddhism originated roughly 2,500 years ago in northeastern India with Siddhartha Gautama, who became known as Buddha – "the enlightened one." Though Buddhism is often seen as an Indian religion, it spread widely throughout Asia and even parts of Europe until it eventually disappeared from its birthplace. Although most Buddhists today are based in East Asia and Southeast Asia, there are still millions living throughout South America, Europe, and North America.

Buddhism's underpinning concepts and philosophy are not relatively so easy to break down, and rather than giving a long, complicated history lesson that may bore you to death, and I'm going to try and paint a picture of what it's all about.

Buddhist philosophy is based on Siddhartha Gautama's teachings, who lived in Northern India between the mid-6th century BC and early 4th century BC. He spent much of his early life as an impoverished palace prince who became dissatisfied with the notion that craving and desire were responsible for an individual's suffering.

Chapter 30. Buddhism and Christianity

Buddhism and Christianity are two religions with great significance in the world. They both have beliefs, doctrines, principles, and traditions that can seem very similar at first glance. However, it is also easy to see where they differ. Buddhism is non-theistic, while Christianity holds Jesus Christ as its central figure.

When observing similarities between these two religious' traditions, it is hard not to focus on the fact that both are founded on a Book, i.e., the Holy Bible for Christians and the Tripitaka for Buddhists. There are five precepts in Buddhism: not harming any sentient being, not lying or deceiving anyone, no stealing, and respect for parents and elders.

Both religions also emphasize the benefit of leading a life of self-discipline and meditation. In Similarly, Christian monasticism developed to include forms like Lectio Divina, where one spends time alone in his cell reading Bible passages for contemplation.

Christianity and Buddhism have differing views on what happens after death. Christianity teaches that Jesus is the only way to salvation. Still, Buddhists believe in an "intermediate state" where beings go through a judicial process that determines if they should be reborn or not. The judgment is based on whether individuals have led a virtuous life full of merit and good behavior. Christian doctrine holds that Jesus died for sinners to free them from their sins, while Buddhist teaching holds that lives are infinite, and beings reincarnate until they become enlightened.

The notion of salvation and the afterlife is reflected in many of their symbols and rituals. In Buddhism, Nirvana is the ultimate goal for each individual. It represents a state of spiritual liberation where all desires are extinguished. Nirvana is achieved when all things are understood to be non-existent, and Buddha was said to have attained Nirvana 2500 years ago before passing it on to others.

The differences between these two world religions can also be seen in their lifestyles. Buddhist monks and nuns practice celibacy, while priests in the Roman Catholic Church are allowed to marry. Christian tradition teaches that Jesus was married to Mary Magdalene and many Christians look upon Mary as an essential figure in their religion. Buddhists also take a firm stance on environmental issues and participate in activities like tree planting on a global scale.

Although there is no doubt that they are different, there is no denying that they both believe in certain fundamental principles that can be found across many other religions.

Similarities of Buddhism and Christianity

Eager for a spiritual journey into knowledge and enlightenment? Want to transcend the mundane, conventional, and superficial ways of life? Were you intrigued by the similarities between Buddhism and Christianity?

If you answered yes to any of these questions, read on! We have compiled two articles that show intriguing parallels between these well-known religions. The first article takes a comparative look at how both religions deal with telling someone that they are no longer a part of their group. Surprisingly, while they may use different methods, their overall goal is the same: To keep on saving as many people as possible by eliminating those who do not fit in with their set standards. The second article takes a comparative look at how both religions define the word "peace," ultimately concluding that peace is something you need to work towards, not an instantaneous reward.

Buddhism and Christianity both have strict requirements for those who want to join their group. However, to ensure that they are keeping only the best members, they have different ways of approaching ex-communication. Buddhism focuses on doing good deeds to keep up with the standards required for belonging to their group (Wallis).

It is referred to as "meritorious action." It was the way Buddhists dealt with ex-communication. The malaise was that "good" deeds were sometimes misconstrued and that people who completed these deeds but did not meet the requirements of belonging to the group were sometimes still granted entrance (Wallis). Therefore, they found a new way to keep up with their standards by doing away with merit and instead focusing on being the right person. It is called the Eightfold Path on Buddha's Wheel of Dharma.

Christianity uses the church community as its primary tool in ex-communication. Those who are kicked out or deny entrance are typically people who have committed one of a few sins. These sins are murder, sexual immorality, theft, and blasphemy (Lowder). The reasoning behind these few serious sins is that they are acts that go against the Ten Commandments. Since Christianity believes all humans are sinners, they think it is necessary to find a scapegoat to explain the reason for their wrongdoings. This scapegoat is known as Satan or Lucifer (Lowder). "The idea of a scapegoat giving up his soul to has been with the Christian Church since its beginning" (Lowder). It was believed that if someone were genuinely sorry for their wrongdoings and confessed them to God, then God would forgive them.

The highest goal of both religions is to get rid of sin. Once they have gotten rid of sin, they will enter Nirvana for Buddhists and Heaven for Christians. The idea behind getting rid of evil is that you are in a state of pure happiness and God's grace (Lowder). However, these rewards are not instantaneous. You cannot just become a better person overnight and expect to gain entrance into Nirvana or Heaven. You must continue to try harder to reach your goals.

The idea behind peace as defined by Christianity is very different from the concept behind peace as defined by Buddhism. Christians believe that peace can only happen once God has been achieved (Roberts). Once you have found God, you will never have to worry about being at war with anyone or anything. "The Prince of Peace" is a term often used in Christianity. Those looking for this type of peace should follow Christ and accept his salvation (Roberts). This type of peace ends up being an instantaneous reward. It doesn't take effort on the person's part, but they must accept that they will not be receiving it until their death (Roberts).

On the other hand, Buddhism believes that those who achieve Nirvana or Heaven will end up gaining a state of peace without ever having to worry about finding it (Wallis). "The peace that the Buddha teaches is not an external peace which crushes resistance: it is an inner peace, which arises from the removal of all desires and cravings" (Wallis). Once you have gained this type of peace, you will have reached Nirvana. The downside to this type of vacation is that we must continue to try harder to achieve it. Therefore, it is a continuous cycle of working towards our goal.

Overall, there are many defining similarities between Buddhism and Christianity. Overall, it starts with understanding each religion's views as a definition for sin and merit/demerit points. Christianity believes that all humans are sinners, but certain sins go against the Ten Commandments. These sins lead to ex-communication of those who commit them, and a scapegoat is used to explain why these sins occurred in the first place (Lowder). If an action is committed, it leads only to suffering. Therefore, Buddhism focuses on doing good deeds to reach Nirvana (Wallis). They believe that once a person has attained Nirvana, they will have achieved peace and will no longer have to worry about being at war with anyone or anything (Wallis).

The Wheel of Dharma also plays a significant role in Buddhism and Christianity. The wheel represents different stages on the path of achieving Nirvana or Heaven (Wallis; Roberts). Both religions must continue to try harder to reach their goals (Wallis; Roberts) eventually. However, if a person believes in Christianity, they think they must do their part on the path to get to God, and it is their sin that prevents them from obtaining him (Lowder). If a person follows Buddhism, they believe that their merit and demerit points determine whether or not they are going the right way towards reaching Nirvana (Lowder).

Differences of Buddhism and Christianity

Buddhism and Christianity have many similarities and differences. Buddhism was developed in India to find enlightenment through self-discipline, which focuses on the self. Buddhist practice is less ritualized than Christian tradition but more individualistic. Buddhist monks live a life of voluntary poverty and are therefore dependent on their lay followers for contributions.

Christianity is rooted in Egypt, focusing on being saved from sin through Jesus Christ's sacrifice to appease God's wrath against humanity. A key difference is that Christianity focuses more heavily on ritual practices such as baptism and communion as part of the faith. In contrast, Buddhism focuses on spiritual practices such as meditation or mindfulness. Buddhism, like Christianity, does not advocate isolation from society but encourages positive action.

They follow his teachings and strive to go to heaven when they die. All life was characterized by grief, and all humans were trapped in what could be called a cycle of suffering. This cycle consists of birth, sickness, old age, and death. The path to be freed from suffering was Noble Eightfold Path: right views, right intention, right speech, right action, right livelihood, right effort, right mindfulness, and right concentration. The historical Buddha did not have a teaching about the afterlife, and there is much disagreement among his followers about what happens after death.

The main difference between both religions comes with what happens after you do achieve your peace. There are many different religions, but the primary way to achieve peace is through Jesus (Roberts). Buddhists do not have a particular direction to follow to find peace. Instead, they believe that there are many ways of getting there. It leads them to the idea of a continuous cycle. In addition to this, other differences between Christianity and Buddhism are the techniques used to obtain Nirvana or Heaven. In Christianity, you have Jesus, who provides an immediate reward once you accept his salvation. In Buddhism, there are many ways to achieve this type of peace. However, none of them can be performed until a person has tried hard enough.

Conclusion

The Buddha's teachings are vast and very profound. Until now, we have treated only some of the fundamental teachings of the Buddha and only superficially. Indeed, it is said that practicing all the basic teachings of the Buddha is difficult even for a monk who lives as a hermit. It is, therefore, no wonder that it is difficult for laypeople like us, who have many worldly responsibilities to face. However, if we can sincerely cultivate and practice even some of the Buddha's teachings, we will have given a deeper meaning to this life. It is also certain that we will find ourselves in favorable circumstances to practice the Dhamma e finally achieve liberation.

Everyone can reach the supreme goal of Buddhism, both laypeople and religion. All that needs to be done is to make an honest effort to follow the Eightfold Noble Path. It is said that those who have realized the truth, like the Buddha Sakyamuni and his main disciples, did not arrive there by chance. It did not fall since sky like rain nor sprouted from the earth like grains. The Buddha and His disciples had been ordinary people like you and me. They were afflicted with impurities mental, such as attachment, aversion, and ignorance. It was only by coming in contact with Dhamma, purifying their words and deeds, developing the mind, and purchasing wisdom, that they became free, heavenly beings, able to teach and help others realize the truth. Therefore, there is no doubt that if we follow the teachings of the Buddha, we too can reach the final goal.

If all of us put Buddha's teachings into practice, there is no doubt that we will benefit significantly from it. If we try not to hurt anyone, if we do our best to help others in every possible opportunity if we learn to be aware and to develop the ability to concentrate the mind, if we cultivate wisdom with study, with careful reflection, and with meditation, there is no doubt that we will get a lot of benefits from the Dhamma. First there it will lead to prosperity and happiness in this life and the next. Finally, it will take us to the ultimate goal of liberation, to the supreme bliss of Nibbana.

Buddhism is practiced by close to 300 million people worldwide. It's an ancient religion that's been around for thousands of years. Buddhism is taken from the word "bodhi," which means "to awaken," and was brought into prominence by Siddhartha Gautama, now commonly referred to as the Buddha. The Buddha became enlightened or awakened at around 35 years of age and spent the remaining 45 years of his life traveling the country, teaching his beliefs to everyone from servants to noblemen. Through the centuries, his teachings have been passed down and developed into Buddhism forms today.

Many believe Buddhism to be less a religion and more a way of life. It's often termed as a philosophy because it seeks out wisdom. In short, Buddhism is usually summarized as trying to lead a moral life, being aware and mindful of your actions and thoughts while developing knowledge and understanding.

Practicing Buddhism and making it a part of your daily life will allow you to understand yourself and the world in new and exciting ways. It will empower you to overcome any tribulations or adversity that is thrown in your direction. It will help to improve your overall sense of well-being while also developing mindfulness. In short, the goal of Buddhism is to help you find eternal happiness.

Becoming a Buddhist is not a change that happens overnight.

So, what does it feel like to end one's Desire and, consequently, Suffering? Naturally, the only way to find out is to experience it yourself. However, the Buddhas often describe it as peace of mind in this life. It's a completeness that leaves no room for want, no space for pride, and no disappointment from what does not happen because there are no expectations. Thus, the Third Noble Truth is that suffering ends.

For instance, let us say you remember the feeling of being disappointed about a canceled trip that you had been looking forward to for months. The cause of your suffering is your desire for the journey. That suffering, in itself, is a manifestation created by your mind depending on what you have taken in throughout your life. Your disappointment or pain can come from any event in your life that has left you feeling that you were cheated of something.

From this disappointment, you are left with a further desire to correct it. You are then caught back in the cycle where disappointment will indeed find you once again. We cling to the positive emotional responses we get without realizing they are self-satisfaction created by our minds, not ourselves.

You might think it is just natural to experience this, and, indeed, you are right. It is why it is considered a reality. In a simple format, the Second Noble Truth is that all suffering has a cause.

Of course, while there is nothing negative about striving for your dreams, clinging too much to them leads to the constant feeling of yearning, which in itself is painful.

Since the world that we live in is ever-changing, we need to accept that we are continually changing too, and sometimes that means moving from one set of emotions to another. We are rarely satisfied with anything because as soon as we derive satisfaction from anything, our mind shifts to the next thing. You will find that meditation and discipline of the mind positively will help considerably cut down the suffering, although the First Noble Truth has to be accepted. There is always suffering from one kind or another in the world. This Noble Truth merely confirms that fact and is often shortened to a very easily understandable format: Suffering exists.

Miracles and Parables

Jesus performed many miracles, including walking on water across the Sea of Galilee, turning water into wine at a wedding feast at Cana, reviving Lazarus from the dead, and feeding 5,000 hungry people with five loaves bread and two fishes. The point of these miracles was to build faith among his disciples and show them he had the power that could only come from God. Christians also interpret these miracles allegorically: For instance, the food is a symbol of spiritual enrichments. Receiving Jesus' spiritual message and accepting the knowledge of him is food for the soul.

Jesus also spread his teaching through parables or stories. Sometimes these are actual stories, and sometimes they are metaphors. For instance, in Matthew 13:31–32:

To most theologians' thinking, Jesus' message is that faith begins as the smallest seed in human beings' hearts. When the source is sown and nurtured, it grows into something bigger, more substantial, and more beautiful. To plant the seed is to accept God's word, which will transform the person from within the same way the source is transformed into a plant or a tree

BOOK 6

Introduction

Intuitive eating aims to achieve where traditional and popular diets fail. It encourages a positive relationship with food. The first principle in intuitive eating is to develop this positive connection with your choice of food and to acknowledge that it provides nourishment that we need to work, exercise and enjoy life. Balance is key and achieving this means paying attention to your body's signals. Often, we lose this balance when we diet, focusing on counting calories, carbohydrates and portions. While this may be successful, we become so caught up in our progress and failures, that we forget about our enjoyment of eating and our mental wellbeing. This is where intuitive eating aims to correct the damage of dieting, therefore restoring our sense of feeling good about how we eat and feel overall.

When you begin mindful or intuitive eating, you learn to become more connected to your body's individual needs and aware of the signals you receive to fulfill those needs. In developing this connection, you will also know when to detect real hunger, as opposed to a craving or non-hungry response to wanting food. During this process, your body will also communicate other needs and in time, you'll find more balance in your approach to eating, exercise and life in general.

Get "In Tune" With Your Body and Your Reactions

The first step to intuitive eating starts with getting "In Tune" with our body so that we are aware of how we feel, think and experience the moment. Learn to appreciate and accept your body unconditionally and all that you can do, instead of focusing on flaws. How many people pick all the least favorite parts of their body in the mirror? It likely happens more than we care to admit. Intuitive eating is more than how we consume, but how we see ourselves first. Getting in touch with our reactions to those perceptions and actions is the next step. Once we are aware of how we react, we can address those thoughts and feelings. For example, when you misplace your phone or set of keys, you may panic and search frantically for them, becoming increasingly more agitated if they are not found quickly. In that very moment, what are you feeling? It may be panic, frustration and eventually, a sense of relief when a lost item is found. A similar emotional reaction, though different, is experienced when we eat something that is forbidden or restricted from a set way of eating or diet. We may feel a sense of disappointment if we eat a large slice of chocolate cake or binge eating at a buffet. This leads to feelings of guilt, shame and anger at oneself for failing at a specific set of rules for eating. In experiencing these feelings, we forget to fully enjoy the piece of cake, which is the reason we choose to indulge in the first place. In the case of the lost key or phone, instead of recognizing our frustration, putting it aside and retracing our last steps to locate an item, we become overrun with the emotional reaction and losing sight of our goals.

Take the Guilt Out of Food and Eating

We all make mistakes, or what we perceive to be an error. It is important to recognize this as part of our being. What if eating didn't require a set of rules but rather, a calm, mindful approach to enjoying a meal. A truly satisfying meal does not leave you frustrated, hungry or disappointed. It is important, in this way, to take the guilt away from food. Honor and respect your hunger. Cravings are natural and everyone experiences them, whether we follow a strict diet or eat freely. Sometimes we might crave a certain food because we pass by a bakery on a busy street or notice an advertisement for a new restaurant. This feeling can be followed by remembering limitations, where we acknowledge the craving, then remind ourselves that our diet must fit within a fixed number of carbs per day or calories per meal. In doing this, we sabotage the enjoyment we could otherwise experience by trying the new restaurant or picking up a fresh loaf of bread. If we skip the experience, does it significantly alter our rate of success? How attached are we to a goal of a specific weight or result of diet so much that our enjoyment of food is stunted by constant feelings of guilt if we even consider cheating?

Taking the guilt out of eating means thoroughly enjoying our meals and choices of food. Choosing to indulge in a full meal, enjoying its taste, texture, and effects on your mood is deeply satisfying, and something a diet does not take into consideration. After a decent meal, your hunger is satisfied and there are no further cravings, without the need to overeat, as taking the time to savor the food triggers your body to recognize it is full. Eating too quickly and hastily only causes more agitation later, as you feel too full once it's too late, leading to feelings of guilt once you experience a stomach-ache. Taking time to enjoy and relax during a meal is the reward you deserve, and your body will thank you for it!

Body Appreciation
If you ask people what they think of their body, most will respond with what they dislike most. Most people are not completely satisfied with how they look. Advertisements, media, and many industries promote an ideal body image: larger muscles, stronger and toned physique for men or a curvy, slender body for women. While there are great strides to accept many body sizes and types, challenging stereotypes and becoming more inclusive, society still has a long way to go. Cosmetics, fitness, and fashion focus on our sense of flaws and wanting to correct them, giving us the ideal or current look to reach for. We may reach our weight goal, then become unhappy with stretchmarks or loose skin. Building muscle may be successful until we become preoccupied with other parts of our body that don't measure up to a set of standards. At some point, we can become like perfectionists, focusing so narrowly on a certain look and forgetting the most important impact: How it impacts the way we feel and think.

Learning to appreciate your body takes time. It requires looking in the mirror without criticism but with acceptance. This doesn't occur overnight and requires a different way of looking at yourself. There is always room to improve, but we can still enjoy our body as it is today. A significant part of showing your body appreciation is eating properly and without a sense of restriction. Maintaining and improving your body can be achieved through mindful and intuitive eating.

Acknowledging that Hunger is Not the Enemy
Diets often treat hunger like the enemy, not something to acknowledge and accept. Intermittent fasting is one such diet, that restricts eating within a certain time that we call "window". There are variations on this way of eating, from 16:8 (eat all meals within eight hours during the day, fast for sixteen hours) to full twenty-four-hour fasts once a week or longer fasts lasting more than a day. Despite a lot of positive testimonials on social media, blogs, and websites that rave about successful weight loss, one major drawback to this diet is the hunger pangs within the fasting window. Even the most self-disciplined people can easily cheat during the fasting time frame with a snack, which is followed by a sense of guilt or disappointment when they realized the fast is broken. Ketogenic and low carb

methods of eating restrict carbohydrates from 100 grams per day or less (low or moderate carb) to under 20 grams a day (keto). These diets were originally developed to treat a number of medical conditions, including diabetes, epilepsy, and seizures. The reduction of carbohydrates can be beneficial, but not realistically sustainable for most people. The Paleo diet aims to align the foods you eat by choosing foods that are less processed and do not require cultivation, though, like other ways of eating, Paleo restricts a lot of options, even without counting calories or carbohydrates. These ways of eating demand a high degree of commitment and tracking of carbs on a daily basis.

When most people feel hungry, they often ignore or put off eating. It can be due to a lot more than the way we eat. Stress, a busy schedule or working day can impact how we react to hunger. If we have a pressing deadline or activity that cannot be easily interrupted, we put off lunch or taking a break. In doing so, we effectively train ourselves to dismiss hunger signals as a nuisance. When we are able to get away, our sense of hunger may contribute to overeating and rushing to eat within the specific and often limited time period, so that we can hurry back to our workplace. When we get home from work, dinner should be a meal to look forward to, but it is often late or not enjoyed as much as it should be. When this is combined with a stressful day, meals might be skipped altogether. Breakfast is commonly skipped, leaving a large gap until lunch time. Hunger is imminent in most of these scenarios, where eating is inconsistent and insufficient. Recognizing the importance of hunger, and its importance is part of intuitive eating.

Hunger Signals: How to Measure and Respond to It?
What makes you hungry? A juicy steak with baked potatoes and salad? Or a fresh plate of sushi and sashimi? The very thought of a delicious meal can make your mouth water, but how intense is it experienced? When we detect hunger or feel the need to consume food, we don't measure it. If someone asks: "Are you hungry?" It's a "Yes" or "No" question, not a sliding scale. Sometimes we experience a sensation that we are hungry, even when we are not. Is this real hunger? Or it is just a feeling because of an advertisement for something tasty? Measuring your level of hunger may seem like a strange concept because we usually respond to all hunger signals similarly: we either plan to eat or ignore them.

Measuring your hunger may take some practice at first, but it becomes easy, routinary and takes only seconds once you master it. When you consider eating, the first thing you should note is your level of hunger on a scale of one to ten, where one is completely full due to over-eating, five is neither hungry nor full and one is feeling famished or extreme hunger. Often when we feel hungry, we don't evaluate the level. This is the first step to connecting your body's needs to food. If you find this challenging at first, consider the following steps:

1. Imagine a large bowl that represents your hunger. If you pour water into the bowl, is it nearly empty, representing strong hunger? Is it half full, quarter full, leaving a sense of hunger but only temporarily? Gauging your level of hunger is helpful in determining how much you will eat. The more hunger you feel, the sooner you should begin eating.

2. *How would you rate your level on a scale of one to ten?*

a.   **Between 8-10:** Almost full (eight) up to completely full (ten)

This is how we feel after we finish a large meal and have a sensation of fullness, either to the extent of no hunger or being overfull and avoiding food completely.

b. From 4-7: Neither full or hungry, where four is closer to being slightly less hungry, and six is slightly more and seven is moderately full.

At this stage, you may feel slightly hungry, if you finished a meal that did not totally satisfy your hunger, though did not leave you famished either. This can vary. Whether or not you choose to eat a bit more or wait until your hunger intensifies, is the individual's decision.

c. From 1-3: Where three indicates moderate hunger, increasing in severity to one, which represents the most extreme case, to the point of feeling pain or discomfort. This is experienced when you go without food (and/or drink) for long periods of time, from working a full day without having lunch or a snack or an extreme deprivation of food for more than a day. If you have not eaten for a long period of time, be cautious not to binge right away, as this will cause indigestion and stomach cramps. Taking time to eat slowly, as difficult as it may seem, will satisfy your needs without pain.

Diets that involve restricting eating to specific hours during the day or calorie restrictions can push the hunger scale towards ten quickly, prompting your response to eat as soon as possible. This is where binge-eating or overeating can occur. The longer you wait, the greater the strain you will experience emotionally, especially if there are long gaps between meals. Your stomach will growl; your mind will visually imagine food more vividly. You will notice family and friends enjoying a snack or meal and feel deprived. This feeling may not seem negative, as you justify the diet and its goals, but it can impact your sense of enjoyment and emotional peace if food is often avoided or restricted.

If you experience a stressful day, you may react emotionally by eating more or less than usual. There are also instances where you feel a compulsion to eat differently in a busy setting, such as a work conference or while you are commuting, where you may literally eat on the go or pick foods that you normally wouldn't like or enjoy, just to have something to fill up on. The opposite can sometimes yield the same results: at a party among friends or family where there is an abundance of food choices and you decide to try them all. These occasions happen and that's perfectly acceptable. As much as possible, try to enjoy your meals when you feel calm and without intense emotion. The important factor in all such instances is to become aware of them and learn how to respond and prepare ourselves for these events.

The Advantages of Mindful Eating

Intuitive or mindful eating is not a diet; in fact, it is considered an "anti-diet." The approach is different in that mindful eating focuses on overall well-being, which includes more than target weight loss goals and losing inches. Intuitive eating takes into consideration the psychological, physical, emotional and mental benefits. This begins in the mind, to acknowledge and accept your body, connect with your feelings and signals, and use these to determine when to eat, how to recognize your hunger and fullness on your own. Once this way of connection is achieved, you will realize your body's potential to know what is good for you and when. This results in greater respect for your body. You'll notice other signals from your body: when to relax, meditate or exercise. Tuning into all of your body's signals will help you achieve a better sense of balance and satisfaction overall.

Advantages of mindful eating include decreased excess weight, maintaining a healthy weight, good cholesterol levels, decreased levels of stress. Intuitive eating also contributes to less focus on weight loss, thinness and more on health and feeling well. Loss of stress will contribute to many other benefits, including better focus, productivity, and enjoyment of life. The very thought of dieting can be stressful in of itself and following specific regimes can be timely and expensive. Certain diets have a social impact on individuals: to conform to eating and following a certain popular diet or breaking from it. It happens during lunch at the office, drinks after work with colleagues or co-workers, and family gatherings; the pressure to join fellow dieters in their plan (such as the latest fad) or to experience guilt and cheat. Imagine not worrying about what you eat but rather enjoying the occasion and enjoying the meal with the company? This has a profound impact on your sense of happiness. Healthy eating can still be achieved, with the right choices, but why should it be stressful?

Chapter 1. Intuitive Eating and Mindful Eating

While in-depth research into Intuitive Eating and Mindful Eating has only been conducted in the recent past, more than 13 studies have already proved that these strategies are truly effective in helping you control binge eating. They can also help you achieve your long-term wellness goals and turn your life around.

To begin with, intuitive eating is all about listening to your body. This concept is based on the premise that your body knows what it needs. When you feel the urge to eat a particular type of food, that is your body pointing to the appropriate nutrition and nourishment it needs. Mindful eating is creating a mental connection with the food that you eat. If you can adopt both these techniques into your everyday diet, you'll be able to avoid binge eating altogether.

Understanding Intuitive Eating

Intuitive Eating is the careful synchronization of your mind and body with food. Food is the fuel that keeps your body and mind functioning and is an important part of your life. The initial step you need to take is to change your mind set. Stop viewing food as an enemy. Stop thinking of it a trigger that turns you into a gorging, overweight monster. Think of it as something you love. Here's what you need to do:

•Let Nature be Your Guide: Nature has programmed your body cells to know what they need and want. Let them have it. Give your body what it wants when you feel truly hungry. You only need to tell the difference whether you're actually hungry or if this is just a craving.

•Eat to Nourish Your Body, Not Your Mind: Recognize the signs of actual hunger. When did you last have something to eat? Did you have an adequate portion size? Should you really be hungry right now? Or, are you just upset your date canceled dinner because of a work issue?

•Stop Feeling Guilty: Don't lay down rules for yourself about what you can and cannot eat. At some time, you WILL end up giving in, and go berserk over the forbidden food. If you're really hungry, you're allowed to eat anything you want. And, let your body tell you when to stop.

Understanding Mindful Eating

Mindful Eating is all about enjoying food. When you eat, turn it into a pleasurable activity and focus your mind entirely on the dish in front of you. Block out the outside world and build a personal connection with your food. Here are some of the steps you need to take to tell your mind and body that food is a friend.

• Eliminate All Other Activities

When it's time for a meal, make it a point to turn off all electronic devices. And, that includes the television, computer, radio, music system, and above all, your cell phone. Never, ever take calls during meals. Letting a couple of calls go to voicemail won't make a difference, but they'll interfere with your meal. Experts also recommend that you don't eat when driving. If you're really, really hungry, grab a bite, but pull over into a parking lot and enjoy every mouthful.

• Savor Your Food

Be aware of every bite and focus your senses completely on the taste, texture, and flavor. Food is mainly about the aroma. Breathe in the scents of the yummy goodness and think about how the ingredients nourish and fuel your body.

• Check in Advance How Hungry You Are

Think of your hunger levels from 1 to 10. 1 being the point when you just cannot eat another bite, and 10 being the level where you could eat a horse at a single sitting. Before beginning your meal, work out the number. You'll find that it is easier to control the portion sizes you eat. And remember, you can eat what you like best.

• It's Not a Race

Give yourself time to eat. Don't rush through your meal with your mind on the deadlines you have to meet or the laundry waiting to be folded. Chew each bite thoroughly and pause now and then. Put down your fork in between bites. Think about how good the food tastes. Considering that your body needs 20 minutes to register that your stomach is full, this is a smart way to control the portion sizes.

• Be Aware of Why You're Eating

Many times, people eat without really realizing what they're doing. And that is most likely to happen when you're stressed out. Think about it. You're worried about how the interview went, and you're waiting for the acceptance call. As you pace the living room, you reach for the cookies and start to eat one after the other. Stop yourself and instead, try to meditate or focus on the highlights of the interview when you excelled with every response. This factor holds true in cases of overeating also. If your mind is on the company layoffs, you'll fill your plate unknowingly with more food than you need. But, if you're aware of what you're doing, you'll choose the right portion.

Stress and scary life situations have the effect of taking the pleasure out of the meals you eat and turning them instead into activities that are bad for you. If you enjoy a cereal and fruit breakfast, that's a good life choice. But, replacing it with coffee and donuts in the morning rush to work is a bad choice. Especially when you end up having absolutely no idea how the donut tasted afterward. You see now? This is why you need to adopt the art of intuitive eating. Read ahead to understand how it can help you to avoid binge eating. And, instead adopt a healthy lifestyle.

Chapter 2. Benefits of Mindful Eating

Here are a few of the most prominent benefits of mindful eating.

Overcoming eating disorders

Ill- eating habits, irregular meal timings, and eating mindlessly can lead to a lot of eating disorders. People who eat mindlessly suffer from over-eating, emotional eating, binge eating disorder, anorexia, and bulimia. They build a harmful and destructive relationship with food. Hence, they either overeat or eat too little. When you eat mindfully, you are aware of your hunger, and body signals. It prevents you from eating unhealthy food items and overeating. It also prevents you from eating for the wrong reasons. Thus, if you eat mindfully, you can overcome eating disorders and build healthy eating patterns.

Significantly lower health risks

Eating in an unhealthy way can lead to many health risks. Eating junk, processed or chemically dense food items can lead to toxicity, acidity, and oxidative damage in the body. Obesity is one of the common symptoms of eating unhealthily. But, it might also lead to cancer, high blood pressure, diabetes type-2, autoimmune diseases, allergies, sleep apnoea, digestive problems, poor gut health, reduced blood haemoglobin levels, nutritional deficiencies, and many other health conditions.

When you are aware of your eating habits and practice, you will choose to eat healthily and avoid eating chemically laden food substances. You then begin to be more aware of your bodily needs and nutritional requirements. Gradually you start to detox the body and enrich it with healthy wholesome food and nutrients. Healthy eating habits lead to a significant reduction in health risks.

Weight management

Many people are unaware of the fact that, when it comes to weight management, food contributes more than exercise. It is indeed true that you can create a fit body in the kitchen by eating right. Many people struggle to lose weight because they have an unhealthy relationship with food. They struggle to maintain a healthy weight because they either make wrong food choices or practice various short-term diets. Weight management is all about eating right. Eating mindfully can help you in managing weight effortlessly. You won't be starving yourself, practicing short-term diets, or restrain yourself from eating. Eating right means to eat food items that are good for your body, fulfil your hunger, and provide fuel (nutrition and energy) to your body. When you eat well, the excess weight will drop automatically.

Better mood and emotional wellbeing

Synthetic and chemically dense food such as junk and processed food, overly sugary drinks, ice creams, candies, etc. give you a sugar rush, unwanted trans fats, triglycerides, cholesterol, and unwanted chemical waste. Your body is not capable of metabolizing and storing these synthetic substances. The sugar and chemicals in processed food give you a sensation of high and happiness, then after 20-30 minutes of eating junk food, you feel sad and low. To stay in a good mood, you begin to eat chemically dense food on a regular basis because you feel that is what makes you feel good. Often feeling emotional distress as you start to reach for food to comfort yourself.

The only way you can sustain a happy mood and emotional wellbeing is via mindful and intuitive eating. Being aware of your feelings and how the food makes you feel is crucial. Real food is not supposed to make you feel low or crappy. Eating nutritionally dense foods make you feel full, energetic, and happy.

A healthy relationship with the body

By practicing to eat in total awareness, it will help you to understand your body in a better way. You will learn how your body signals for hunger, emotional stress, sleep, and fatigue work and most importantly you will be able to recognise these signals and act upon it correctly. You will discover that food is the answer to hunger and not to any other signal. You will eventually understand what your body needs. Eating mindfully will help you to love your body and heal the broken relationship.

A fulfilled life and longevity

I can say this without a doubt that the problems cause by mindless eating can be reduced by eating mindfully. You will no longer deal with stressful eating, over-eating, emotional eating, the guilt of eating unhealthily, and the weight issues. You can live a fulfilled and long life by eating mindfully. It is quite surprising that a simple activity can contribute so much to your life. Just by eating right you can transform your life, and it is correct to say that food indeed is the medicine.

Chapter 3. The Side-effect of Mindless Eating

I am sure you know that mindless eating deteriorates the mind body and soul. You have already read about a few side-effects of mindless eating. Without going too much into detail, let me explain to you the adverse effects of mindless eating.

Eating mindlessly takes away your control over the eating habits. You are no longer aware of anything related to the eating habits. You lose control over the following things when you eat mindlessly.

What are you eating?

The quantity of food that you eat.

How frequently do you eat?

The excessive eating that you do.

Food is an integral part of our life, and when we mess up the eating habits, it can lead to poor well-being. It hampers our overall mental, emotional, and physical health.

Eating disorders – You are more prone to having an eating disorder such as binge eating disorder, bulimia or anorexia.

Weight issues – it causes you to struggle with weight loss and maintaining a healthy weight.

Increases in health risks – Mindless eating makes you more susceptible to diseases such as diabetes type-2, hypertension, infertility, allergies, and autoimmune diseases.

Fatigue – The constant feeling of tiredness throughout the day. You wake up tired and feel fatigued without any reason.

Mental Fog – It is a state of mind where you feel confused and puzzled. The mental clarity, creativity, decreases when you have mental fog.

Low stamina – Irrespective of the amount of food you eat and rest you take, you feel like you have no energy. You get tired quickly and fail to build stamina.

Emotional distress – Anything can set your mood off or make you feel emotionally unstable. You get angry, cry, or are irritated easily.

Mood swings – Similar to the emotional distress you experience erratic mood swings. You can get sad or feel low without any reason with short bursts of good mood.

Anxiety, stress, and depression- People who practice mindless eating often suffer from anxiety, stress, and depression. It is mainly caused due to not being able to express emotions, feeling fatigued, having mental fog, and other ill-effects of mindless eating habits.

Low self-esteem and self-hate – All the side-effects of mindless eating often sum up and lead to self-hate, guilt, and low self-esteem.

Poor gut health – Digestive issues, bloating, constipation, diarrhoea, stomach aches are a common sign of poor gut health.

Mindless eating can hamper your ability to live a happy and fulfilled life. Some of the side-effects might not seem dangerous, but these symptoms are interdependent. Thus, if you are feeling fatigued, you will probably have low stamina, mental fog, and irritable mood. I hope you can understand that it is imperative that we eat healthily by being aware of our eating practice. So, without waiting any longer, let us now learn how to begin eating mindfully.

Chapter 4. What Really Is Binge Eating?

To binge eat doesn't just mean that you eat too much. That is called overeating. To binge eat means to eat excessively in a short period – normally several hours. Now, to be clear, to eat too much occasionally is perfectly normal and shouldn't worry you. We all have a tendency to overindulge on special days, like Christmas or Thanksgiving. If you occasionally find yourself lying on the couch groaning that you really shouldn't have had that last helping, that does not mean you're necessarily a binge eater or that you've raised it to problematic proportions.

It's when you've got an uncontrollable urge or compulsion to eat to excess which you can't stop yourself from indulging that you might be a binge eater. Binge eating disorder is the most common eating disorder in the US, with 3.5% of women and 2% of men affected [1]. It can lead to serious health and mental problems.

What's more, binge eating can escalate in a self-reinforcing spiral where binge eating leads to more serious symptoms, which in turn leads to more binge eating. Obviously, that's not a situation anybody wants to find themselves in, but it can be a hard one to avoid. This is because binge eating is often done to fight feelings of both stress and anxiety and in the short term can certainly help a person feel like they've got better control over them. Unfortunately, in the long run it can do quite the opposite. In that way it's a great deal like drug addiction.

All that might make you feel anxious, which ironically might lead to you wanting to binge eat, just in order to feel better. Before you head off to see what the fridge has to offer know this! There is hope. There are ways to defeat binge eating and return to a normal life! We will be looking at proven methods to help you contain and ultimately defeat the disorder. But first let's explore the condition itself, as the first step to defeating a problem is to understand it.

Disclaimer
At this point it is important to put in an official disclaimer. The information presented in this guide isn't official medical advice, we are not doctors or medical professionals. Yes, we offer tips and guidelines that might help you, but we are in no way suggesting that you should rely on what is written here to diagnose and treat your illness. Binge eating is a serious medical condition, with serious consequences and often needs serious medical attention. That is not to say that this information hasn't helped some, but that does not mean it will automatically help you. Everybody is different and everybody needs different treatment.

What Causes Binge Eating?

Alright, with that out of the way, let's tackle the nature of binge eating. What is it exactly? It's a good question that we don't exactly know the answer to. That said, we do know a number of the underlying factors that make us more prone to binge eating behavior.

These include:

- *Family history:* If other family members suffer or have suffered from eating disorders then you are more likely to suffer them as well. This might in part be down to genes, though it could also have something to do with exposure, with which I mean that you've seen other people behave in a certain way and are therefore more likely to copy it.

- *Psychological issues:* A lot of people who binge eat suffer from low self-esteem and similar low self-regard. They might hold themselves up to very high standards and then feel that they haven't met them, which then makes them feel like they aren't accomplishing or haven't accomplished enough in their lives. This can lead to high stress, anxiety or tension and the binge eating, in this regard, might be a form of self-comforting.

- *Dieting:* Dieting has been shown by many studies to lead to a disconnect between your hunger systems and eating. What this means is that you might no longer know exactly when you feel full and should stop eating, due to you spending so much time suppressing your hunger urges. This, in turn, can break the system in the other direction as well, leading to you to continue eating when you're already completely satiated.

- *Your age:* Binge eating can manifest itself at any age, but is most likely to start during a person's late teens or early 20s.

Symptoms of A Binge

So you think you might be binge eating but you're not quite sure? Here is a list of the symptoms that can indicate you're suffering from this disorder. These are both useful for people who are afraid they suffer from binge eating as well as for people who are afraid a loved one might possess the disorder. Note that rarely is only one symptom indicative of binge eating syndrome. Instead, you should look for a constellation of different symptoms before getting worried.

- *Though not everybody who is overweight or obese binge eats, many binge eaters are overweight or obese.* In fact, up to 2/3rd of binge eaters fit into this category. That does not mean, however, that if a person is not overweight, they don't binge eat. We've got different types of metabolic rates and some people can eat tremendous amounts without actually gaining much weight. Importantly, if a person belongs to the category of non-overweight binge eaters that does not mean that they're escaping all of the negative health implications associated with it and it does not mean they shouldn't tackle the problem.

- *Eating unusually large amounts of food over a short period of time –* something like about two hours. Also indicative of a problem is that they person does not feel they can control the behavior. Quite often people that suffer binge eating episodes promise and vow that they will not engage in this type of eating, only then to break their promise and engage in another period of binge eating.

- *Eating too fast* is another sign that indicative of binging. With binge eating the person is not trying to savor and enjoy the food, but rather trying to consume as much as possible. Therefore, if a person is eating so quickly that they barely seem to take time to chew, this could be indicative of a problem.

- *Eating past the point of satiation.* This means that even though your body is sending signals that a person has had enough they continue to eat. In part this might be down to the fact that it can take a while for your body to actually signal to the brain that you don't need any more food (this can take up to 20 minutes). This, combined by the high speed of food consumption, then leads to drastic overeating.

- *Feeling ashamed, guilty or depressed about episodes of binge eating after they happen.* If a person frequently feels bad about their binges, that can be a pretty good indicator that they're binge eating. Alternatively, it could also mean that they're suffering from other eating conditions not least of which is anorexia. So though this can be very indicative of binge eating disorder, it should not be the only symptom for you to look at.

- *Eating alone and in secret.* This reason is often related to feelings of shame that people that binge eat experience due to their binge eating habits. They understand that their behavior is abnormal and therefore work to conceal it. Of course, this might not be a conscious process, with a binge eater instead giving in to subconscious triggers. For others the best way to see signs of secret eating is the sudden disappearance of large amounts of food as well as finding a large amount of empty food containers and wrappers.

- *Frequent dieting*, particularly when there is no weight loss, can also be symptomatic of binge eating. The lack of weight loss is down to the fact that the person is engaging in binge eating episodes, which defeat their weight-loss strategies.

- *Not eating very much during scheduled meals.* This should particularly be a worry signal if the person has a great deal of weight and even though they don't seem to be eating much, they don't seem to be losing any of it. Of course, it could mean that they've got a physical condition that makes weight loss difficult, so again don't jump to conclusions.

- *Being all or nothing and perfectionistic.* People that suffer from binge eating episodes frequently have trouble seeing they gray between the black and white. They feel they're either succeeding or they are not. They're either controlling their eating habits or they're not. This, coupled with a tendency towards perfectionism can lead to serious guilt and shame issues when things go wrong.

- *Control issues and difficulty expressing emotions.* It is possible that a person who has binge eating craves to be in control of situations and/or cannot communicate their emotions well.

Other Eating Disorders

Though binge eating is the most common of the different eating disorders, there are quite a few more and it is useful to be familiar with them so that you don't end up focusing on curing something you don't actually have. This is not to say that the cause of the different eating disorders might not be the same – still different disorders do seem to have different cures.

- *Anorexia Nervosa*: In a round-about-way anorexia is the opposite of binge eating (though it would be more accurate to say that it is the polar opposite of overeating, but let's not get too technical, shall we?) People that suffer from anorexia have a disturbed body image, which is an actual mechanism in the brain which tracks how you see yourself. It is the same system that makes you capable of grabbing things with your eyes closed in that it lets your mind track the position of your hand. People that are anorexic believe that they are overweight when they are in fact not. This makes them diet unnecessarily and as a result starve their bodies, which can be incredibly devastating on their health.

- *Bulimia Nervosa:* This disorder leads people to eat food, but then feel the need to vomit or use laxatives to get it out of their system as fast as possible. Though this might sound like a good idea, vomiting and laxatives are very harmful for the body and should not be engaged in on a frequent basis – certainly not after every meal! What's more, as the body does not get enough time to digest the food taken in, here too there is a risk of malnutrition.

- *Other disorders:* Sometimes people only suffer a milder condition of the conditions you see here. Sometimes they might restrict what types of food they're willing to consume to where it becomes unhealthy. Still, even though you might not be able to fit these problems into neat little categories, as eating is so inherently important to us, those who have eating problems can do themselves a great deal of harm. What is more, they can be indicative of psychological problems. It is important not to let any of eating related condition worsen.

Chapter 5. The Use of Medications in Treating Binge Eating Disorder

There are some types of medication that can be used in treating binge eating. Remember though those medicines are not to be relied on as the sole means of treating the problem. It can help in relieving some of the symptoms and effects of the disorder, but it can never be used in treating the cause and reversing it.

With that in mind, here are some of the common medications prescribed for treating Binge Eating Disorders:

Appetite Suppressants

Appetite suppressants are some of the most common drugs used for treating binge eating. One of the reasons this drug is used is because most patients who suffer from BED would also like to lose weight.

The psychotherapy that they are undergoing might do nothing for you when it comes to weight reduction. Appetite suppressants on the other hand promise some weight loss. Though you need to eat less as well.

This type of drug was first used for treating BED during the 90s. The problem was that one of the first appetite suppressing drugs used for this purpose was found to have some very harmful effects on the body. The risks included a high rate of cardiovascular diseases and other unwanted side effect.

Learning proper protion control and choosing healthier foods is the best approach and even if you use appetite suppressants you'll still need to choose your foods wisely.

Current Drugs

Today the most common drug used for treating binge eating by suppressing appetite and causing weight loss is Orlistat. This drug affects the ability of the body to absorb fat which in turn prevents the body from gaining weight.

In reality it really is not an appetite suppressant. Orlistat works by binding to the molecules of the fat in the food and preventing it from being broken down by the stomach into components that are easier to absorb.

There are other drugs currently being considered for use in controlling the appetite of those who are suffering from binge eating disorder. There are problems though with the side effects caused by these drugs. Some side effects include impairment of the patients cognitive ability. Another side effect that has been reported is that of tingling and numbness of the skin. This is not to say that Orilstat doesn't have unpleasand side effects, and if you are thinking about using it, you'll want to discuss this carefully with your doctor.

Topamax

Topiramate which is another name for Topamax is a drug that was originally intended for treating seizures. Some studies have suggested that it can help curb binge eating and that it could help jump start or increase weight loss.

Certain studies indicate that people suffering from Binge Eating Disorder might benefit from taking Topamax. While this use of the drug is not an officially approved or recommended use of the drug it does hold a great amount of promise for those who are suffering from this form of behavioural problem.

History of Topamax
Topamax was created for treating epilepsy and seizures. The drug was created in the late 1970s. The effect of the drug was meant to stop the convulsions of those who suffer from epilepsy.

Aside from the treatment of epilepsy the drug has also been used for other types of diseases. It has been used to treat bipolar disease and to counteract the weight gain in other diseases. Its use for treating bipolar disease has stopped since it has been shown to offer too few benefits for that problem.

Other Uses
The drug has been used to treat other problems as well. It has been used for treating migraine and severe headache. This use is due to the effect the drug has on blood vessels in the brain. It helps to widen them. Another reason why it is effective as a migraine treatment is because it has very few side effects.

It has been used for fighting the effects of alcoholism and other behavioural problems. There are other diseases and health problems for which this drug is being used but the one that we are most interested in is its effect on those who have Binge Eating Disorder.

Topamax for Binge Eating Disorder
Although the use of Topamax for BED is not really recommended by experts there are some very positive reviews on its effects. Studies conducted indicate that people who are suffering from BED were able to control their eating and their appetite by taking Topamax.

Those who used the drug had less attacks of binge eating, lost weight and even experienced a great amount of loss in their BMI. People who used the drug were able to lose as much as a pound per week over a 14-week period. Though this is not an officially approved use of the drug it does show a lot of promise for those having to cope with binge eating.

Topamax Usage
There are some reminders about Topamax usage I'd like to share:

- 1.   Anyone taking the drug should stay away from activities that require a certain level of mental alertness. The drug might impair abilities in that area.

- 2.   The use of the drug can affect the way that the body regulates heat so if taking Topamax, you should refrain from activities that can increase body heat.

- 3.   Topamax can decrease the effectiveness of certain contraceptives.

- 4. The sudden discontinuation of the use of the drug should be discouraged because it might cause a sudden increase in the number of seizures.

There are cases of overdose of this drug but they are very rare. The more serious cases of problems with the drug were instances where it had been used in conjunction with other medications. Overdose can cause several symptoms and they might include depression, blurred vision, problems with speech and thinking.

Before taking Topamax or any drug for that matter, in order to treat your Binge Eating Disorder make sure that you consult your doctor first so that s/he can give you the best advice.

UNDER NO CIRUMSTANCES SHOULD YOU TAKE ANY DRUG WITHOUT YOUR DOCTOR'S PERMISSION AND CONSENT.

Antidepressants
Another type of drug that is often used for treating BED are antidepressants. Recent research has proven this effect of the drug although long term studies are lacking.

There were seven studies conducted where the results showed promise that antidepressants might be able to help those who are suffering from BED. Over 40% of people who suffered from BED and took part in the studies had positive results after taking in anti-depressants.

The Use of Anti-Depressants
Antidepressants are used for alleviating the mood of those who suffer from depression and other forms of mood disorders. This kind of drug can have an alleviating effect on those with mood problems, but they do not have the same effect on normal people. Usually, this kind of drug has delayed effect of about 3 to 6 weeks and its use is usually prescribed for a period that lasts for months to years.

Side Effects
There are certain side effects that come with the use of antidepressants. These side effects include nausea, dry mouth, dizziness, constipation and sleepiness. There are other types of side effects as well depending on the drug taken.

Use of Antidepressants in Fighting BED
The use of antidepressants when it comes to fighting the effects of Binge Eating Disorder seems promising, but you need to keep in mind that it has not been officially recommended for that use. There are also some risks involved including relapse if you discontinue using the drug.

Self-Prescriptions
The medications listed here have shown indications that they can be beneficial when it comes to treating Binge Eating Disorder. However, you should never use them on your own. Even if these are not officially prescribed as medications for binge eating you should still consult a doctor before you take any of these medications.

As you have seen, some of the drugs have some adverse side effects. This information I have researched on these drugs is offered to you so you can talk to your doctor about your options in your specific case. You always seek the guidance of a physician before you use any drug.

Chapter 6. The Battle is About to Begin

It is important to remember throughout this journey that you are not alone. You will get through it, if you follow the steps that we are laying out in this book. That was the hardest part for me, in my journey. I always wanted to see myself as strong. I wanted to be in control, and I didn't want to have to depend on anyone else.

What I really needed was help, however, which is why it took so long for me to recover. I was too embarrassed to go to my family right away, so instead, I went online where I could meet strangers that wouldn't know who I was or that I had this problem. That was certainly helpful, but really talking out loud to other people was something that gave me the strength to know that I can do this on my own. But first, I needed some help to get started.

A major root cause of emotional eating comes from an emotional trigger, usually established during childhood. Our brain development slows significantly when we hit our 20s, and what we learn before that will stick with us basically forever.

You might remember the childhood friend you played with next-door for a year when you were seven years old more than you remember a college roommate you shared a dorm with for a semester, because you were developing more back then. We aim to teach kids about general topics like math and science during these developmental stages, so hopefully, that information sticks with us. Young minds are more susceptible to change and knowledge, but unfortunately, that also means they are more likely to hold onto trauma.

Childhood Triggers

Identifying your trauma is a crucial part of overcoming your triggers and fighting this battle. When we're able to look back on a specific time in our lives and identify that it might have been the reason, we are a certain way today, it is much easier to understand our reactions and emotions now, as adults.

There are three forms of trauma: complex, chronic, and acute. Acute trauma is from one instance, such as witnessing a death, a car accident, or something else that happened one time. Chronic trauma is more prolonged and will have occurred consistently throughout someone's life. Complex trauma is when multiple traumatic events have caused a person to hold onto a lot of pain. You don't always have to know the differences, but it can be helpful when diagnosing certain mental health disorders with a professional. It is also important to remember that trauma isn't just something that occurs after one scary event. We typically think about traumatic events in the form of acute trauma, such as getting mugged or breaking a bone. It can be much more in depth than that and can spread throughout someone's childhood and into their life.

A huge trauma might be bullying. Bullying makes the victim feel as though they have no value. These people will often start to believe what their bully says and take on the roles they were assigned. Bullying can cause a lot of people to binge eat, especially those who were made fun of for the way that they looked.

Anyone who has experienced disasters, accidents, or medical trauma might find that they struggle to deal with their emotions. If you were exposed to this kind of trauma as a child, it is especially challenging because you didn't understand what it meant, as a kid. As adults, we have trouble wondering why someone might cause others to hurt, or why we live in a world with natural disasters like hurricanes or tornadoes. Being a kid makes it even more challenging to comprehend. As a result, you might start to binge eat as a way to numb the pain you feel, rather than trying to deal with its complexities.

Violence and physical abuse are also very triggering for different individuals. It can make children feel helpless, giving them the sense that they don't have control. As a result, they might start to binge eat because they want to take that control back.

We have to remember that neglect can be very traumatic for children, as well. Any form of abandonment, whether a parent died or a single parent had to work two jobs, can be very traumatic for children. This kind of abuse, as well as mental abuse, will be the most common for those who suffer from a binge eating disorder. We were likely made to feel less than others at one point, destroying our self-esteem. Having someone belittle you makes you question your own thoughts; therefore, it gets hard to trust your instincts.

Racism, sexism, colonization, genocide, and war are all types of historical trauma that can be very triggering, as well. What's most important to remember with trauma is that we will usually carry the emotional intelligence with us that we had at the time of the trauma. For those with serious PTSD issues, they will likely still have a mentality that happened at the time of their trauma because that instance caused them to stop developing. Though it is easy to see as an outsider that abuse might have led to the eating disorder, when you are in the middle of it, you can't get that same perspective.

The Need to Reprogram
If your body has become accustomed to binge eating for years, you will need to reprogram it. Not only will your stomach have physically stretched, but your mind will have, as well. You likely no longer see regular portions as acceptable anymore, and instead think a plate full of food is the only way to go. We were wired to hide our feelings, too. Rather than telling other people we need help and looking for ways to improve our lives and habits, we fall into patterns where we need to keep secrets and feel ashamed for the things we've experienced.

We have to get to the root cause of the problem, so we can prepare for the fight of our lives.

Coping Mechanisms
A coping mechanism is anything that you do in order to alleviate stress. Coping mechanisms present themselves in different ways in all people. Some people will cope by writing music, others will cope by smoking cigarettes. Whatever the problem is, there is usually an unhealthy coping mechanism behind it if the problem is not being properly managed. Emotional eating is a very common and very serious coping mechanism.

Your binging alleviates some of the symptoms of the problem, but it doesn't actually cure what needs to be fixed. There is always a reason that you binge eat. It's obvious that food tastes good and that's why we like to eat it, but binging is more than that. Why can't some individuals just have a slice of cake and not the entire thing? There's a psychological reason, usually trauma, and eating is the way to curtail that emotion. However, after the binge has ended, it is just going to come back. It is providing a feeling, not a function.

It's a coping mechanism that halts the feeling. It doesn't go away. It is like taking Tylenol to fix a brain tumor. You might be able to take a pill to make the pain go away, but the reason that the pain is there won't go away unless you specifically address that.

It will get easier. It gets easier because you can look back on your binges and see why you did that, why it happened. When you know why something is occurring, it is easier to solve it and prevent it from happening again. Next time you have a binge, you can say to yourself, "well I'm just stressed about this thing," and then you'll find a way to alleviate that stress without food — and realize you don't want to binge at all.

Action Step #1

Start by identifying your obvious trauma. This might be the death of a parent, a sickness, or a major accident. Whatever traumatic experience you can come up with from your past, write it down. From each of those experiences, write down other trauma that might be related, and how it affects your thought process. This is going to be the groundwork for your recovery and will form the basis for the thinking patterns you'll need to break.

Chapter 7. Still Life

No book on overeating is complete without including a look at the place of physical activity in our lives. If you have the dieting mindset shared by most Americans, you might assume this is about working off more calories or about more effective health management in general. Those effects do matter, of course, but there is a more fundamental reason why overeaters in particular need to think hard about this:

There is a powerful connection between regular exercise and the ability to maintain focus with food. It's hard to maintain one without the other; if you lose track of one, the other tends to fall away soon after. Deep down, you probably already know this. For that reason, I urge you to read on and consider the information that follows.

The Loss of Movement in Modern Life

It is only recently in American history that most of us have had the ability to choose a sedentary way of life. From 1910 to 2000, the majority of our workforce shifted from brute force work like farming, mining, and manufacturing to professional, technical, clerical, and sales jobs.[1]

It was a sign of progress and improving quality of life that we were able to create work that was easier and safer than much of what had come before, but it did result in the removal of much physical activity from our lives.

We have mirrored this shift in our leisure time as well. Many of us have left behind the more physically oriented hobbies of the past in favor of many hours now spent online. It's hard to know whether we're losing interest in being more physically involved in our lives or whether it is simply a matter of competing interests which are incompatible with being up and moving around.

In any event, most of us now spend our lives sitting, often punctuated only by brief strolls to get to another room or to get to and from our cars. We move some for basic household tasks and errands and that may feel like being busy, but that doesn't usually translate into much actual physical activity; the fact is that we move dramatically less than has any previous generation. It took a great deal of innovation to create a way of life in which it is actually possible to move too little, but as soon as we had that choice, we seized it.

Physical activity has become such an oddity in our lives that we have a special name for it now—"exercise"—and we do it mostly in specially designed places—fitness centers, health clubs and gyms—rather than experiencing it as the natural part of daily life that it always was until the late 20th century. We now have to make a point to think about it, plan for it, and schedule around it, which would have been inconceivable to people from just a couple of generations ago.

Every physical system we have, it seems, operates more effectively when regularly used.[2,3] Your body shows you this when you feel better as a result of having moved around even a little more than usual if you are normally sedentary.

It is very easy in our fast-paced world, however, to overlook how little we move on most days. It is also easy to feel that there is just no time to fit it in anywhere. The price that we pay for these creeps up on us incrementally, causing our quality of life to dwindle without us even noticing it until the losses have become quite pronounced.

The High Price of Low Activity Levels

The most obvious cost of moving too little is that far fewer calories get burned. This is particularly damaging when combined—as it usually is—with the overconsumption of high-calorie foods. The outcome of that particular math is terrible but is barely the beginning of the price we pay for being too still.

Our bodies operate on the use-it-or-lose-it principle.4 The less we move, the harder it becomes to move, for a variety of reasons. Range and ease of motion are compromised as muscles and tendons get tighter and shorter from lack of use. Aerobic condition falls, reducing endurance. Muscles lose condition, reducing both strength and endurance. Coordination and balance degrade due to simple lack of practice, in addition to the normal losses to those systems which occur with aging.5 Immune system function is compromised as the body falls further and further out of condition,6 thus being less able to protect, repair and maintain itself (By the way, isn't it amazing that our bodies can actually fix themselves?!).

You start spending more of your time coping with opportunistic infections, more time getting over them, and more time just feeling "off." Pain levels tend to increase on more sedentary days; this dampens interest in moving, fueling the vicious cycle of escalating and longer-lasting pain.

Options for managing and enjoying life are severely reduced if you are less able to move. There are fewer ways to make life interesting, challenging, and fun. There are fewer ways to share memorable bonding experiences with friends and loved ones. There are fewer ways to blow off steam when you're stressed. There is simply much less of most things that make life worthwhile.

Being sedentary into your 50s and beyond will steal your ability to walk without assistive devices many years sooner than necessary. It can become the factor that determines whether or not you remain independent as you age.

Brain health suffers far more than most people might realize. Physical activity is now recognized as one of the most powerful tools you have for maintaining your brain as you age.

In short, moving too little means a less enjoyable and more stressful life today, and sets the stage for senior years that are unnecessarily limited, painful, and frustrating. This means that you live with a higher baseline stress level at all times which, whether or not you are aware of it, creates a nagging need for emotional relief. That leads, of course, to frequent urges to eat for comfort.

And that is why you need to keep moving if you want any hope of controlling your drive to overeat.

A Dangerous New Syndrome

There is a specific element of moving too little which deserves special mention, and that is the issue of sitting too much.

Unfortunately, you cannot compensate for this additional risk with regular exercise if you spend most of the rest of your time sitting,9 and those who try have even been referred to as "active couch potatoes."10 Every year, millions of people die prematurely due to chronic diseases that were triggered or exacerbated by an overly sedentary way of life. We lose so many people this way that Sedentary Death Syndrome11 is the term often used to describe the cause of such deaths.

Whether or not you ever adopt a consistent pattern of actual exercise, the hazards of sitting too much can be avoided simply by incorporating more general movement into the rest of your day. Get up often, stand when you can, walk when you can, stretch when you can, and create opportunities for these simple acts all day long. Seldom in life will you encounter a problem so serious that is so easy to solve.

Scientific research and new buzzwords aside, we probably all have life experience that shows us we feel better when we are more active than we do when we are more sedentary. In the end, that is all the information you really need.

Living Longer, Aging Faster

Longevity statistics might not feel like the most fascinating topic in the world, but they provide an important perspective at this point in our story. Lifespan here in the US, for example, has increased steadily throughout our history.1

We've gotten this far by stabilizing the availability of food and clean water, improving general sanitation, vaccinating against infectious disease, smoking less, and developing a variety of medical advances that have extended and improved quality of life.2 Today's longevity is a product of changes and innovations from the past, slowly rippling their way forward through time.

What we do today then, will ripple forward through time to create the longevity experienced by our descendants. It can be tempting to think that we will always live longer and things will always get better no matter what simply because in our lifetimes, that's been true.

The recent spike in obesity rates,3 however, is now reversing many of the health gains we previously worked so hard to achieve. It is obesity and its medical consequences that threaten the lifespan of today's children,4 along with degrading the general health in most other age groups compared to just 15 years ago.5 We are now in the novel position of witnessing the first large-scale reversal of public health in our history.

Our population has begun to experience accelerated aging even as our longevity—for now—continues to rise. We see increasing incidence of disability in younger and younger adults,6 which means that while we're gaining years of life, we're simultaneously losing healthy years. The costs in terms of reduced quality of life and increasing medical expense promise to be staggering for most of us now in adulthood, but what about our kids?

We see children developing diseases previously known only in adults: conditions like cardiovascular disease, type 2 diabetes, bone and joint problems, sleep apnea, fatty liver disease, and depression.7,8

We are in uncharted territory as pediatricians scramble to become more conversant in medical issues they weren't supposed to see, and we begin to find out the hard way what it means for human beings to be treated for these conditions beginning in childhood rather than in middle or older age.

How does it affect us to take the necessary medications for these conditions decades longer than was ever intended or studied? What happens when we use adult medications on children during crucial times in their development?

We don't know, but we are forced to try it and see how it plays out over time. However grim the eventual disability risk for today's adults, it is considerably worse for today's children. It can't turn out well when you're saddled with coronary artery disease or type 2 diabetes before you've finished high school, for example, and we now have lots of kids on exactly that trajectory.

This is clearly not a position we want to be in. Nobody meant for it to turn out this way, yet here we are.

While our current way of life sets the stage for this mess, few of us (with the noteworthy exception of children) are forced to choose it. Most of us have access to better food than we usually eat and more activity than we usually pursue. Most of us have the personal experience to know that we feel better when we make higher quality choices for ourselves, yet we don't make them with much consistency.

On the surface, this makes no sense at all. That just means that the surface is not the right place to search for an explanation.

Chapter 8. Difference between Emotional and Physical Hunger

You need to learn to differentiate between emotional hunger and physical hunger. Emotional hunger can often be so powerful that you easily mistake it for actual physical hunger. You have to become more conscious about identifying it and not indulging in emotional hunger.

• Physical hunger usually comes on slowly and is not so noticeable unless you haven't eaten for quite some time. You don't feel the need to urgently eat when you are physically hungry but just become aware that your body needs food.

• Emotional hunger has a very sudden onset and works like a craving. You feel an urgent need to satisfy it. It's not related to the body actually needing food.

• Physical hunger can be satisfied with any form of food. Your body will be satiated with anything from vegetables to meat.

• Emotional hunger is sated only with specific kinds of food. These are the comfort foods we reach for when we feel down. Only junk food that gives you a rush—usually in the form of sugary food or junk like pizza—will satisfy emotional hunger.

• When you eat from physical hunger, you are more aware of the food. Your stomach will feel satisfied once you eat enough.

• Emotional eating is quite mindless, and you just keep eating without being conscious of it. You don't feel satiated for a long time, and you stop only when you have filled yourself with food from your stomach up to your throat.

• Physical hunger is felt from your belly. Your stomach growls or hurts if you haven't eaten for too long. This subsides once you eat a meal.

• Emotional hunger is not related to the stomach but to the mind. This hunger arises in the form of thoughts and cravings where your focus is on your comfort foods.

• When your body is physically hungry, you feel good and satisfied after a proper meal. You don't think about it later.

Emotional hunger gives you momentary satisfaction when you indulge it, but later you feel guilty and ashamed. This is because you know that you didn't eat because your body needed it and that it's actually bad for you to eat that way.

All of these are some basic ways to differentiate between when you are physically hungry and when you are emotionally hungry. Your body only needs food when you are physically hungry. Overindulging in emotional hunger can be detrimental to your physical and mental health. Start to be more conscious of identifying what type of hunger you experience and eating only when you need to. Physical hunger will be satisfied with some food. Food will satisfy emotional hunger temporarily, but the feelings and problems will still remain and make you feel worse later.

Chapter 9. The Cycle of Emotional Eating

Many times, you will notice that food cravings are at their strongest when you're emotionally weak. When you're stressed, bored, or facing some difficult problem, you tend to turn toward food as a source of comfort. This emotional dependency can sabotage your efforts to lose weight and also prevent you from actually solving the real issue at hand. Emotional eating is a maladaptive way to cope with negative emotions like stress, boredom, and fear. Many events in your daily life—conflicts in your relationships, excessive workload, financial problems, health issues—can easily trigger this unhealthy craving for food. There are some people for whom such issues curb their appetite so that they lose a lot of weight, but others turn toward food to deal with emotional distress.

Over time, your emotions become tightly tied up with your food. Every time you feel sad or angry, you automatically reach for comfort food to make yourself feel better. This food just serves as a distraction and does not solve any problems. Instead of dealing with painful situations, we turn our focus to the food and avoid dealing with what is actually important. When someone we know goes through a breakup, we might encourage them to go ahead and eat that tub of ice cream, even though we know it's completely unhealthy. The same thing is repeated over and over again—every time something upsetting happens, you turn toward food.

Regardless of the trigger, the end result of overeating will always be the same. You are harming your body, gaining extra weight, and not solving your real problems. In fact, the guilt of this emotional overeating just adds to the burden. All this leads to an unhealthy cycle of a trigger making you eat too much, feeling guilty over it, and feeling bad again. The negative emotions are temporarily suppressed, but they arise again. It is important to break out of this cycle and get back on track.

Here's how you can start keeping track of your eating habits:

- Start paying attention to and differentiating between physical and emotional hunger. If you just had lunch or dinner, your cravings are not from physical hunger. Drink some water and focus on something else when you get such cravings.

- Start practicing ways to deal with your stress in a healthy way. Many people recommend yoga or meditation as an effective way to manage stress.

- Reach out for support in your journey. Find people to share your feelings with who will support and encourage you through it.

- Don't allow yourself to get bored. Find a way to occupy yourself when you have nothing to do. Don't lie in front of the TV and reach for a ton of junk food. Take a walk or play with your pets to occupy yourself if there is nothing to do. Mindless snacking can develop into a very unhealthy habit.

- Get rid of all the excess junk food in your house. Having it around will just tempt you to reach out for it every time something triggers your emotional eating habit. You are less likely to indulge in it if you have to make a trip to the grocery store for it. By the time you get there, your craving will probably have subsided.

- Just because you are starting a healthier diet does not mean you have to deprive yourself of all the food you like. Most fad diets fail because they deprive you of all the food you like to eat. Eat more healthy foods but allow yourself to enjoy some occasional treats.

Don't stick to the same treat but instead add some variety so that you don't start making associations with that food again.

- Start snacking in a healthier way. Mindless snacking is one of the fastest ways to gain extra weight. Keep some healthier snack options available so that if you suddenly feel hungry, you have something to munch on. Keep some cut fruit in the fridge or have a handful of nuts. These are much better options than eating a whole box of cookies or a bag of chips.

- Forgive yourself for any setbacks. Just because you could not control yourself that one time does not mean you can't the next day. Think about what made you fall off the wagon and try to deal with it better the next time. One bad day does not make everything fail for you. Just stay focused and keep trying to reduce the number of bad days. You can only improve if you learn from your bad experiences. Don't give up and fall back on binge eating to deal with the stress. This will only make all your efforts futile.

All these are small and simple steps you can take to deal with your emotional eating. If these fail, you can try a more intensive method or consult professionals for guidance and treatment. There is more on this later.

Chapter 10. Listen to Your Body and Trust Its Language

Begin by learning to trust your body. Once you do this, you are not going to schedule a 2,000-calorie meal at 1pm when that could be all you needed for an entire day. In fact, you may not even need to eat anything at that hour. Probably hunger will have struck at noon and you satisfied it with a 500 calorie healthy snack. Or maybe you will feel hungry much later than the scheduled 1pm.

Another thing is to allow yourself to enjoy what you are eating. Even if you do not like the fact that you are 70kg or more, if you decide to eat, please do let yourself enjoy what you are eating. And you register enjoyment by concentrating on the food. And because your mind is set on the eating and how you are feeling, you will easily tell when the hunger is gone. That point is where you let go. The minute you cease to enjoy eating, avoid pushing an extra mile because soon you will begin speaking ill of either the food or yourself.

What we have just recommended is an attunement of your food, your mind and your body. That way you will be able to tell the foods whose taste and smell you like and enjoy, your mind will tell you when there are issues you need to sort out outside of eating, and your body will tell you when you need to feed it and when you need to stop loading it with food it does not require.

At the end of the day, you will be a happy person, and your health will stabilize at a nice place without you even thinking about it. And by happy place we mean you will neither feel sluggish from too much sugar, nor too heavy for your bone structure to carry around. You will also not have your heart beating too fast from strain of too much bad fat and salt, your skin will glow, and you will generally feel good about yourself.

This is what we are suggesting you do:

Allow yourself to eat when you are hungry regardless of the hour.

Allow yourself to eat what you are longing for without invoking feelings of guilt.

Pay attention to your hunger as well as satiety level to determine when to stop eating; or simply how much to eat.

Once you follow these tips, you will be able to build a great relationship between your body, your choice of food, and the amount of it. What you are seeking to develop, essentially, is mindful eating. Soon, you will develop an eating environment where you are no longer in doubt about whether to eat or not. The answer will be so clear because you know you need to eat when you can truly savor the food; and you can only do that when your body needs it – when you are truly hungry; not very hungry, mark you, but sincerely hungry.

How to create a favorable eating environment
1)   Slow down your eating pace

Experts say there is a delay of around 20 minutes between the time you put your food in the mouth and literally swallow it, and the time your body registers it has actually been fed. So if you are a fast eater, you run the risk of eating too much and getting uncomfortable later. And within that time two unfavorable things will have happened.

You will not have savored the flavor of your food, because when you eat quickly it is like you are trying to get rid of your food as opposed to taking your body through an enjoyable session.

You will, very likely, have loaded your body with calories it does not require; calories it may have to look for ways of storing.

2)   Try to learn your signs of hunger and satiety

We keep hearing that each person is unique and that is true, but we often think this ends with abilities and talents; but it does not. You are unique in how your body communicates to you, and that is what you need to heed. As you continue settling into the habit of being present as you eat, you will notice those cues and soon deciding how much to eat will no longer be ambiguous.

You will find yourself eating in response to hunger – genuine hunger – and not to your cry for emotional nourishment. In short, eating makes you healthy when you consistently eat solely to satisfy your physical need. The more you think about what we have said about intuitive eating, the more you will realize how much sense it makes.

Think about it – are there not counselors to deal with emotional deficiencies, and religious leaders for spiritual nourishment? Yet they will not purport to regulate your feeding. That is all up to you, because only you can read your body in an accurate way and satisfy your physical need. How many times have traditional grandmothers insisted to their grown children that they should eat more only because their bodies did not seem to have a lot of muscle, yet those were quite healthy people?

On the flip side, how many times have figure-conscious people remarked that one needs to cut down on eating, even when the person in question was in tip-top shape, BMI and all? In short, the responsibility of feeding your body with the ideal portions and the right type of food lies with you. You just need to listen to its language, the one only you can comprehend.

3)   Eat the right portion size each time

Which is the right portion size? Well, it is the one your body demands as opposed to the one you think you should give it. If all your senses are alive to your needs, you will pick up the relevant cues from your body, primarily your taste buds and your tummy.

4)   Avoid distractions as much as you can when you are eating.

That is linked to the strong suggestion that you be always present when you are eating. With distractions, you tend to put food into your mouth and chew in a kind of routine, not particularly coordinating your senses. If it is the TV you are concentrating on, you will more alive to the sense of sight and imagination than those of your tummy saying it has had enough, and your taste buds saying they have had too much of the flavor.

Remember it is true there is such a thing as too much of a good thing. Even if food tasted nice when you began to eat, if you eat too much, it is not only your body that will register complaints; your taste buds also will.

<u>5)   Savor your food</u>

By that is meant you have allowed all your senses to focus on your food and the eating process. So, you can tell how the food looks, how it smells, how it tastes, and even how it feels in your mouth and subsequently in the stomach.

If all those senses together agree you need to continue eating, then you will be doing the right thing. If one or two begin questioning the reason for your eating, you probably should halt and confirm if you actually are not really full. This point emphasizes the assertion already made in this book that you need to ensure you are eating in an enjoyable environment – when everything about you says it is good you are giving your body this food.

Chapter 11. Overcoming ignorance and offering hope

Real knowledge is to know the extent of one's ignorance.

Confucius

- Help for sufferers and careers

- I have worked with clients who have suffered with problematic eating for over twenty years, and in the past fourteen years I have been intimately involved with this issue in my current role as a clinical supervisor and trainer for a charity known as Eating Disorders Support.

This charity provides a daily telephone and email helpline, along with the facilitation of fortnightly self-help groups for sufferers, careers or those from any walk of life who wish to learn more about the experiences of those who live with problematic eating. Working with this charity has made me painfully aware of the lack of help available for many sufferers of problem eating. We are frequently contacted by people from all over the world who sadly are unable to get the support they need from their own continent. In reality there is often a serious dearth of support for sufferers of eating distress.

But as well as treating sufferers of problem eating, I frequently work with the parents, partners, colleagues, friends and adult children of sufferers. They, like the sufferer, need support, since the emotional demands placed upon them can be very intense. They often feel that they can't do right for doing wrong when trying to offer help to the sufferer. Many family members describe the household dynamics when living with someone with problem eating as being like permanently walking on eggshells.

Friends and family can be terrified that they might make matters worse by commenting on changed behaviours, such as excessive exercising or the refusal to eat various food groups. The mere mention of weight loss or gain can lead to tears and tantrums. Mealtimes can become a dreaded battleground causing distress and anxiety for the entire family.

Being in a family with someone suffering from problem eating, particularly if you are the primary carer, can be a lonely journey, fraught with frustration, despair and isolation. Sometimes you might feel that there is a glimmer of light at the end of the tunnel, only to have your hopes cruelly dashed by a relapse.

In many cases, problem eating can become the focal point of the entire family's existence, causing their regular social life to dwindle as it becomes difficult to invite people to the home. Holidays may be put on hold, food and menus dominate, arguments become a regular occurrence and family members feel permanently tense and bullied.

Problem eating doesn't just affect the sufferer. Relatives, partners and friends all suffer too, but they can also offer valuable support when it comes to recovery.

- A need for increased awareness

- It still shocks me to discover that many members of the public who have not been personally touched by an eating disorder perceive these mental health illnesses in a pejorative and highly inaccurate fashion.

I have frequently heard eating disorders being described as: voluntary lifestyle choices, evidence of a greedy disposition, manifestations of vanity, proof of lack of self-control and attention-seeking. All of these beliefs woefully miss the mark and undermine the seriousness of these dangerous conditions.

People suffering from an eating disorder have a serious mental illness and are deserving of the same level of respect, support and attention as someone seeking help for a physical condition. If you think you might have a problem, you deserve and need help in the same way you would if you were injured or physically ill.

- A need for a culture change

- The ignorance and misunderstanding surrounding eating problems is further compounded by the fact, in my sad and frustrating experience, that a considerable proportion of the medical profession does not possess a solid grasp of the aetiology, process or treatment of problematic eating. Problematic eating has long been the poor relation within the mental health field, perceived by many as self-inflicted.

Obviously there are many good doctors out there, and I don't want to put you off seeking medical help, but it is shocking that this dismissive attitude persists, especially since there is compelling scientific evidence that genetics plays a significant role in eating disorders. For example, there is a 55 per cent concordance of anorexia in identical twins compared to a 5 per cent concordance in fraternal twins.

Brian Lask, President of the Eating Disorders Research Society, has discovered a very interesting phenomenon, which sheds light on the theory that some people have a genetic predisposition to develop an eating disorder.

When someone starves themself, all major organs in the body shrink, including the brain. By using neuro-imagery, Lask discovered that once a healthy body weight has been restored, everything goes back to normal except one crucial area of the brain: the insula. The insula plays a key role in how we perceive taste, control anxiety, maintain an accurate body image, receive hunger and satiety cues and sense pain.

A dysfunctional insula explains why a severely emaciated person can feel that they are hugely fat when clearly they are not. It also explains how a malnourished person can push themself to exercise, despite physical injuries, since their pain tolerance threshold has shot through the roof.

This neurological research casts light on why some people who diet develop an eating disorder while others do not. Whether it is because someone is born with a faulty insula, or whether extreme starvation causes permanent damage to this essential part of the brain, remains to be decided. Whichever of the two hypotheses is correct, it clearly demonstrates the perniciousness of starvation diets.

To my absolute horror, I recently heard the following statement on a morning TV programme from a GP who was responding to a caller who had enquired if an eating disorder would remain on her medical record. He replied:

Yes, it will be in your medical records; it's on your medical history forever. It will be there as a black mark, as a stigma … it shouldn't be but it is.

This thoughtless comment would, I'm sure, have undermined the likelihood of this caller seeking help and would have deterred many sufferers from coming forward for help rather than risk being stigmatized.

- Be determined and persistent when seeking help

- In fairness to GPs, one should not expect them to be specialists in every field. However, even though it is accepted practice, I think it's awful that in the case of eating disorders patients are told that they need to become sicker before they will be entitled to treatment. If you were worried you were an alcoholic, you wouldn't expect your doctor to tell you to come back when your liver was sufficiently damaged.

That's why early diagnosis of problem eating is key – the longer the unhealthy eating habits prevail, the harder it is to dislodge them, and the more damage is done.

The mortality rate from eating disorders is the highest of all mental illnesses. This is partly due to physical reasons such as heart failure, malnutrition or other organ failure. However, a huge proportion of deaths are due to suicide. Early intervention is absolutely crucial.

It is my belief that the younger generation of doctors and other medical professionals is much more aware of how eating disorders can ravage lives. This is due to many of them having experienced the damage caused by these disorders first-hand, within their own friendship circles or among fellow classmates at school, college and university.

However, there are still a number of dinosaurs out there. If you do not get the response you need, do not give up. I suggest that you make another appointment immediately, but this time take someone with you for moral support or to act as an advocate in expressing your right to have timely and effective help.

If you're worried about your eating habits, have you ever spoken to your doctor about it? If not, book an appointment now. You might be pleasantly surprised by the outcome.

- Message of hope

- I know this all sounds a bit doom-and-gloom, but one of the most important things I want you to take away from this book is that problematic eating – from inconsequential pregnancy cravings to acknowledged serious mental health disorders such as binge eating disorder or anorexia – can be overcome.

However, people with long-standing and deeply entrenched eating disorders can still make a full recovery, providing they are given the appropriate treatment.

Sufferers can move on to lead full, healthy, joyous lives, freed from the enslaving shackles of the eating disorder's tyranny. For many, the reign of an eating disorder can be terminated permanently, although some practitioners would have you believe otherwise.

I have often heard people claim that there is no total cure to an eating disorder and sufferers remain susceptible for the rest of their life. It is a similar philosophy to the expression 'once an alcoholic, always an alcoholic'. However, Janet Treasure, a professor of psychiatry at Guys, King's & St Thomas Medical School in London, recently stated that eating disorders 'can be completely cured, especially if they are treated during the first three years'.

Each sufferer is unique, and while one treatment might work well for one person, it may prove to be unsuitable for another. In fact, I am aware of many cases where people have needed a range of professional treatments before achieving recovery. In other cases people have overcome their problem eating without professional help and have achieved recovery through self-help books, coupled with the support of family and friends.

Problem eating in the 21st century

• Today, there is no doubt that the number of people experiencing problem eating has escalated enormously, which is both alarming and disheartening. However, on the positive side, the number of sufferers who are now openly admitting to having experienced an eating disorder is on the increase too.

Suffering from problem eating can be extremely isolating, since many people feel embarrassed about sharing their habits and behaviours with others. To know that you are not alone is very empowering, particularly for younger people who worry more about being different from their peers.

A gradual cultural change is happening and rather than denying that mental health issues such as eating disorders exist, people are coming forward and sharing their experiences. This openness helps to educate the general public to be vigilant in recognizing the symptoms, and encourages them to take action at the earliest stage to get help.

• Don't wait until tomorrow; take action *now*

• If you are suffering from eating distress, I strongly urge you to take the necessary steps to address the problem now, in order for you to start living your life with you at the helm. This might mean confiding in a friend, picking up the phone to call a helpline or making an appointment to see your GP.

Taking these first steps to seek help takes courage, but the rewards in doing so are quite spectacular. Having conquered an eating disorder, survivors are confident in the knowledge that they possess the resources to overcome whatever challenges life may throw at them.

Chapter 12. Identifying Binge Eating Disorder in Adolescents or Children

In Western society, childhood obesity is on the rise and binge eating is becoming more prevalent for our youth and adolescents. A combination of factors leads to the problem, including stress, inactivity, and poor food choices in the home. The result is disastrous as children consume alarming quantities of food on a regular basis. A vicious cycle begins as weight creeps up, self esteem goes down, and young people continue to turn to food for comfort.

Symptoms of Binge Eating

In most cases of binge eating, parents are not even aware of the problem. Victims of this eating disorder tend to go on eating sprees in private, hidden from the prying eyes of others. It might happen on the walk home from school, when Mom and Dad are still at work, or after everyone goes to bed. Children and adolescents who have begun binge eating may feel like they have no control over their actions. They often are embarrassed by the cravings that force them to eat large amounts at one sitting. Bouts of binge eating may take place more than once a day. They can be in response to stress, problems at school, bullying or peer pressure. Family members may be at a loss, seeing a child gain weight with no explanation of how it's happened.

Who is Most at Risk?

Binge eating often strikes during the teen years when young adults confront body image issues and go through many changes. It's a point when life seems out of control. Many children turn to food, consuming large amounts in a short period of time to the point of feeling ill from overeating. Individuals who have difficulty dealing with stress or their emotions are likely to fall prey to an eating disorder as well.

What's the Answer?

Parents need to pay attention to their children. If they see any signs of binge eating, it's time to seek professional help. A doctor can provide guidance and may point families to counseling as well. It will take a concerted effort of all family members to deal with the problem. A teamwork approach works best as everyone becomes a support system for children who have a binge eating disorder. Encourage children to talk about problems, rather than bury them in food.

Make Lifestyle Changes

Families should make changes at home to assist a child in overcoming binge eating. Stock the fridge and cupboards with healthy options. Limit the time spent on the television and video games. Get involved in active pastimes as a family. Everyone can get out on their bicycles or start a game of backyard football. Go on outings together and help children to stay active. If young people are occupied, they are less likely to get into trouble of any sort, including binge eating. Eating disorders can be conquered when families work together.

Chapter 13. How to Approach Your Child or Teen who has a Binge Eating Disorder

If you suspect that your child or teen has a problem with an eating binge disorder, approaching him or her will be sensitive. The child or teen will have a multitude of guilty and shameful feelings associated with the disorder. Therefore, any attempts to bombard him or her will cause an immediate shut down. Persuading a young person to open up about an imperfection such as an eating disorder requires quite a bit of patience and resilience. The following are some tips that can help you to approach your child about binge eating:

Open the Lines of Communication

The first step in speaking to a child about binge eating is opening the lines of communication. It may be wise to avoid letting the child know about the subject of the conversation until later. Wait for a moment that the child is not involved in school activities, work or any other activity that distracts the thought processes, and then ask for a moment of his or her time. Wearing a smile and having a calm tone is helpful, because it sets up the foundation of trust. A welcoming look tells a child that you are not angry or disappointed in him or her.

Tell a Story

The best way to approach a problem that may make another person feel low about him or herself is to align with that person. Think about a story that you can tell the teen or child about a time when you were not perfect. The story could include something that you did that was against the rules or something that you tried to do that did not work. Explain how you overcame such trials and tribulations. Using this tactic, you may be able to lead the child into coming forward about the binge eating.

Reassure the Child of Your Affection and Support

At this point, you have hopefully convinced the child to come forth about the binge eating. The next step after you opens the lines of communication about the subject is reassuring him or her. Let your child know that you will stand by him or her no matter what crisis he or she may be facing. Tell the child that you will stand behind him or her during the journey to come back to emotional and physical health. Begin to present the idea of entering a rehabilitation facility or signing on with a support group.

Handle the Outcome

Even with the right tools and the right attitude, some attempts to speak to a person about binge eating may not work. The key is to keep the lines of communication open and reiterate that you will always be there for your child. True recovery will not occur until the person is ready to change. This may involve getting professional help for your child, as well as family therapy. Binge eating can sometimes stem out of family problems, so as a parent, you may need to be willing to change yourself as well. However, you can increase health within your family by coaching, nurturing and continuing to fortify your child's self-confidence and esteem. Binge eating is not an easy subject to approach, but with enough patience and compassion, anyone can be successful in clearing the path to healing.

Chapter 14. What are the Ramifications of Emotional Eating?

We all have different reasons why we've decided it's time to stop binge eating. A big reason for many people to decide there's a problem is because they are gaining weight. Many people with faster metabolisms or purging problems might not be as ready to admit there's an issue. When everything looks fine on the outside, we start to feel like we don't need to admit that something is really wrong on the inside.

Your size, weight, or shape doesn't matter. What matters is how you eat, and how you cope with stress. If you're a size 22 and you binge and purge, that's just as bad as being a size 0 that only binges. We have to remember, throughout our recovery, to separate our bodies from our disorder. You might have gained or lost weight as a result of your unhealthy eating habits, but right now, whatever size you are, don't let it affect your recovery.

Should overeating persist, there are a lot of long-term problems that can end up coming along.

Health Problems of Binge Eaters

Binge eating is going to have many potential long-term effects on your body. First and foremost, we have to remember that it is what we do as a result of our binge eating that can alter our health, too.

Mentally, when binge eating isn't managed, it will lead to more serious health issues down the line, such as anxiety and depression. Ignoring your issues and suppressing them with food is only going to make them more dangerous later on. You might end up suffering from chronic anxiety and consistent panic attacks because of an inability to manage stress. Depression can come from endless cycles of unhealthy behavior, and when that's not managed, it can lead to self-harm and even suicide.

If you choose to purge yourself of your food, it can cause you to become bulimic, which has its own serious health issues. Being bulimic will cause most of your organs to suffer because they are being deprived of the basic nutrients they need to function. You will also end up having health issues with your throat and intestines because you are causing them to undergo activities that they shouldn't, such as constant throwing up or having to poop too often from laxatives.

If you do not purge yourself and begin to gain weight, it could lead to more serious health issues should you become obese. High cholesterol, type 2 diabetes, gallbladder disease, cancer, sleep apnea, and overall aches and pains are common. Being overweight isn't necessarily unhealthy. Though we see plus size people as unhealthy, that's just a result of our society. When you are obese, however, and weight a lot more than your body intended for you to, then it can lead to more serious issues. The extra weight will put stress on your bones and muscles, and your heart will have trouble functioning properly, as well.

Diet Mentality

A big reason that we got into these unhealthy patterns in the first place is the diet mentality many young girls have. How many times a week, or even per day, do you hear someone reference a diet, or needing to go on a diet? At any given time, you can go to any store and see a magazine with a cover about how to lose weight, usually more than one. I suffered from having a mom who was diet-obsessed, as well.

Luckily, she didn't tell me that I needed to go on diets often or tell me I needed to lose weight. Still, she would often discuss how she needed to diet, making me think that was the only way to be healthy. She would often try out new diets, and we always had at least one of those women's lifestyle health magazines laying around with a before and after picture on the cover. Dieting is, more often than not, unhealthy because of how we look at diets and our relationships with them.

Know the difference between eating healthy and dieting. When I'm talking about dieting, I'm referring to people thinking they can only have one meal a day, or those who will only drink smoothies in place of eating an actual meal. It's important that we don't overeat, and that we avoid sugary foods as much as possible. Many people I know who talk about dieting, however, usually discuss a point of starvation, or at least depriving their body of something they actually want.

We should all strive to eat healthy. Diet mentality is toxic because people get this idea that you can go on a diet of nothing but cabbage soup, and the next week, go back to eating Taco Bell for dinner every night. That's where the toxic mentality forms. Sometimes, you might want to reduce your weight or train your body to build muscle, and yeah, you will have to go on a diet and alter the food you eat. However, this is something that should be done with a professional or a trainer, to ensure that you aren't crash dieting or putting yourself through something unhealthy.

Eating healthy means avoiding foods that are high in fats, carbs, and empty calories. What's more important than dieting is getting to a place where you eat whole foods, more veggie-based foods, and meals that supply you with all the nutrients and minerals you need. This is a lifestyle, not a diet, and that's what we should all try and achieve.

Giving yourself the foods that you still want is going to be very important. Moderation is key. You can have cookies, but you have to make sure that you're not eating the entire bag in one sitting. You can eat fast food, but it should be once a month or less, not every other day. If you can get to a point where you can have three healthy meals a day and maybe one "bad" snack, that's a good pattern. When you can do that, you'll find you never need to diet again.

Diet culture is out of control. You'll see "nothing ever worked for me," or "the diet that finally sticks." Eating healthy and living a lifestyle with an emphasis on food that's good for you — this is what finally works. Because it is not about the food. It's your mentality.

Feeling Like a Failure

For a person who feels like they often need to diet, they might find that they are consistently setting themselves up for failure. I would do this to myself all the time. Like I said on Monday was my diet day. This is when I would wake up and say, "Now I'm going to diet. I'm never going to eat a Whopper Jr. again and am instead going to only eat salad." That kind of thinking got me stressed out!

I had an "all or nothing" mentality with food. I thought I needed to quit junk food cold turkey and eat only healthy food. Then, when I would go back to my old ways and eat junk, I thought that I had already failed, so it didn't matter what I did next, and I would simply eat as much food as I wanted because I had given up. I felt like a failure when I couldn't diet, so I would eat more. Then, I would gain weight and once again feel like I needed to diet — it was an endless cycle that left me exhausted.

Then I started to realize the benefits of eating healthy beyond just losing weight. No longer did I worry about eating healthy to lose weight, as I realized I needed to do so just so I would physically feel better. I had crash dieted in the past, and I would lose 20 or so pounds, until I could fit into something I thought I had to give away. Though I thought I looked good, I felt miserable. I was still unhappy and not managing my anxiety, and I was also depriving myself of food that I loved!

Once I started to dedicate my life toward a healthy lifestyle, I lost weight without even realizing. It wasn't just that, either. My skin was clearer and more radiant. My hair was healthier and grew longer, faster. I woke up early and wasn't exhausted after a few full sleep cycles. I could walk up three flights of stairs without running out of breath, and even when I was still overweight, my self-esteem was incredibly high — something I thought would only be possible if I were a size 2. My body ached less throughout the day, and I had levels of energy I thought I had abandoned in my childhood. I was feeling better than ever, and most importantly, my anxiety and depression were reducing.

I still eat bad sometimes. I'll go out to dinner with friends and get a meal that's made up of only fried food. I'll order a pizza on a night I don't feel like cooking, and I'll go through a drive-thru when I'm short on time. The difference between then and now, however, is that these are special occasions, not my way of life. When I order a pizza for myself, I can get a small and eat a few slices rather than having to get a large and eat it all by myself. It's not about the food for me, it's about what I choose to do with that food.

Action Step #2

Identify how emotional eating has affected your body. Have you gained weight? Do you purge to the point where you're underweight?

Identify how emotional eating has affected your mental health. Do you feel more anxious having to keep this secret? Has hating your body caused depression?

Identify how emotional eating has affected your personal life. Are there people you shut out because they tried to help? Do you keep toxic relationships around because they support bad habits?

Identifying this should give you more insight into how emotional eating plays into building your identity.

Chapter 15. Free from the Gluten-free

In 2011, the tennis player Novak Djokovic revealed that he was following a gluten-free diet and a great part of his numerous successes was due to that diet. A year later, Miley Cyrus also declared in the social networks that she was suffering from gluten intolerance. And if you type the word "gluten" in Google Trends, you will see that, accidentally or not, the term has increased its popularity and the peak of its web search there was exactly in that year.

Of course, the term "gluten" has been known for many years before that, but you can see how something which is relatively unknown to society could become vastly popular just because of a few famous people mentioning about it – especially if it's put in an unfavorable light. Logically, the bad name of gluten led to the reveal of much more information (and, of course, misinformation) about it – in particular, it was the main topic of many culinary and health shows, a lot of cooking books with gluten-free recipes were published, many documentary movies were shot, and magazines and social networks helped a lot in spreading its bad fame, as well.

Actually, let me clarify something really important here – for some people gluten could be extremely dangerous indeed! Following a gluten-free diet is not only strongly recommended to those people, but in most cases – it's absolutely mandatory. The reason for that is the insidious autoimmune disorder called celiac disease. In short, it primarily affects the small intestines mucosa and has catch-all health consequences. Usually, some of the first symptoms are noticed in early childhood and include abdominal bloating and long-lasting constipation (or the vice versa – diarrhea). Many people who suffer from the disease have those basic symptoms for a long period of time and at some point, they could be followed by new ones – anemia, chronic fatigue, malabsorption syndrome, lack of concentration, often mood changes, depression, aphthae and so many more.

Unfortunately, there is still no cure for celiac disease – following a strict gluten-free diet for a lifetime could secure a normal lifestyle but only if the possible health damages aren't at a progressive stage. In case the individual has any concerns, immediate doctor's assistance should be sought – blood test for anti-gliadin and anti-endomysial antibodies is taken to aid the diagnosis. If these antibodies are found in the blood sample of the person, then most probably we're talking about celiac disease. A very common doctors' mistake is to advise the patients to go directly on a gluten-free diet, even before having the results from the blood test in – that is inappropriate as the antibodies will quickly disappear and the diseased wouldn't be diagnosed correctly – very often the results would show incorrect data for good health. Of course, the diagnosis isn't easy to be made – additional secondary care, an endoscopy test, and extended medical tests are required in order to confirm it.

Another thing to point out is that a lot of people don't suffer from celiac disease but they're still sensitive to gluten in some form. Advising those people to stop gluten is not necessary but it's considered highly recommended.

The positive effects of the gluten-free diet on many people is not a myth – it's indeed the basis of quality life for a considerable part of the world population. The real problem, however, is the too much overexposure of the issue and looking at it in a single point of view only, with lack of facts and numbers. Now, do we all need to throw away pasta from our kitchen? Should we stop eating bread once and for all? What about cakes? Biscuits?

Pizza? And beer? Banned forever! And what are the odds to have celiac disease? All about that is coming next.

But before that, let's just briefly review what gluten is – basically, it 's a composite of proteins found in foods made of wheat and similar crops - barley, oats, rye and etc. All wheat cultures contain gluten. An interesting fact is that this substance is responsible for the elastic texture of the dough and helps it keep its shape while rising.

And after we've clarified what the problems of gluten consumption might cause us and what is the gluten itself, let's review some facts and statistics now.

First of all – what is the percentage of people who suffer from celiac disease? Truth is that it's not precisely known but the figures vary between 0.5 and 1% of the world population. Let's repeat – it's less than 1%! Of course, we are talking about dozens of millions worldwide, but still – the chances that we could be just fine are so much greater. Talking in numbers, an estimated 1 in every 133 Americans has celiac disease which means that no more than 2-3 million Americans suffer from that illness. The figures date back from the end of 2016, so we could suspect that there is no significant difference in them as of now.

Fine, people who suffer from celiac disease are not a lot at all (again, when we consider the total percentage rather than talking in numbers only), but we did mention about those who aren't ill but still suffer from similar symptoms and have gluten sensitivity, correct? Interestingly, most scientific resources report that between 5 and 9% of the world population has some kind of form and degree of gluten sensitivity. You'd say this is a way too higher percentage, right? But honestly, these percentages could be considered very inflated as in most of the studies the volunteers that had participated, reported too common health problems which could but also could not have their roots in the gluten intake – most of the examined volunteers had headache, constipation, diarrhea, bloating, joint pain, fatigue – all of those are indeed too common symptoms, aren't they? That's why it's completely possible the real percentage to be around or even below 5%.

So, what's the conclusion? We read or hear about how unhealthy gluten is and decide to go on a gluten-free diet and we give up a dozen of foods which we have always liked… But now it turns out that there is no need to do that at all – at least not in about 95% of us. We wrongly believe that when we stop gluten, we would have a healthier menu and we would manage to fight those extra kilos, but we don't realize that the quality of our diet is not determined by its presence or the lack of it. I have met so many people who tried to convince me that once they had stopped bread and pasta, they immediately felt better, refreshed and toned and quickly lost some kilos – well, that's completely normal and expected – it's natural to feel an improvement in your health when you give up high-calorie foods that lack micronutrients and replace them with fruits and vegetables that are so rich in them. So, is gluten the real culprit in that example or the causal relationship which was misinterpreted yet again?

Even though the fact that the percentage of people who have been diagnosed with any gluten problems is proven low, there are still nutritionists who fiercely defend the gluten-free diet. One of their most common arguments is that in Asia the gluten-rich food products aren't that popular and people there eat a lot of rice and whole unprocessed foods and live long years in good health. But think about it – food products that have gluten are typically rich in calories and relatively poor in vitamins and minerals. And what could be the outcome if you consume vegetables and fruits instead of bread and pasta? Better health, of course. It seems easy on paper – eat more whole foods and quit those containing gluten.

But in reality, in order to follow the true gluten-free diet, we must deprive ourselves of so many other things – so much more than we think, in fact...

First and foremost, the gluten-free diet has nothing in common with the detox diets that last only for several days or for a few weeks. Gluten-free is and should always be about total avoidance of all products that contain gluten… forever. If you're considering to go on that diet just for a certain period of time, you'd better don't start at all. You can ask someone who suffers from celiac disease what the real gluten-free diet is – it's not only to give up calorie-rich pasta, pizza and biscuits. That diet, for instance, prohibits beer – that could strongly influence your social life and gatherings with other people. You may also find gluten in products which you have never thought of containing it – processed meat, supplements, medical goods, toothpaste, and even cosmetics (mostly in lipsticks and lip balms). In general, you would be doomed to read every food label when shopping and to be very careful what you order in restaurants.

Apart from the difficult choice that we have to make when buying any type of product, avoiding certain foods that contain gluten might lead to a deficiency of different nutrients and minerals in our bodies. Again, we decide to give up a whole group of foods after all. And some of the most common deficiencies when following a gluten-free diet are of iron, calcium, riboflavin, folic acid and last but not least, fibers. That, on the other hand, is a prerequisite for buying all kinds of supplements and multivitamins which should fight the deficiencies. Just want to bring to your attention again that gluten could be found in these products, too, so their labels must be read slowly and carefully.

We shouldn't underestimate the financial factor, as well. Having also in mind the more expensive price of the special gluten-free products and supplements, such a diet could actually cost us a fortune in the long term.

So, the gluten-free diet is extremely restrictive, time-consuming, and expensive, and requires really strong will power. It's vitally needed for people who suffer from celiac disease, it's recommended to those who have gluten intolerance and, let's say it out loud, it's useless for anyone else. If you're misfortunate to be part of that 1% of the world population who suffers from celiac disease, perhaps you already know everything that has been written so far, most probably even in more details. Still, if you have any doubts that gluten isn't good for you and you often have bad health experience after the intake of gluten foods – don't determine the nature of the condition on your own, but visit a specialist who will be able to help you. And if you feel completely fine physically after you have eaten a slice of bread or a few biscuits or after you had a beer or two, then you hardly have any reasonable motives to start that diet. Not only would you save yourself the trouble of reading food labels and restaurant menus in details, but you'd also save some money from not buying unnecessary supplements and, even more importantly, you'd definitely have a more delightful time with relatives and friends.

Chapter 16. The Emotional Effect of Overeating

Overeating is often called emotional eating because we're more likely to overeat and binge eat over emotional reasons. Along with this, we often establish other emotions when we overeat as we start to feel ashamed or angry that we "let ourselves go" and had another binge eating episode. The emotional effects tend to be the same general emotions for the majority of people who suffer from binge eating. But, because we're all individuals, other emotional effects can pop up in a person that doesn't pop up in the next person. No matter what your emotions are after a binge eating episode, they contribute to the cycle which can make you continue to binge eat.

One of the biggest accomplishments when you work on overcoming your binge eating is breaking the cycle. Without breaking the cycle, none of the other steps you're accomplishing would be possible as a cycle tends to keep us going around and around within it. Cycles usually have a deep grip within people that are hard to escape. I feel it's important for you to understand how vicious the cycle is because once you do escape that cycle, you should be proud of yourself. You should note this accomplishment because cycles are very hard to break, especially after you've lived within them for a long period of time.

Nausea

Whenever we overeat, we tend to feel a little nauseous as this is our body's way of telling us we ate too much, too fast, and it's working hard in order to process the calories. Because we ate too much, it would take longer for our body's organ to work through all the food.

Nauseous is never a good feeling for anyone. Even if we don't have any other symptoms, like you would if you had a stomach bug or flu, it tends to make us feel more miserable than before. Some people become sluggish, and due to not feeling well, they go to lie down. These effects of nausea contribute to people's vicious cycle who just had a binge eating episode. Because they're aware that they ate too much and made themselves not feel well, they tend to have other emotional effects of eating too much.

Guilt

Guilt is one of the most common emotional effects of binge eating. When we start to feel guilt over our actions, we allow our negative emotions to take over our thoughts. We start to feel the way these negative emotions tell us we feel. For example, we start to feel bad about what we just did to ourselves and wonder how we could be so stupid to be able to let this happen again. We start to tell ourselves that we should know better and wonder why we didn't learn from the last time.

When you start to feel guilty about your emotional eating, you start to put yourself down. You start to tell yourself that you knew better. You're stupid for falling for that trap again. You start to emotionally beat yourself up because of the guilt you're feeling. This causes you to have low self-esteem, which holds you in this vicious cycle of binge eating as you feel that you won't ever overcome it because you're not good enough.

Humiliation and Embarrassment

Embarrassment, humiliation, and shame are other emotional side effects that tend to keep you in the cycle of binge eating. These feelings are similar to guilt for they give us low self-esteem because of the negative emotions we feel and the way we see our bodies. When you start to become embarrassed over your binge eating episode, you start to become ashamed of what you did to your body. In return, you start to become ashamed of your body and the way you believe other people see your body. You start to view yourself as obese, ugly, and feel that people laugh at you because of your size.

It's a proven fact that binge eating causes us to gain weight, and if you're a binge eater, you already know this, and you've already seen it. It's these body images that not only keep us in the cycle but can lead others into developing different eating disorders, such as bulimia and anorexia. Instead of working toward losing weight a healthy way, we often keep ourselves in this cycle due to the emotional effects of binge eating.

Another way people become embarrassed about themselves is when they realized they have an eating disorder. They feel ashamed because, as millennials, we feel we should know better. How many of us went to school and learned about eating disorders? Because of this, we feel that we should have known better and not fallen into the trap, or we should have known better to be able to stop our overeating sooner, so it didn't become a problem.

Depression

Depression is another common emotional effect to recurring binge eating episodes that can lead into much bigger, sometimes life-threatening, problems. Before I get any further into depression and binge eating, I want to tell you that if you feel so depressed that you've considered harming yourself, others, or taking your own life, please seek help immediately. I realize that this is a very sensitive issue and touchy subject for many people, but I want you to know that you are loved by so many people. You're loved by your parents, your friends, your coworkers, other family members, and people in your community and college classrooms. Your life is a precious gift, and you have so many amazing gifts that you can share with those around you. If you're not sure where to start, you can call any suicide hotline as there are many that remain open twenty-four hours a day, seven days a week, 365 days a year. You can also go into the emergency room, and a doctor will help you with the next steps. If you're a college student, your counselor's office is a great place to start. I also want you to know that you're not alone, and you don't have to fight the battle alone. Call a friend or family member as they will find ways to help you too.

Depression starts to occur as an emotional effect of binge eating due to the negative way we talk to ourselves. The more and more negative statements we feed to our self-esteem, the more likely we are to become depressed. When we start to talk down to ourselves, we start to believe ourselves, and we start to believe other people feel the same way about us. Because we aren't lifting ourselves up in positive ways, we're not going to feel positive about ourselves.

There is a difference between depression and sadness. Sadness usually only lasts for a few hours to a couple days, whereas depression can last longer because it's a stronger emotion. There's also a difference between clinical depression, which we need treatment to overcome, and depression that lasts for a short period of time. Without spending too much more time on this effect of binge eating, I just want to take a few moments to give you some of the major symptoms of depression. It's very important to get help for depression as soon as you notice you hold some of these symptoms as just with any other disorder, such as binge eating. It continues to get worse, and before you know it, it's controlling your life instead of your controlling your emotions in your life.

Symptoms of Depression

- Loss of interest in doing things you used to once enjoy

- Sleep disturbances, such as insomnia or sleeping much more than usual

- You always feel hopeless, sad, and tearful

- People with depression often have angry outbursts and suffer from anxiety

- You have trouble concentrating and thinking

- You stop eating as much or start to eat more

- You have suicidal thoughts, think about death, or attempt suicide

Reality of Your Emotional Effects

People who struggle with binge eating show these emotional effects for many reasons. One of the reasons is because society has not only stereotyped people with eating disorders but anyone who suffers from a mental illness. The reality of this is nearly everyone in this world has some type of mental illness they suffer from. It's just some people suffer from a mental illness more severely than others. The negative stereotypes society has placed on people who battle mental illness has changed over the decades, but there are some that are still hanging on. The bottom line is, your life, the way you feel, and the way you take care of yourself are way more important than any negative stereotype you've heard from society because you are more important. You matter in this world along with everyone else.

The other reality of your negative emotional effects to binge eating is they're not correct. You shouldn't feel guilty or embarrassed because you had another binge eating episode. You shouldn't put any of these thoughts into your head and believe them because you had a binge eating episode. One way to overcome eating disorders is to be kind to yourself. Instead of telling yourself that you should be ashamed for having another binge eating episode, work on telling yourself that it's okay you had another episode because you will do better next time. For every time you have a negative thought about yourself, turn around and give yourself two positive thoughts. For example, if you tell yourself that you're dumb for allowing yourself to binge eat again, stop and tell yourself that you're smart for recognizing that you had another binge episode again. Then you can tell yourself that because you recognized this. You can overcome binge eating because you're a strong person who can establish a healthier life for yourself.

In order to help you start turning your negative thoughts into positive ones, you can use a few of the steps we will talk about later in this book, such as journaling. We often think that journaling needs to be focused on our negative thoughts, but we should write down our positive ones too. Another step that will come in handy is your vision board, which I will talk about, and you will make one later in this book.

Chapter 17. Contraindication of Intuitive Eating for Binge Eating Disorder

Even though the strategy of intuitive eating is so very straightforward and easy to follow, it may not be as simple for everyone to adopt. This chapter will talk to you about the many people who may not be able to benefit from this philosophy. If you think, some of these characteristics talk about you; maybe you need to take a good, hard look at what your preconceptions about food and eating are. You might also want to check with your doctor for a clean bill of health before you begin.

Conviction that Following Diets Works

Considering the incredible hype about different kinds of diets and the multi-billion-dollar industry that has been created around weight loss and fitness fads, it's not going to be easy for most people to follow the simple technique of intuitive eating. When the media tells you that you need to be pencil thin to look hot and desirable, it's difficult to accept that you can look attractive even if you're not a size zero. As you flip through the magazines and couture sites, it's normal to want to fit into those elegant clothes and look awesome in them.

You might have always been of the conviction that following diets can turn you into a model and keep you looking like that for the rest of your life. But, the trouble with diets is that their restrictive rules about what you can and cannot eat are just not sustainable on a long-term basis. After a point, you will revert to your regular eating patterns and possibly, even begin to hate the so-called foods that are right for you. Can you actually go through the rest of your life without carbs? Or, can you have only a vegetable smoothie for lunch forever? There will come a time when you're going to begin hating the very look of smoothies. And, one day, you'll have an impossibly generous serving of your favorite pasta and then go on this massive guilt trip.

Why not instead choose an eating habit that you and your body loves? And, why not focus on feeling fit and healthy? Change your mindset and you can be happier with who you are.

Medical Conditions
Many people develop certain disorders because of which their body can no longer tell them when it needs nourishment. In fact, certain medical conditions could cause your body to signal that you must eat way more food than you actually need. Let's talk about a couple of them.

Insulin Resistance

Diabetics and people with insulin resistance typically experience hunger when they have high levels of insulin circulating in their blood. This insulin lowers blood sugar levels making the body crave more food to make up for the deficit. If you're diabetic, you might also feel this excessive urge to eat more and more sweets. In this case, listening to your body could be detrimental to your health.

Unnatural Dieting

Your body needs different categories of food in perfectly proportioned amounts. These include fat, carbohydrates, vitamins, minerals, water, and protein. As long as you feed it the foods it needs to function normally, you'll feel okay. But, when you begin to cut back on a specific food group, your body continues to signal the deficiency even after you have eaten. And, you're likely to continue to feel hungry even after consuming all the foods that are on your accepted list.

Anorexia Nervosa

Anorexia nervosa is a condition where patients go to utter extremes to deny their hunger and thirst instincts. They will ignore the signals their body gives them to the point where they may not stop to rest or even use the bathroom. Patients need careful therapy and rehabilitation to cure them of this disorder. Only after they learn to resume regular eating habits can they adopt intuitive eating practices.

Insomnia or Irregular Sleep Patterns

People that suffer from insomnia or disturbed sleep patterns tend to feel hungrier than normal people. The body relaxes and repairs itself when you sleep. Getting adequate sleep is also very essential for the mind to relax and calm itself. But, if you're unable to sleep the necessary eight hours regularly, exhaustion and depression creep in. To compensate for the tiredness and sadness, the body could urge you to eat more.

Medications

Certain medications that you take can also make you feel hungrier than usual. If you have ruled out all the medical conditions above, you could consult with your doctor and check the composition of the medicines you take regularly. Ask for substitutes if any of them have side effects.

Having ruled out medical conditions and changing your mindset, you're probably convinced about the benefits of intuitive eating. If you're ready to make the important changes in your diet, there are a few factors to keep in mind. Understand that intuitive eating is not an overnight process, but a habit that needs to be carefully cultivated over time. Listening to your body and mind, and learning to decode the signals is a slow process. When you suddenly crave ice cream, all your preset notions are going to scream, "NO!" But, intuitive eating will tell you to ask your body, "Are you famished?" If the answer is, "Just a little!" you might choose to indulge in just a small scoop and enjoy every bit of it. If you don't answer the craving, your mind will continue to focus on it until you do. There will come a time when you'll snap and end up eating a whole tub. So, what's your choice? A scoop and enjoyment? Or, a tub and guilt?

Chapter 18. How to Succeed at Intuitive Eating and Avoid Common Mistakes

Are you ready to begin your journey to intuitive eating? The process is straight forward but takes some practice to adapt to your body and needs. Set goals for yourself: learn to read your body's signals and communication. Review your schedule to make sure you have enough time during the day to eat if you feel hungry, and set aside room for exercise, relaxation, and meditation. This section will focus on errors and common mistakes that can hinder your progress in maintaining a healthy success with mindful eating.

Avoid Skipping Meals

This is good advice for anyone. Skipping meals is sometimes inevitable, especially if your schedule doesn't allow much time to take a break. If you expect this to happen and can prepare ahead, get up early to start breakfast early. Pay attention to your level of hunger in the morning, to determine how much you want to eat. Bring a light snack to work or school, just in case there is an opportunity to satisfy your hunger, should you feel this way and need to prolong or skip lunch. Whether you eat small or large meals, ensure that you have something nutritious and tasty, just in case. Even the best-planned schedules can change at the last minute and being prepared can alleviate a lot of unnecessary stress.

Not Drinking Enough Water

Hunger can be a symptom of dehydration. If you feel hungry, drink water first. Being hydrated is one of the most important ways to stay healthy. It can also regulate your hunger signals so that when you feel like eating, it is a response to hunger and not for other reasons. If drinking water during the day doesn't appeal to you, try adding lemon, lime or cucumber. Sparkling water can be another alternative. Herbal teas are great during colder months, to ensure you are hydrated. Fruit contains a lot of water and natural sugar, which can provide a boost in energy in between meals if needed. Coffee is acceptable in moderation, though alternate drinking coffee with water, as it can have a dehydrating effect.

Setting Unrealistic Goals

Many of us set goals when we diet, and often, they can be unrealistic. Magazines, advertisements and diet programs promote quick fixes and sure-fire ways to lose weight fast, but this is only good in the interim. In extreme cases, where weight loss is necessary for health reasons, a medical professional or nutritionist may provide a specific guideline for eating. Even within this plan, mindful eating can be practiced, by noticing how the food you eat impacts you and when you eat. Choosing healthy foods can be counter-productive if we eat when we're not hungry or too much when we are, therefore not listening to our signals.

Focus on one goal at a time, if necessary, to avoid discouragement and disappointment. In other words, don't expect to lose a lot of weight, reduce your anxiety and lower your sugar levels all at once, though if you eat relatively healthy and exercise, even moderately, you'll likely see positive results within a few weeks. The key is not to expect overnight transformations that you can post on social media for a shocking response. Even the most successful people, when it comes to losing one hundred pounds or becoming athletic, must dedicate months, even years, to achieving their goals. When the goal is reached, maintenance is still needed and must continue. Mindfulness can instill that level of maintenance from the very beginning so that it becomes part of your everyday way of living.

Obstacles to Intuitive Eating: Emotional Response to Food and Changing Habits

We all have habits that are difficult to break or change, and it's not something that can be achieved overnight. Recognizing a negative habit is a start to making an improvement, as it shows we are aware of it. Habit forming traits often happen as a response to something else in our life. For example, we may overeat when we feel emotionally upset or as a way to make ourselves feel better when we have a challenging experience. This can happen when someone is grieving or feeling a sense of loss. Food can often take the place of that loss in order to cope. When you are going through a difficult time, it's important to not blame yourself, especially for eating habits. Realize that it is temporary, and in time, when you are ready, you can change the way you think about eating. The key is awareness. A helpful approach is a meditation, to give yourself that space to reflect, without judgment, and set realistic goals.

Avoid Multi-Tasking When You Eat

Meeting a deadline, chatting online or in person, and getting work done are all activities that many people try to accomplish during a meal. This happens most often during lunch break, as a "working lunch" or as a way to save time and alleviate the stress of having to complete the work after lunch, though the opposite will occur. As you try managing both tasks, you're eating habits and connecting with your body's signals will interfere. This breaks the connection between your food and you. It is during this multi-tasking that you may feel more anxious to rush back to work from lunch, or in a more social and conversational atmosphere, lose that sensation you experience when you enjoy your meal alone and without distraction. Even if you are pressed for time, leaving a minimum of twenty minutes to enjoy a meal is a good start. Put down the files, leave the computer screen and go for a walk in a quiet and serene place. Meals, whenever you choose to enjoy them and when you can find adequate time and space for them, should take center stage, and all other events put on pause until you are finished.

If you enjoy eating with co-workers, family, and friends, make it an enjoyable event. Keep it positive and fun. If a working lunch is what you want to do, find that enjoyment in your food when you can and chew, savor every mouthful. Keep multi-tasking to a minimum, if you have to keep tasks in motion during your break. Your team may notice how you slow down to eat and enjoy the taste of your food. It may be appropriate to talk about the food and appreciate what you have. This may encourage others to see how you approach intuitive eating and could motivate them as well!

Conclusion

In conclusion, you need to remember that adopting a healthier way of life by listening to your body is not something that can happen overnight. To begin with, it's going to be a bit difficult to let go lifelong perceptions of what food is good for you and what is not. Unfortunately, these ideas have been ingrained in us since what seems like forever. You'll also take time to begin to understand what your body can and cannot tolerate properly. And, what it really, really needs. As for the weight loss issue, you will begin to see a difference. You only need to be patient for it to happen. That's because your body will take time to accept that starvation is not always around the corner, and it doesn't need to shore up on the calories in anticipation.

Give intuitive eating a chance. Your health and happiness depend on it.